MEN'S HEALTH TODAY 1998

MEN'S HEALTH 1998 TODAY

The Most Important, Current Tips and Tools for Healthy, Strong Living

Edited by Michael Lafavore, Men'sHealth® Magazine

Rodale Press, Inc.

Emmaus, Pennsylvania

ISBN 0–87596–493–1 hardcover
ISBN 0–87596–494–X paperback

Distributed in the book trade by St. Martin's Press

2   4   6   8   10   9   7   5   3   1   hardcover
2   4   6   8   10   9   7   5   3   1   paperback

OUR PURPOSE

*"We inspire and enable people to improve
their lives and the world around them."*

Notice

This book is intended as a reference volume only, not as a medical manual. The information given here is designed to help you make informed decisions about your health. It is not intended as a substitute for any treatment that may have been prescribed by your doctor. If you suspect that you have a medical problem, we urge you to seek competent medical help.

Contents

CURES

SLEEP

HEALTH MANAGEMENT

Introduction

It's about Time

What's your most precious resource? What's the one thing you wish you had more of? Sure, more sex, money, or power might be nice. But whenever the staff here at *Men's Health* asks men what they really want, at some point nearly everyone says that they could stand to have a little more time. To be with their families. To be by themselves. To do their jobs better. To head off illness. To squeeze in workouts. To get a better night's sleep. To catch their breath. To enjoy life to the fullest.

That's what *Men's Health Today 1998* is for. As a time-saver, you couldn't do better. It would take you months to assemble the most current news and health information for men. We know, because it took us that long to sift through the Everest of data, research, and advice that makes up the ever-growing field of men's health. We culled the best of it and loaded it in here. If it's in these pages, it's the most actionable, useful information men can get. The most timely, too.

But this book will do more than save you time. It can help you gain time, too, throughout your day and throughout your life. This year, in addition to covering the key health topics that concern men the most, we're including a special report on something we call The New Science of Age Reversal. At the heart of this book, you'll find 40 pages of fresh advice and tips for turning back the clock on your life. No matter what your age, we'll show you ways to look,

feel, act, and think like a man 20 years younger. We'll give you the lowdown on anti-aging treatments and why some of them may be the latest but not the greatest. You'll find short-term strategies for things you can do tonight to start feeling younger as well as long-range goals you can achieve over the many years that lie ahead. Instead of worrying about the future, you can start looking forward to it again.

In addition to this bonus section, we offer plenty of other vital news and information, much of it provided by our friends at *Men's Confidential*, a newsletter that offers the latest on male health, sex, and fitness. We've excerpted from new and noteworthy books covering all the topics important to guys. We also bring you up to speed on the newest tools; the best (and lamest) health and fitness fads; and the most comprehensive resources you can reach by picking up a phone or surfing the World Wide Web. If you're on the lookout for time-saving, time-gaining advice and wisdom, here's a sample of what you'll find in these pages.

No time to head to the gym? Then head to our Fitness section. With the total-body workout we offer, you can follow a routine in your own basement that exercises all the major muscles in less time than the usual health club routine takes.

Among men, the number one thief of time is heart disease. But medical researchers bring news of a vitamin that can reduce your risk of heart attack by two- or threefold. It's in Eating.

Does hunting for that G-spot seem like a colossal waste of time? In Sex, we'll tell you where to find new erogenous zones that'll make her knees buckle. And if you've ever spent time wondering what women *really* want from their men, you'll appreciate our exclusive interview with a researcher who spends his time hanging out in bars, studying male and female interaction to determine exactly what women respond to when men make their move (ah, science is a cruel mistress).

You don't need us to tell you that one of the best ways to maximize time is by trying to do two or three things at once. In Weight Loss, you'll learn of a simple plan for losing fat while building muscle.

Don't lose precious time battling colds, flu, and illness. Instead, marshal your immunologic forces now to fight off any microscopic invader. See Disease-Proof for the full details on these and dozens of other ways to beat every kind of health problem, from skin cancer to salmonella.

Preserve your quality time with daylong strategies for hamstringing stress, whacking business woes, and breaking negative thought cycles, all courtesy of our Mental Toughness section.

Want to feel better fast? When time is of the essence (when isn't it?), turn to Cures for instant headache relievers, super stomach remedies, and dozens of other ways to fix what ails you. And is your downtime rife with the sort of tedium that has you channel-surfing until the wee hours? A leading expert on

boredom tells us how we can all make our lives a little more interesting.

Make the most of your sleep time with four before-bed exercises designed to ease daily tensions and promote better slumber. And for an investment of about 20 minutes, you could reap nearly all the benefits of a full night's sleep. We'll tell you how in (what else?) Sleep.

The Health Management segment of this book is devoted to news from the forefront of personal care and health issues, including time management. An expert in that field has some sobering news for you: You can't control time, he says, but you can make friends with it. He tells you how.

Consider that a mere smidgen of the cool stuff you'll find within. And you'll find it with ease. Knowing you're a busy, action-oriented guy, we've designed this book for maximum readability—no dense table of contents or inscrutable index here. At a glance, you'll be able to find your way to the topics and information you need the most.

But we hope you'll also spend a little time pondering, laughing, and lingering over what we've dished up for you. We don't want you to feel that you have to rush. Take all the time you need.

Michael Lafavore
Executive Editor,
Men's Health Magazine

1

FITNESS

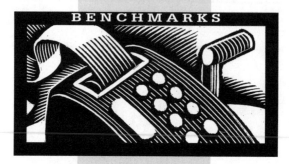

AVERAGES

- Number of pounds a bowler lifts in a typical three-game series: 700 to 1,000 pounds

- Number of people taken to the emergency room each year for sports-related eye injuries: more than 40,000

- U.S. city with highest percentage of completely sedentary people: Washington, D.C.

- Number of golf balls for every man, woman, and child in America: 3.2

- Number of situps you'd have to do to lose 1 pound of fat: 14,000

- Distance a man walks in his lifetime: equivalent to four times around the world

- Number of pounds you'd burn if you walked 45 minutes a day, four times a week for one year: 18

- Percentage of body weight that the average guy can bench-press: 88

- Number of sweat glands in a man's body: 2 million

- Amount of moderate exercise per week that may cut a man's diabetes risk in half: 40 minutes

- Percentage of professional football rookies who consider themselves their favorite athlete: 28

- Resting heart rate of a well-trained endurance athlete: about 40 beats per minute

- Resting heart rate of the average American: about 69 beats per minute

EXTREMES

- Most pushups done throughout a year: 1,500,230

- Most squats performed in 1 hour: 4,289

- Highest number of consecutive chinups: 370

- Odds that you'll die falling into the Grand Canyon while hiking in the inner canyon: 1 in 410,000

VITAL READING

The Total-Body Workout

Give your routine a jolt with this complete free-weight workout.

Nothing can bore you into inertia more completely than trying to stick to the same old exercise program. So we tapped Liz Neporent, co-author of *Fitness for Dummies*, to help design an interesting and challenging full-body workout for you. The following routine includes lower- and upper-body exercises; you can do them all in one workout or split them to work your upper and lower body on different days. If your goal is building muscle size and strength, shoot for 6 to 8 repetitions for each exercise. If you're in the market for definition and muscle endurance, use lower weights and try 12 to 15 repetitions.

HALFWAY SQUAT (works the quadriceps, gluteal, and hamstring muscles)

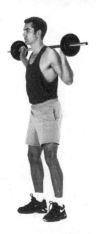 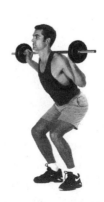 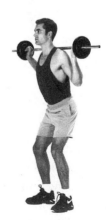

1. Stand with a light barbell across your shoulders and feet hip-width apart.

2. Slowly squat until your thighs are almost parallel to the floor.

3. Slowly push up, but rise only about half the distance. Do three sets.

STIFF-LEG BARBELL DEADLIFT
(works the hamstring, gluteal, and lower back muscles)

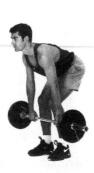 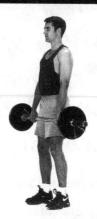

1. Stand in front of a light barbell with your feet hip-width apart. Keep your knees unlocked throughout the exercise. Bending at the waist, grab the barbell with one palm up and one down.

2. Keeping your back flat and legs straight, raise yourself back into a standing position, with the bar in front of your thighs. (Don't lean back.) Your arms should stay straight. Lower the bar to the floor. Repeat for three sets.

ONE-ARM ROTATION ROW (works each side of the back)

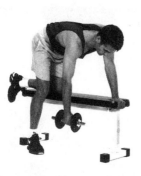 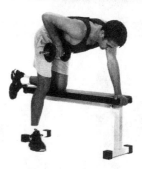

1. Stand with a weight bench to your left. Hold a weight in your right hand. Rest your left hand and knee on the bench and bend forward until your back is almost parallel to the floor. Your right arm should hang straight down, palm facing the bench. This is the starting position.

2. Slowly pull the weight up to the side of your chest while simultaneously rotating your right hand inward. Your palm should end up facing behind you. Lower the weight back down, rotating your hand outward so your palm once again faces the bench at the end of the movement. Repeat for a set, then switch positions to work your left side. Do two sets for each side.

REVERSE OBLIQUE (works the abdominal muscles)

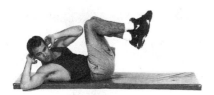

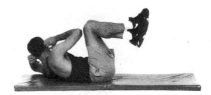

1. Lie on your back with your legs bent at a 90-degree angle, feet flat on the floor. Cross your ankles and lift your legs until your thighs are perpendicular to the floor. Touch your hands lightly to the sides of your head, elbows up.

2. Lift your shoulders off the floor, twist your body to the left, and draw your knees toward your elbow. Pause. Return to starting position; repeat the movement, twisting to the right. Alternate sides for 15 to 20 repetitions.

OPEN-HAND FLY (works the chest, shoulder, inner upper arm, and upper and outer rib cage muscles)

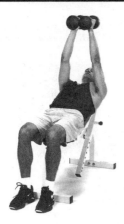

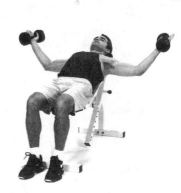

1. Lie on an incline bench with a light dumbbell in each hand and feet flat on the floor. Raise your arms so the weights come together directly above your chest. Bend your elbows slightly; lower your arms slowly out to the sides until your elbows are just below chest level.

2. As you go, open your hands slightly so the weights are balanced in your palms. Hold this position at the bottom for a second. Slowly draw your arms back up, wrapping your fingers around the weights so you have a tight grip on the handles when they're over your chest. Do two sets.

REVERSE RAISE (works the shoulder and upper back and neck muscles)

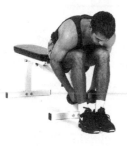 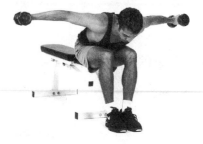

1. Sit on the edge of the bench with a light weight in each hand. Your arms should hang straight at your sides, palms facing each other. Now lean forward until your chest is an inch or two from your thighs. Your back is straight, not rounded.

2. With arms straight, slowly raise the weights up and back until your arms extend behind you, parallel to the floor. Pause for a second. Slowly lower your arms until the weights are again hanging toward the floor. Repeat for two sets.

HANGING CONCENTRATION CURL (works the biceps muscles)

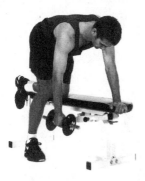 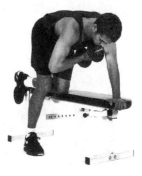

1. Stand with the bench to your left. Hold a weight in your right hand. Rest your left hand on the bench; bend forward until your back is almost parallel to the floor. Your right arm should hang straight down, palm facing the bench.

2. Bending only at the elbow, curl the weight up until it reaches your right shoulder. Your elbow is pointing at the floor. Squeeze your biceps for one second. Slowly lower the weight. Repeat for one set; switch sides. Do two sets for each arm.

TWISTING KICKBACK (works the triceps muscles)

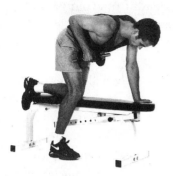
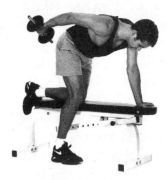

1. Stand with the bench to your left. Hold a weight in your right hand. Rest your left hand and knee on the bench and bend forward until your back is almost parallel to the floor. Next, bend your right elbow and lift your upper arm up and back until it extends behind you, parallel to the floor. Your arm should be at nearly a right angle, with the weight toward the floor. This is the starting position.

2. Keeping your upper arm stationary, straighten your right arm behind you. As you go, twist your wrist inward so your palm ends up facing the ceiling. Hold for a second, then bend your elbow to lower the weight back down, twisting your hand outward so that your arm is again angled toward your body. Do two sets for each arm, switching sides every set.

Build a Better Back

Prevent injuries and look slimmer by doing
these back-strengthening exercises.

Life-management rule number one: If you neglect something long enough—be it a rattle in your engine, a leak in your basement, or a cold, dark frown creasing the face of your beloved—eventually you're going to pay. Oh, you'll cruise along safely for a while, sure, but the end result will inevitably be a crack in your engine block, a crack in your foundation, or a crack in your heart.

The same is true for your body. And when it comes to neglected body parts, your back is at the top of the list. You don't see it, you don't worry about it, you forget it. Until, one day...crack!

Try thinking about this way. The back extends from your neck all the way to your buttocks. That's a pretty large piece of real estate to leave weakened and ineffective. What you need is a program that works your back from top to bottom.

Ours was designed to do just that. And not only will it help protect you from injury but it'll make you look better, too. A well-shaped back gives the illusion of wider shoulders and a slimmer waist. You might even look taller, thanks to improved posture.

Try doing one set of each exercise, or just add one or two to your normal routine to mix things up. Pay a little more attention to these mucles, and people won't be talking about you behind your back. They'll be talking about your back, behind you.

BEHIND-THE-BACK SHRUG (works the upper back and neck muscles)

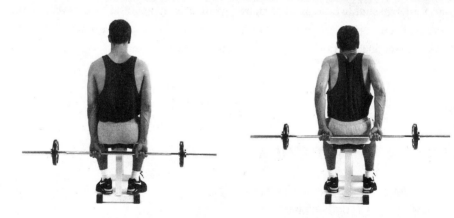

1. Sit on the end of a bench with your back to a barbell, arms hanging straight behind you. Have someone give you the bar and grab it with your hands about shoulder-width apart, palms facing away from you. The bar should hang just below your buttocks.

2. Keep your back straight and slowly raise your shoulders as far as you can. Resist the urge to bend your arms to help. Pause at the top, then slowly lower your shoulders, dropping them as far as possible. Do 8 to 12 repetitions.

CLOSE-GRIP PULLUP (works the mid and lower back muscles)

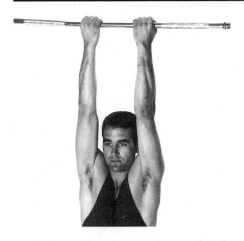
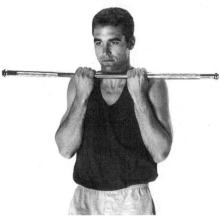

1. Grab a pullup bar with your hands spaced about 6 inches apart, palms facing you. Hang from the bar with your arms straight. Slowly pull yourself up until your chin is directly over the bar.

2. Contract your back muscles at the top for a second; slowly lower yourself until your arms are straight. Build up to 10 repetitions. Then add ankle weights or hold a dumbbell between your feet.

ONE-HAND BENT-OVER BAR ROW (works each side of the back)

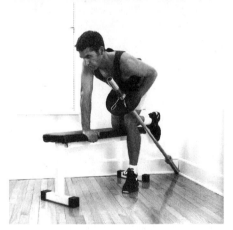
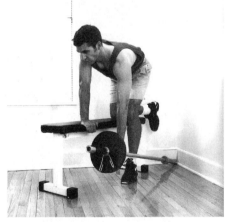

1. Place a weight bar on the floor with one end in a corner. Attach a few light plates to the other end. Stand between the bar and a weight bench and bend forward so that your torso is almost perpendicular to the floor.

2. Grab the bar directly behind the weights with your left hand. Slowly pull it up toward your left side until the weights touch your chest. Lower to within an inch of the floor. Do 12 repetitions for the left side, then switch for the right.

America's Best

The country's cutting-edge gyms offer these top tips.

A gym is a gym is a gym. It has weights. It has really bad aerobic music. It has some leotard-clad lass named Brenda who is a sweetheart when she signs you up but is otherwise occupied two weeks later when you're trying to figure out how to use the pituitary press. That's just the way most gyms are. But some gyms are clearly above this type. After we identified the best gyms in America, we sat down with their trainers and grilled them for their favorite fitness tips. Even if your gym (or basement) isn't in the same league as these heavy hitters, you'll walk away with the same top-notch exercise advice available to members of these clubs, without paying the $100-an-hour consulting fee.

Workout for a Busy Man

If you're trying to build muscle between workday meetings, heed the advice of Jordan Shay, the San Francisco Bay Club's top trainer. "Most people wait too long between sets," says Shay. To shave time off your workouts, cut rest time to no more than a minute. After 60 seconds, your muscles are as recharged as they're going to be to perform the next set. "Waiting more than that won't make your workout better as much as it'll make your workout longer," he says.

Shay deals mainly with highly stressed executives, most of whom are lucky if they find time to work out at all. Here's what he tells his clients.

Make workouts a secret. For highly motivated men, leaving an important meeting or event to go exercise is hard to justify. Other executives won't accept it, and neither will your conscience. The solution is to make every workout a standing appointment, says Shay. No one needs to know where you're going or what you're doing. All they need to know is that you have an important meeting somewhere else. That way, you don't feel like a non-team player by leaving early.

Fold three into one. "One way to save time is to connect three exercises for the same body part into a circuit," says Shay. This method, called tri-setting, lets you hit a muscle group from several angles in one concentrated burst, rather than simply doing one exercise, resting, then doing it again and so on. With this routine, you perform each exercise 8 to 12 times, then move to the next exercise without resting in between. Run through the routine for two sets to thoroughly work the muscle group you're focusing on that day.

Change in Novel Places

A big exercise mistake that men make is doing their favorite exercise at the beginning of the routine and their least favorite (do we hear crunches?) at the end. The result: You either put little effort into these last few exercises or, if you're pressed for time, you just skip them entirely. "Doing what you hate first assures that you'll give these muscle groups the attention they deserve, and saving your favorites for last helps you recharge when energy levels are on the decline," says David Smith, the top trainer for the East Bank Club in Chicago.

Once you've gotten the miserable stuff out of the way, Smith has some more advice for you.

Take care of the quiet muscles. The muscles of the rotator cuff (the shoulder muscles involved in throwing motions), lower abdominals, lower back, and tibialis anterior (in the front of the calf) may not bulge out of your clothes. But imagine them acting as motor oil for your body. "Exercising them regularly is like keeping the oil changed, leaving you injury-free from month to month," says Smith. Be certain to hit each of these areas twice a week.

Think in quarters. Your muscles are composed of millions of fibers. When you lift, your muscles call upon a certain percentage of muscle fibers to raise the weight. And the more fibers you use in an exercise, the more the muscles strengthen and grow. One way to maximize the number of muscle fibers used in an exercise is to employ the "one-and-a-quarter principle."

"For machine exercises, start in the contracted position. For example, with the leg extension, start with your feet extended in front of you," says Smith. Do one full repetition, lowering the weight and returning to the starting position. Next, perform a quarter-repetition, lowering the weight only a quarter of the way, then raising the weight. Continue to alternate between full repetitions and quarter-repetitions throughout the exercise. This keeps the muscles in a contracted state longer and forces them to recruit more fibers to do the job.

Follow Some New Exercise Rules

"The body adapts quickly to what you throw at it," says Dion Laquinn Nichols, one of the top personal trainers at Colorado's Athletic Club at Denver Place. He urges his clients to change two things about their exercise routine at the start of each week. This can range from trying two different exercises to changing the number of repetitions or the amount of weight that you use. "Keep the muscles guessing, and you'll keep the muscles growing," says Nichols. And the simplest changes you can make will go against some standard exercise rules. Here are some examples.

Visualize it. To ensure that you're exercising a muscle correctly, you have to understand how it's working as you lift. Closing your eyes frees you of visual distractions and can help you visualize the muscles in action. This technique is especially helpful with exercises for posterior muscle groups such as the back, hamstrings, and buttocks since you can't see them as you exercise. (It doesn't work for every exercise, especially those that require balance.)

Shun the mirror. Yes, your biceps look rather Samsonesque when you pump iron in front of the mirror. Who cares? "A lot of guys stop pushing themselves because they become distracted by what they see in the mirror," says Nichols. Better to ignore the mirror, or throw on a light sweatshirt when you're doing exercises that require you to check the mirror for form.

Lift the heavy ones first. Many people start exercising with a weight less than they are capable of lifting, then raise the amount as they go through an exercise. This is a colossal waste of time. Most people don't work as hard at the beginning because they're saving energy for the heavier weights, so there's little if any benefit to the first set or two. To maximize your efforts, try working out in reverse. After two very light warmup sets, do a set with the heaviest weight you would normally work up to. Wait no more than 30 seconds, then jump into the next set. You won't be able to do the same weight as before, so lower the weight by about 20 percent. (This can vary, depending on your strength.) You'll end up doing the same number of repetitions with each weight class, but you'll feel the lighter weights challenging the muscles instead of merely warming them up.

Using Your Head

As the training center director of The Marsh in Minnetonka, Minnesota, the top mind-body health club in the country, Tim Mortenson advocates a holistic approach to fitness. He believes that you can't teach your body to perform at its best unless you understand exactly how it works. Here's how to get in sync with your muscles.

Brush up on science. Pick up a copy of any anatomy book and learn about how the body works. "The best drivers know what's under their hoods," says Mortenson. Understanding what areas of the body you're working will also prevent you from overuse injuries, since you'll notice if you're focusing too much on a certain area.

Lend a hand. If you're not too shy, have someone touch the muscles as you work them. This will help you build a higher awareness of the muscles and can help you focus as you go. This may be more fun if you try the following tip.

Work out with the opposite sex. "Opposite-sex partners can clue you in to problem areas about your body that you may not recognize," says Mortenson. It also precludes the need to compete with your workout partner, a bad habit that some guys fall into.

Log it. "To make muscles grow, you need to work them harder," says Mortenson. "To work them harder, you need to remember what you did the day before." Unless you're Rain Man, keep a log of what you do each week and challenge yourself to beat those numbers every month.

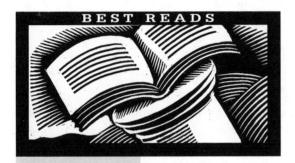

BEST READS

The Blended Workout

Any good workout program contains three parts—strength training, aerobic exercise, and stretching. Problem is, all three take time. And one thing we guys don't have is lots of time. One solution is to combine two workout elements into one. That is what John Abdo and Kenneth A. Dachman, Ph.D., suggest in their book Body Engineering: How to Reinvent the Way You Look and Feel *(Perigee Books, 1997). The book looks at the body as a machine and gives rational, logical ways to adjust performance. What follows is their method for combining strength training and aerobic exercise into one, which they call integrated training. The benefits, by the way, go far beyond time savings: Combining an aerobic activity with short spurts of intense, muscle-challenging exercise has big benefits for your body as well (can you say "maximum weight loss"?).*

An Integrated Training Approach—a technique by which the body engineer combines aerobic and anaerobic exercise every time he or she works out—is the most effective method ever devised to increase muscle development, promote cardiorespiratory endurance, and accelerate fat reduction. No matter what specific activities you choose to incorporate into your workouts, combining complementary exercises is a basic cornerstone of your Body Engineering process.

Depending on the workload at hand, the body's operating systems select one of two energy sources for use as fuel. If the activity the body is asked to perform includes powerful and explosive movements interspersed with short rest intervals, the body chooses carbohydrates as its primary fuel source, triggering a process called anaerobic metabolism. If the activity the brain requests involves long, uninterrupted movements, the body chooses oxygen and fat as its primary fuel source—aerobic metabolism.

Sustained activities are fueled with fats and oxygen because these energy sources are abundant in the body. Unlike steady, low-stress movement, a powerful burst of accelerated and strenuous action can only continue for seconds because the carbohydrates (stored as sugars in the body) that are being used for energy are depleted quickly.

In terms of fuel management, the human body resembles a rocket ship. When a rocket is launched, a high-octane, volatile power source enables the craft to explode from its launching pad. Once the rocket is airborne, initial power boosters are disengaged and the rocket relies on a slow-burning but more stable fuel supply to carry it through the remainder of its mission. The body's initial power boosters are forms of anaerobic energy; its long-term fuel supplies are provided by aerobic energy. When any physical activity begins, your body relies on immediate and fast-burning fuel sources—carbohydrates. If you repeat this activity after a replenishing rest, your body will once again use carbohydrates to fuel its movements. But when an activity persists without interruption—as is the case in aerobic exercise—carbohydrate supplies are depleted or bypassed as the body automatically shifts to a fuel mixture of oxygen and fat for its energy.

The sequence of this internal activity has obvious implications for the body engineer. *The body does not start burning fat until all its available carbohydrate and sugar sources are depleted.* Approximately 40 percent of most conventional workout time is spent burning sugar as fuel. Almost no fat is converted into energy until these supplies are exhausted.

The astute body engineer can take advantage of the body's fuel-management protocols to design and implement an Integrated Training Approach that effectively taps both energy sources. The Integrated Training Approach is the best way to combine aerobic and anaerobic activities. The body engineer will also use strength training and flexibility exercises as part of the Body Engineering process.

Regardless of what you choose to do at the gym, or in the den or the garage, your anaerobic activities should precede your aerobic workout. Anaerobic exercise will quickly deplete your carbohydrate fuel stores before you begin the aerobic phase of your training. Because there are no carbohydrates readily available, you will be burning fat continuously—from start to finish—during your aerobic activities.

Generally speaking, your aerobic workout should last at least 20 minutes, with sessions over 30 minutes being ideal. During aerobic exercise, you should aim to reach 70 to 85 percent of your maximum heart rate to achieve the best results. This is known as your aerobic range.

Scientific data indicate that the amount of energy expended after low-intensity aerobic exercise tends to be minimal. Conventional aerobics is effective in burning body fat only during a portion of the actual workout. Most aerobic exercise does little to stimulate your postworkout metabolism rate. That's because aerobic activity does not stress the muscle tissues to the point where they must be repaired or rebuilt after the workout ends. Your internal systems have no need to work to convert stored energy sources (fat) to rejuvenate cellular-level muscle tissues.

The way your body burns fuel accounts for the difference in physiques between the lean, muscular sprinter and the chubby aerobic maven. A sprinter's training sessions almost always include a series of explosive body movements. While training, the sprinter will race like crazy, rest, then sprint again, then rest again. (Sprinters rest by walking or jogging.) This cycle repeats itself over and over again until the training session is complete. In comparison, an aerobic athlete may train for the same amount of time as the sprinter (or any other anaerobic athlete) but will work steadily and continuously instead of intermittently and explosively.

The difference in training methods makes a difference in the physiques of the two athletes because aerobics puts stress on the heart and lungs and rarely challenges the body's muscular system. Anaerobic exercise, on the other hand, works the muscles vigorously. During an anaerobic activity, like sprinting, the tissues in the muscles are severely stressed. The body reacts by rebuilding and strengthening the muscular system's lean-tissue compartments. This reparation period continues long after the anaerobic workout is completed. In fact, the postworkout reparation of damaged tissues stimulates metabolic activity for several days after each workout, utilizing many energy sources—notably stored fat—to fuel the remodeling.

This is why the sprinter finds it easier to stay lean than does the aerobicizer. The sprinter's metabolic rate is much higher, even at rest.

The secret to maximizing the benefits of your Body Engineering process is to use aerobic and anaerobic activities via integrated training. In addition, I recommend that your aerobic activities be conducted at interval intensities and that you incorporate some resistance training into all your workouts. You will be using aerobics to condition your heart and lungs and anaerobic activities to strengthen and stimulate your muscles. By combining the two forms of exercise, you will develop quality lean tissue that will burn fuel from all of your energy sources—carbohydrates (or sugars), oxygen, and fat.

Interval intensity means that you will design your exercise plan to allow yourself to move in and out of both your aerobic and anaerobic energy ranges during the same workout. For example, if walking were your aerobic exercise of choice, you'd employ the interval aerobics approach by first strolling at a comfortable pace. You would increase your speed and upper-body movement gradually until you felt warm and loose. Then you'd accelerate to a power walk (or even a slow jog) and drop back to a pace you can endure comfortably for a few minutes before you restarted the cycle. You would continue these rest/power walk intervals until your workout was completed.

The interval aerobics approach can be applied to walking, jogging, running, stairclimbing, biking, rowing, and all other forms of aerobic activity. Do whatever you enjoy doing, but—frequently during the course of your workout—do it hard! Some aerobic training devices (bikes, treadmills, cross-country skiing machines, and the like) have preset computer prompts that make interval training principles extremely easy to follow.

What you must keep in mind about conventional aerobics is that the only time you are benefiting from the activity is *during* the activity. Not much is being accomplished on the days you don't work out. In contrast, integrated training (combined with interval aerobics) will be reshaping your body not only when you are working out but when you are resting as well.

To complement this integrated training approach, body engineers will also use resistance training and flexibility exercises.

Setting Goals

We know. You don't want to hear about goals. Exercise is about doing—it's running and throwing and lifting and going fast and breathing hard and strutting like a demigod. Goals are about thinking—they just kind of float around, if abstract thoughts can be said to do anything at all. But if you want to get results with any fitness plan, you'll need both exercise and goals. In this chapter from The Men's Health Guide to Peak Conditioning *(Rodale Press, 1997), Richard Laliberte and Stephen C. George tell you how to do exactly that.*

Everyone begins an exercise program with something in mind, even if it's vague. Maybe it's looking better, maybe it's feeling better, maybe it's living longer than your father did. There are as many motives as there are people. Setting goals is just a way of making what's in your head translate to your body, while keeping your head interested for as long as it takes.

If you don't make decisions up front, you're more likely to give up when you don't perform as well as you'd like, because you don't have a tangible, realistic plan in place to get there, says Kate Hays, Ph.D., a sport psychologist and founder of The Performing Edge, a performance-enhancement training company for athletes, performing artists, and business people in Concord, New Hampshire. Not exactly a prescription for success. Goals give you the motivation to keep going when you start feeling bored, lazy, or impatient with your progress.

"The main reasons people don't stick with exercise is that they either don't set goals or they can't meet the goals they do set," says Bess H. Marcus, Ph.D., associate professor of psychiatry and human behavior at Miriam Hospital and Brown University School of Medicine in Providence, Rhode Island. We're not talking five-year marketing proposals here—we're talking a few basic decisions on the actions you're going to take.

Scoping Out Your Life

Goals start with a reality check. If having impossible goals is almost as bad as having none at all, you need to take stock of your limitations and opportunities. You can make exercise work around reality, but not vice versa. According to Dr. Marcus, some of the more crucial considerations are:

Which twitch? Some men excel at sprints, others excel at marathons. Both sports involve running, but success depends on what your muscles are made of. There are two types of muscle fiber: fast-twitch and slow-twitch. Fast-twitch fibers contract rapidly and burn energy in short periods; they're used for anaerobic activities that require quick bursts of force, like sprinting and powerlifting. Slow-twitch fibers contract less rapidly and burn energy more gradually; they're used for aerobic activities like cycling and long-distance running. Your muscles contain a mix of both fibers, and both can be developed with training, but one type dominates. Bottom line: You'll get better results doing exercise that plays to your physiological strengths.

A crude way to tell which fiber type dominates your muscles is to look in the mirror, says Wayne Westcott, Ph.D., strength-training consultant to the YMCA in Quincy, Massachusetts. Generally, men who are *ectomorphs*—long and thin, with little fat—have more slow-twitch fibers and will do better with aerobic exercise. Men who are stocky, beefy *endomorphs* have more fast-twitch fibers and will do better with weight training. Still, there's another category of body type, the *mesomorph*, that's in between.

Your funhog quotient. One of the more noxious myths about exercise is that it has to be something you hate. Totally wrong. People who study exercise adherence, like Dr. Marcus, say you're only likely to succeed over the long term with activities you like. That doesn't mean exercise will ever feel like sipping mint juleps under a palm tree. You will work, you will sweat, but you will still enjoy it. How you'll do it depends on what you already consider fun. It's not just a matter of choosing inline skating over rock climbing. "Fun could be socializing with others or enjoying an opportunity to spend a rare moment by yourself doing what you want," she says. Either way, "if you enjoy it right then, you'll feel a lift afterward, and that's what will keep you going," she adds.

Time constraints. Some types of exercise require more time than others—or demand rigid schedule commitments. If your goal is to lose weight, for example, Dr. Marcus says you'll need to do fat-burning aerobic workouts for at least 20 minutes almost every day of the week. If you want to build strength and muscle at a gym, your workouts (including travel to and from) may take more time, but you'll have to do them only two or three days a week, she says. Pertinent questions to ask: If you elevated exercise to the status of a business meeting, where could you create openings in your schedule? Do you travel a lot? If so, try to choose an exercise that's easily done while on the road (like running) or that you can make arrangements for ahead of time (by, say, booking yourself into a hotel with an on-site gym).

Glory days. In some respects, a man with a long history of fitness finds it tougher to start a new program than someone who has never exercised in his life. "Men in particular may have really strong memories of who they used to be, and that can be a snag," says Dr. Hays. We often assume we can pick up our physical prowess wherever we left it last, especially if we were, say, captain of the football team or state cross-country champ in high school. Why is that a problem? We expect—and try—to do too much too soon, which can lead to injury or discouragement. One strategy Dr. Hays suggests: If you're going to start an activity you excelled at in the past, make sure your current expectations and goals relate to your present lifestyle—fitness, time, and energy.

Making Goals Work

At some point in your program, you'll ask yourself why you're doing this. Goals are for answering that question with reasons strong enough to keep you going. "Being healthy or fit or losing weight are really good reasons to exercise, but as primary incentives they're not enough," says James Gavin, Ph.D., professor in the department of applied social science at Concordia University in Montreal and author of *The Exercise Habit*. Here's how to make soft goals more firm.

Be specific. Unless goals are concrete, it's tough to tell when you've met them, says Dr. Marcus. Without that sense, there's no feeling of accomplishment or progress—reinforcements that are crucial for continued motivation. Instead of saying you'll take up running, say you'll run two miles twice this week.

Talk action. The best goals are about what you will do, not what you will accomplish by doing it. "Outcome goals can jump the gun or be unrealistic," says Dr. Hays. For instance, deciding you'll lower your resting heart rate to 60 beats per minute is specific, but it's not action-oriented. Focus more on process than outcome by deciding, for example, that you'll take three half-hour walks every week.

Think short-term. It's perfectly fine to have a dream or ambition like "I want to ride 100 miles on my bike in a day." But to realize long-term goals, you'll need to concentrate day-to-day on accomplishing smaller objectives, which offer immediate gratification all their own, says Dr. Hays, as well as a sense of progress toward the big enchilada.

Seek control. What you're after in the ongoing process of improving your skills and making progress is a sense of mastery, which eventually becomes a source of enjoyment and a motivating force. You won't get it by dwelling on things you can't control. Don't aim to bench-press as much as any other guy; keep your comparisons centered on how you're better than *you* once were, suggests Dr. Hays. Don't run a race to win; run it striving toward achieving your personal best. Don't bemoan your lacking the skills of someone more experienced in your sport; focus on how you enjoy the skills you have.

Measure your progress. How can you improve if there's no benchmark to tag it to? If you're weight lifting, keep track of when you add plates and how many. If you're running or biking, figure miles traveled and the time it takes. Write it down. Whenever you find yourself wondering what the use of exercising is, take a look at the record and see just where it's gotten you, recommends Dr. Hays.

Change when needed. You could set your goals all the right ways but still get bored. When that happens, start doing things differently. No need to start from square one with a totally new exercise. Just follow the FIT formula, says Dr. Hays, which entails making one of the following changes, but not two or more at once.

- **Frequency:** Change how often you do a particular activity or the number of repetitions at a given weight level.
- **Intensity:** Alter your speed or change the amount of weight.

• **Time:** Do a given exercise for a longer or shorter period or change the number of sets.

Set multiple objectives. You want to keep focused, but it doesn't hurt to have more than one goal going at once, as long as they don't conflict. You could aim to bike three times a week and also to do a 100-mile ride in four months. "If you bomb on one goal, you might still accomplish another," Dr. Hays says.

Cut yourself some slack. Remember, exercise accumulates. "There used to be this all-or-nothing thinking where if you couldn't get in your run, you figured, 'Why bother with anything?'" says Dr. Marcus. "Now you can get in a 10-minute walk at lunch and the day is not a loss. Our studies find that you need goals but you also need to give yourself some flexibility in meeting them."

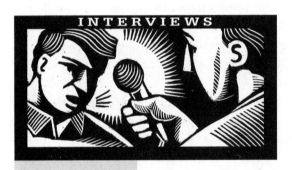

INTERVIEWS

Bob Lefavi on
Strength-Training Foundations

While lots of exercise scientists certainly sound like they know what they're talking about, they don't exactly look or act the part (maybe it's the white lab coats and lack of muscle tone). And then there's Bob Lefavi, Ph.D. Not only is Dr. Lefavi a sports training specialist at Armstrong State College in Savannah, Georgia, but he was also the 1990 International Federation of Body Builders North American bantamweight bodybuilding champion. We figured: Who better to explain the science of building muscle for beginning and experienced weight trainers?

Suppose a guy has never really worked out with weights before. Would 20 minutes or a half-hour in the gym three times a week give him strength or muscle gain over time?

No question about it. Between the first and third month you really do see a good bit of growth. In fact, if you're weight training for three months and you don't notice your muscles getting bigger, you're doing something wrong. Way wrong.

Would you take us through the changes that occur for a beginning weight trainer?

Right off the bat, the muscles start responding. Immediate strength increases are impressive. These increases, however, stem from the neuromuscular learning that occurs with every new activity. In other words, just to learn how to do a squat or a bench-press in a way that efficiently activates the nerves and muscles takes skill; it takes learning. It's not a whole lot different from learning to swing a golf club—you have to swing it just the right way in order to activate the nerves and muscles. A dramatic increase in strength would take place in the first weeks simply because of that learning. After your strength increases, you see real muscular changes, what we would call protein synthesis, going on within the muscle cells. It's real growth—the increase in muscle cell size as a result of new muscle protein being formed. When all of this starts to happen, postexercise soreness becomes standard, and you begin to experience the "pump"—that feeling of fullness immediately after training a muscle.

Then you have to start looking at doing some things differently to keep that curve continually growing. Growth can taper off as you get closer to your potential.

What causes muscle growth?

Muscle growth is the by-product of a stress response, not much different from the general response your body has to any stressor—mental or physical. There has to be what's called the alarm stage. Here, your muscle has to be exposed to a stress that it wouldn't normally be accustomed to. Let's say that you walk on the beach one day, after you haven't been there in a while. By virtue of the fact that your toes sink into the sand and you're challenging your calves in a new way, you're sore the next day. That's an alarm. If you play in your company softball game over the weekend and Monday you feel all these muscles in your back and your shoulders that you haven't felt in years, that's an alarm. Bodybuilders and elite athletes recognize this, too. If you're going to keep moving up that potential scale, you have to continually challenge your muscles with something they're not used to.

Are you suggesting that this alarm principle guides more advanced weight training, too?

Exactly. The most important thing that everyone—from neophyte, a new weight lifter, to elite bodybuilder—needs to keep in mind is that every day that he walks into the gym, he should ask himself the questions: What can I do differently today? What have I not done in a while? What would place an unaccustomed stress on my muscles? You are always trying to keep variation in mind and always do something differently. And that makes it fun.

After the alarm stage, your muscle goes through the resistance stage. And this is the good part: It's as if the muscle cell says, "You've given me a stress that I'm not accustomed to and you've injured me—that's the soreness you feel— and I don't ever want to go through that injury again. And so this time, not only am I going to repair myself but I'm going to repair myself a little bit better and a little bit bigger with protein so that the next time you give me this stress, I won't have to go through this stage again." And that's how growth occurs.

Are your muscles a little more forgiving when you start working out? Do they adapt easier and grow more quickly?

Yes. You can overtrain in the early stages, and still you are going to see tremendous growth. I can take a new weight lifter, put him on the worst routine in the world, and overtrain him like crazy and he will probably still make gains because it's such a new experience for his muscles. He is increasing his muscles' ability in a number of ways, but I think that after a while the importance of rest and recovery becomes more critical.

For beginners, especially, how long should you let your muscles rest and recover between each session?

We think that muscles are able to repair themselves within two to three days. In the early stages, it could be five to six days before a muscle is ready to be stimulated again and undergo another alarm. How do you tell? One subjective way to tell is to notice the amount of pain that is still there. If your muscles are sore to the touch, that's an indication that the repair needs to continue. The re-sistance stage has not completed itself. If upon contraction the muscles are sore and you feel a sharp pain, particularly deep in the middle of the muscle, that's another indication that the muscle is just not ready to be tested again. But if it's the fifth or sixth day and you feel that the muscles are tight, that's a different sit-uation. Muscle tightness, stiffness, even a little a bit of muscle soreness is really fine. After an easy warmup, your muscles will be ready for exercise.

So are you suggesting working out every other day to start?

For the most part, yes. But keep in mind that beginners usually follow rigid routines, so they may find out that two days later they're not ready for another workout for that particular muscle. As a lifter begins to learn and incorporate new exercises into his routine, he may want to break up his workout into two parts. For example, he'd train his upper body one day and his lower body the next. And with a day of rest here or there, he may not train the same body part for three to five days.

How long should someone who has just started working out go before dramatically changing his routine?

I'd say about three months. After that, use your own intuition to gauge when your body has adapted to a particular routine. You can always make small changes, like altering the order of your exercises.

In order for a beginner to achieve his goals, how much weight should he use and for how many repetitions?

Try to think in terms of reps and not weight. And depending on what your goals are, you'll want to do different things. If you want a general improvement in physique, the ideal is to pick a weight at which you can do between 8 and 12 reps. That doesn't mean that you should choose a weight at which you can do 20 reps and stop at 12. Of course, once you're consistently able to do 12 reps at a certain weight, increase that weight by 5 to 10 pounds.

If your goal is for your muscles to look streamlined with less mass, then you should stick with doing high reps of a lighter weight, say, a weight at which you will fatigue at 15 to 20 reps. But if you want to build strength and power, you'll want to lift heavier weights for a lower number of reps, namely, a weight at which you'll fatigue at 3 to 6 repetitions.

Is it ever a good idea to try to do more than 12 reps?

Sure, some days you may feel like you have been under a lot of stress and you just don't want to get under any heavy weight. Great—that's a perfect day to throw some light weight on the bar and burn out a bunch of reps. Use a 15- or 20-rep range. That's a great way to incorporate variation and get your muscles adapting to something new.

What about low reps? And how often should we try to max out—to lift the most that we possibly can in one rep?

There are definitely those days when you simply feel strong and you want to stack weight on the bar and try a maximum attempt. Unless you're in a serious power- and mass-building cycle, you don't want to try to max very often because that can result in injury. For a beginner, the lion's share of the time, try to be around an 8- to 12-rep max weight if you want to make changes in your physique. One to two sets is probably best for a beginner. As you get better at it, and you're able to withstand more training and become more interested and you want to test it out a little further, I think that three or four sets is most efficient for stimulating muscle growth.

William J. Evans on
The Myths of Muscle-Building Supplements

Few areas of fitness are fraught with as much misinformation as body-building supplements. In this candid interview, William J. Evans, Ph.D., director of Noll Physiological Research Center and professor of applied physiology and nutrition at Pennsylvania State University in University Park, destroys some myths while providing some helpful tips to build your body.

Is it fair to say that a lot of so-called muscle-building products are better at reducing the size of your wallet than building your biceps?

That's absolutely the case. And I think it's even a little more insidious than that. They play on the fears that most people have or should have about the unsafe use of anabolic steroids. It's well-known both by the scientific community and by weight lifters and bodybuilders that anabolic steroids will clearly enhance muscle building but that they also can cause serious, even deadly side effects. And then you see these ads that say "steroidlike effects" and people will buy them thinking that they have steroidlike effects without the risk. They play on the legitimate fears that people have.

Can you name some of the biggest offenders, in your opinion?

Products that contain sterols. These are plant-derived compounds, but they are not anabolic steroids and they don't have anabolic muscle-building properties. But the word *sterols* sounds like *steroids*, and that makes people believe that they act like steroids. Product labels often list stearic acid and magnesium stearate as ingredients, which are nothing more than sterols. Another ingredient to be wary of is desiccated testes. They could be bull testes, monkey testes, you name it. They're touted as having steroidlike properties, but they don't.

There's some suggestion that antioxidants like vitamin E reduce the amount of muscle damage experienced during heavy exercise. Would vitamin E ever reduce soreness or recovery time from heavy training?

We have done some studies on vitamin E, and the evidence suggests that vitamin E doesn't reduce the amount of muscle damage. The damage probably occurs as a result of mechanical forces on muscle, which can happen in weight lifting—*not* when you lift the weight, but when you *lower* it.

What vitamin E may do—and this is a big "maybe" because it's not proven—is help in the repair of that damage. Essentially, what happens during strength training is that you do some damage to your muscle and then the muscle repairs itself and makes itself stronger than it was before. So there is some evidence that vitamin E may help repair that damage, but it's very preliminary. There haven't been any real studies done on people who train that would demonstrate a clear connection. But I think that taking 200 to 400 international units of vitamin E a day certainly wouldn't hurt.

Would taking an antioxidant like vitamin E reduce soreness?

It probably wouldn't because soreness is caused by another phenomenon—an inflammatory response to the damage. And, in fact, that inflammatory response is part of the repair process. So I don't think that vitamin E would help in reducing soreness, but it may have some positive effects in helping with the repair process.

Are there other vitamins that we may need to supplement when we're training?

I don't think so. Our research hasn't shown any real change in vitamin status or any kind of influence of vitamin intake on muscle building. The thing that probably contributes most to muscle building is getting enough nutrients like dietary protein. That's more important.

We hear all the time that most men eat enough protein. Do we? Will eating more help build muscle?

I think there is good reason to believe that increased dietary protein intake will enhance muscle building. How much extra isn't very clear, but I would hazard a guess that 60 to 70 grams of high-quality protein a day over and above the normal 10 to 15 percent of your total caloric intake will probably be of benefit to people who are trying to build muscle.

How would you define *high-quality*?

It could be soy protein if you don't want to eat meat. Or casein, which is the protein found in milk. By the way, many of the protein supplements that you buy in your local health food store are nothing more than casein, very high quality milk-derived protein. You can buy this protein without paying the jacked-up prices of the supplements. So if you want to increase the amount of protein that you get each day, buy some nonfat dry milk and have it in a daily milkshake. It's far less expensive than what you would pay for some weight gainer that you would buy in a health food store. Or eat any other low-fat animal protein sources such as tuna or chicken. These foods are fairly high-quality proteins.

There's a variety of products on the market now—like HMB (beta-hydroxy beta-methylbutyrate monohydrate) and creatine—that are touted as being anabolic agents or muscle builders. They have taken the fitness and bodybuilding world by storm, but how solid is the research behind these products?

I haven't seen much on HMB, so I really can't comment. But the research on creatine and creatine phosphate is very, very interesting. Studies show that creatine phosphate supplements increase your ability to perform high-intensity exercise like sprinting and weight lifting. And if that's true, then the next logical step is that if you are doing more work as a result of taking these supplements, your muscles will be able to get stronger and your muscles will get bigger. It's an incredibly promising supplement that may have a positive effect.

Where is creatine found?

It's in meat.

Lots of guys who are into bodybuilding have been claiming for years that they need to eat more meat to get the protein to build muscle. Could it be that they were actually getting creatine?

That's an interesting question. One of the things that we have seen is that when we do controlled feeding studies and we eliminate meat from the diet, we never see the same amount of muscle growth as we do when the subjects are eating meat. It has kind of led us to believe that there might be a meat factor, and I don't know whether it's creatine or some of the iron-containing protein. It's very hard to say. But there is at least some reason to believe that meat may help. We are about to begin a study that will directly compare a group that is not eating meat to a group that is eating meat, and we will be able to say more definitively if it's the creatine or something else.

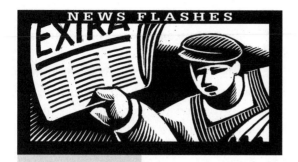

Inline Skating Yields Same Benefits as Running

AMHERST, Mass.—New research has turned up a way to get all of running's aerobic pluses without the joint-jarring minuses: inline skating.

In a nine-week study at the University of Massachusetts, researchers saw that 35 people's aerobic fitness and endurance levels were the same whether they consistently skated or ran. The runners and skaters were put on similar training programs of three 20- to 40-minute sessions per week at 80 to 90 percent of their maximum heart rate.

These results suggest that inline skating can be used as an alternative to running without any decrease in aerobic benefits. What's more, the side-to-side motion of skating makes it a much easier exercise on the body than the up-and-down pounding of running. Keep in mind, however, that the skaters in this study were skating continuously—a leisurely glide around the park won't produce the same results. If you haven't skated since your junior-high days at the roller rink, get some lessons first. The U.S. Amateur Confederation of Roller Skating (call them at 402-483-7551) can tell you where to find certified inline skating instructors in your area. And lessons or not, always wear protective gear when skating—that means a helmet and wrist, elbow, and knee guards.

Aerobic Power: A Matter of Timing

DENTON, Tex.—The time of day that you choose to exercise does have an effect on your overall aerobic power, according to a study from the department of kinesiology at the University of North Texas.

The researchers studied 24 college students as they participated in intense aerobic training sessions within about a four-day period. All of the exercise tests were performed on stationary bicycles and began with a 5-minute warmup followed by a 5-minute rest period. The students then pedaled at the rate of 80 revolutions per minute (rpm) and continued until they couldn't pedal at that speed anymore. Tests were scheduled at approximately 8:00 in the morning and 4:00 in the afternoon.

The results: When they exercised in the afternoon, the participants' hearts and lungs responded faster than when they exercised in the morning. They had more power in the afternoon, too—it took exercisers 9 percent longer to pedal themselves to exhaustion. What's more, their maximum oxygen consumption, or max VO$_2$, a measure of endurance and stamina, was 7 percent higher in the afternoon than in the morning sessions. If you prefer to work out in the mornings, don't let this news stop you. If you're curious about tapping your top aerobic power, though, give an afternoon workout a try.

Exercise May Help Avoid Knee Surgery

MEMPHIS, Tenn., and WINSTON-SALEM, N.C.—Exercise should be part of the treatment for people suffering knee osteoarthritis, conclude researchers at the University of Tennessee and Wake Forest University.

More than 350 adults with knee osteoarthritis were studied to determine the effects of different exercise programs on their symptoms and mobility. Those who did aerobic exercise (for 1 hour three times a week) reported a 12 percent reduction in knee pain. In fact, aerobic exercise was found to reduce pain and disability so much that osteoarthritis sufferers considering knee-replacement surgery may be able to put it off for several years, according to study leader Walter Ettinger, M.D. In some cases, exercise may even eliminate the need for surgery altogether, he says.

A weight-training regimen can also ease osteoarthritis symptoms, the study found. Participants who followed a weight-training regimen instead of aerobics reported 8 percent lower pain. Both exercise groups showed increased mobility when walking, climbing up and down stairs, and getting in and out of cars.

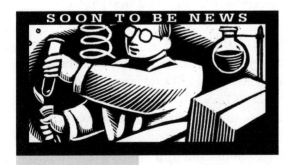

SOON TO BE NEWS

Can the Mountain Come to You?

Soon, you won't have to head for the mountains in order to get the athletic benefits of high-altitude training—you can just head for the gym. Members at the Crunch fitness club in Manhattan are already getting that opportunity by experimenting with high-altitude training in the world's first "Hypoxic Room."

This 9- by 9-foot vinyl chamber is filled with air that is filtered to provide just 15 percent oxygen—same as what you'd inhale at 9,000 feet above sea level. The concept behind high-altitude training goes like this: When you work out in the thinner air common at higher climbs, less oxygen is supplied to your muscles and other body tissues during exercise. That means that your body has to make more red blood cells to carry the oxygen. It's those extra red blood cells that help you gain greater athletic performance when you return to normal environmental conditions.

While just hanging around in the Hypoxic Room seems like a workout in itself to some, training sessions on the stationary bike and the treadmill inside the chamber are intended to quickly increase the members' aerobic fitness.

More fitness clubs are expected to follow Crunch's lead and acquire their own hypoxic-type chambers. Meanwhile, trainers from NFL and NBA teams have expressed their own interest in the Hypoxic Room.

Is Exercise Good for the Soul?

You know that your regular workout is good for your body but it could be doing wonders for your soul, too. Spiritual exercise is a new and growing area of interest in the world of health and fitness, and it has been associated with a whole host of benefits.

In response to an increasing demand for exercise that goes beyond the physical, Canyon Ranch Health and Fitness Resort in Tucson, Arizona, has created a spiritual fitness department. According to Rebecca Gorrell, director of movement therapy and fitness development, the new department offers a wide range of yoga, martial arts, relaxation, and meditation classes, all of which are becoming more and more popular with the clientele. "All of the classes in our spiritual fitness department have shown a sizable increase in attendance, while our more traditional aerobics and weight-training classes have shown somewhat of a decrease," says Gorrell.

Exercise for the soul can include just about any kind of activity, be it running on a treadmill, going on an outdoor hike, or doing yoga. The point is to concentrate on fully experiencing the present moment—don't think about your weekend plans or even the report that's due tomorrow. Instead, focus on merging body, mind, and spirit to achieve "complete mindfulness" during your exercise session.

Whether you add this spiritual dimension to your current fitness routine or you join a power yoga class, the psychological and physical benefits can be substantial. Having your body and mind work as one during exercise can reduce stress and increase focus, while creating a new physical awareness that can allow you to get a better workout while avoiding injury. "If you are detached while you are exercising, there is no feedback loop where the body can tell your brain when it's working too hard or not hard enough. This inattention can either lead to an ineffective workout or to injury," says Gorrell.

With a rising interest in the benefits of spiritual fitness, expect to see more clubs around the country offering such classes.

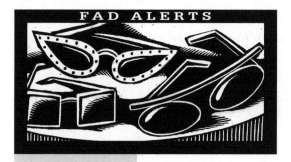

Creatine

 It may be the biggest thing to hit weight training since Arnold Schwarzenegger himself. But if this wonder supplement keeps generating documented results without side effects, it will probably be around the iron game a heck of a lot longer.

The supplement in question? Creatine. And study after short-term study shows guys making big gains while using it. In bench-press studies, men were able to boost their one-rep max—the maximum amount of weight they could lift in one bench press. Sprinters bested their 300- and 1,000-meter times. Cyclists pedaled faster for short distances. And in at least seven studies, all of the guys using creatine gained weight—from about 2 pounds to 4 pounds.

"One of our graduate students did the same kind of study here with baseball players, and in one week they gained nearly 5 pounds," says Melvin Williams, Ph.D., professor of exercise science at Old Dominion University in Norfolk, Virginia. "After that we put them on a maintenance dose for two weeks, down to 5 to 10 grams per day, and they maintained the weight gain. Then they went off creatine supplements for another week and still maintained it."

So how does creatine work? More research needs to be done, of course, but this much we know: Creatine is found naturally in your muscles and in almost all animal meat—beef, pork, chicken, turkey, fish, and others. Unfortunately, you'd need to eat about 10 pounds of meat per day to get the same dosage in the study: 20 grams.

After you eat creatine, studies show, it's stored in your muscles as what is called phosphocreatine—a ready fuel for high-intensity exercise like weight training. On the other hand, heavy lifting apparently depletes your muscles' creatine phosphate stores quickly unless, it seems, they've been saturated with extra creatine.

Once your muscles reach that saturation point, research shows that you're able to work out harder with more weight—a prime builder of muscle tissue over time. And that's a key point because it's likely that much of the muscle size and weight gained in a week when you're using creatine is water being drawn into your muscle fibers. But it's probably only a matter of time before those strength gains and more intense training sessions produce even more muscle, says Peter Lemon, Ph.D., director of the Applied Physiology Research Laboratory at Kent State University in Kent, Ohio. "It's as if you're training as hard as you can and I somehow give you a magic potion that enables you to train 10 percent harder. It almost sounds too good to be true," says Dr. Lemon. "I think we're going to be looking at this stuff for a while."

Luxury Bikes

 We have to wonder how long luxury car manufacturers like Mercedes-Benz, BMW, and Porsche will be making posh mountain bikes when the prices seem so darn high. Sure, the Porsche FS has an aluminum frame and front and rear disc brakes. But it costs $4,500.

Then there's Mercedes-Benz's 24-pound offering, complete with self-adjusting disc brakes and hydraulic rear shock. If only its price ($3,300) also collapsed, as does the bike, into a convenient carrying case. Even motorcycle manufacturer Harley-Davidson has gotten into the act, creating a street cruiser priced at $2,299. BMW seems to be the only outfit among the group that isn't trying to give us serious sticker shock—their price tag ($795) is downright rock-bottom in comparison.

Speaking of comparisons, you should know that bike manufacturer Cannondale makes several aluminum-framed bikes in the $500 to $800 range. Trek makes a bike with front and rear suspension for less than $1,000. Green Gear Cycling, the premier maker of Bike Friday travel bikes, custom-builds foldable bikes you can stuff in a suitcase or even a carry-on. Their prices start at around $995.

Ab Machines

 No doubt you're as sick as we are of those blasted ab machine commercials. Seems like you can't even watch a little mindless TV without some pitch person trying to sell you some apparatus that's supposed to give you the abs of your dreams—and all for just three easy payments of $19.95.

What that televised shill isn't telling you is that if you perform crunches and other ab exercises properly and on a regular basis, you'll get the same or better results—without having to buy the abdominal exercise device they're selling, says John Jakicic, Ph.D., an exercise physiologist and assistant professor at the University of Pittsburgh School of Medicine.

"They offer no physiological advantage over doing crunches with good form," says Dr. Jakicic. If you want great abs for free, here's the plan: Reduce the number of calories you eat, especially fat calories; get regular aerobic exercise; and turn back to page 5 for a good abs exercise you can do without the aid of some injection-molded plastic doodad. You don't need any special equipment. You already have the best machine money can buy: your muscles.

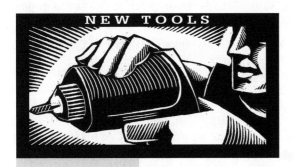
NEW TOOLS

Combined Strength and Aerobic Training

Rowbike

Bored with biking, ready to retire from rowing, but like the benefits of both? Consider the Rowbike. Designed by Scott Olson—the same guy who designed the Rollerblade inline skate and founded the company that sells it—the Rowbike is being touted as "the first total-body outdoor fitness machine." Although not recommended for use in traffic, the Rowbike's rowing and riding action can work glutes, quads, and calves as well as pecs, back, shoulders, and biceps simultaneously, Olson claims. And for those days when you don't want to leave home, the Rowbike comes with an indoor stand. Made in Minneapolis, the Rowbike costs $599. For a free Rowbike video, or to order one for a free 30-day trial, call (612) 442-7049.

More Efficient Fat Burning

Heart Monitors

Checking your heart rate during aerobic activity is as old as Richard Simmons—and only slightly less annoying. But there's a better way to keep tabs on your ticker during exercise than stopping to take your pulse. It's called a heart monitor. Now we know what you're thinking: Aren't those things for super-serious triathletes and other hard-core fitness buffs? While it's true that lots of competitive athletes use them (like the entire Colorado Avalanche hockey team), using a heart monitor may be just what you need to lose that last 10 pounds. By keeping track of your heart rate and telling you when you're pumping hard enough to get some fitness benefit from your exertion, a monitor lets you train smarter. More to the point, it helps you burn more fat. Strapped inconspicuously around your chest, the monitor's results are broadcast to a wristwatch-type device for at-a-glance readings without breaking stride. A typical heart monitor sells for about $100 in most any sporting goods store or department store.

Better, Stronger Calves

Otomix Bodybuilding Shoes

If you're bullish on sporting bigger calves, you have to try a pair of Otomix Bodybuilding Shoes. Feather-light and super-comfortable, they have thin, flexible soles that allow full contractions when you're performing leg presses and calf raises. In fact, after you've tried them, you'll feel like you've been doing your leg workouts in a plaster cast. Some old-timers who swear by them had to settle for black high-tops that gave them a distinctive Johnny Unitas look. Sharp new styling makes them as attractive as any athletic shoe on the market. Prices range from $60 to $100. For a free catalog, call (800) 701-7867.

Ultimate Chinup Bar

The Door Gym

And you thought a home gym had to be a big, elaborate affair with handles and pulleys, gobbling up both your floor space and your salary. Enter the Door Gym. This removable bar attaches to your doorway in seconds without screws, hooks, or any other wood-marring fasteners. And when you're done with your pullups, you can hook it under the door for several sets of crunches—the Door Gym will help lock your legs in place. Or even flip it over to use as pushup handles. Just make sure to perform those pullups slowly. Even the Door Gym can dislodge if you don't use proper technique. $40 from Kanak Enterprises at (717) 629-5357.

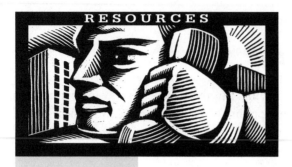

On-Call Experts

The Fitness Connection
(800) 318-4024

No matter where you happen to live, a massage therapist, personal trainer, or sports-specific trainer (a golf or tennis pro, for example) is just a phone call away. This service can arrange a session for you with a certified and prequalified professional who'll bring equipment to your office, home, or hotel (if you happen to be on the road). You only pay for the session, which averages $50 to $60 an hour. If you like the instructor, you can arrange for regular sessions. Mention *Men's Health Today* and receive a 5 percent discount on services. Outside the United States, call (201) 996-1618. Services are available in Canada and in some European countries.

Online Training

Biofitness Health Club Web Site
http://www.biofitness.com

Now you can use your personal computer as your personal trainer. Just point your browser to the Biofitness Health Club. This interactive site, operated by award-winning weight lifter, health club coach, and trainer Steven Zeigman, will assess your strength, aerobic capacity, and body fat (which it determines through your measurements and activity level). Just enter your vital statistics and you're on your way to fitness. Then, if you want a personal workout plan, Biofitness can generate one for the modest sum of $19.95. Plan options include bodybuilding, power lifting, weight lifting, sports training, or general fitness and are updated in four-week segments to take your progress into account. You can also watch expert demonstrations of several exercises.

Fitness Finder

The Fitness Zone Web Site
http://www.fitnesszone.com

Whether you're traveling or relocating, you can find a health club anywhere in the United States on this Web site, which keeps track of more than 13,000 gyms nationwide. And is your stationary bike encased in dust because you'd really like the challenge of a cross-country ski machine? You can buy and sell used exercise equipment at the Fitness Zone, too. The site, an online shopping catalog run by Beta Interactive Marketing, offers complete warranty coverage and will deliver and set up equipment virtually anywhere on Earth. If that's not enough, you can post fitness questions to experts and read articles on the latest fitness topics and equipment reviews.

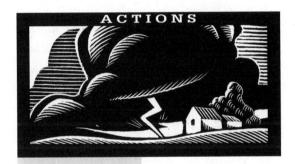

At their worst, gyms can be voracious devourers of your precious time and, ironically, they can rob you of a good workout. Long waits for popular equipment force you to cut the rest of your workout short or leave you wandering aimlessly to whatever is available. Or the guy on the next treadmill wants to compare workout routines and suddenly you're talking up a storm when you should be working up a sweat. To help make the most of your club membership, we interviewed dozens of exercise physiologists and personal trainers to come up with 15 time-saving strategies that you can incorporate into your routine right now. These tips were designed to help you maximize your strength and fitness gains while slashing gym time. And if you're lucky enough to have a weight bench in the basement, don't turn the page yet—many of these tips will help ensure a speedy home workout, too.

1. Practice some fancy footwork. Simply changing your foot placement from exercise to exercise can turn a simple leg press into a total leg workout, says Courtney Barroll of Equinox Fitness Club in New York City.

Placing your feet as close together as you can without them touching, for example, fires the center part of the quadriceps a little more. Placing your feet a little wider apart, about hip distance, and putting pressure on the outer part of the feet emphasizes the lateral (outer) part of the quadriceps. Positioning your legs on the outer corners (toes on a slight angle out to take stress off your knees) also works your buttocks more.

2. **Attack the opposites.** Train opposing muscle groups during rest periods. For example, after you get done doing bench presses, which work the front of your body, switch to seated rows to train your upper and lower back. Just finished doing your biceps curls? Do triceps extensions. "This is a really time-efficient workout that I do regularly," says Steven Wheelock, fitness co-director of Canyon Ranch Lifestyle Resort in Lenox, Massachusetts.

3. **Stay focused.** You've heard it before: He who fails to plan, plans to fail. Add this corollary: He who walks into the gym and wanders around wastes massive amounts of time, says Rebecca Gorrell, director of movement therapy and fitness development at Canyon Ranch Health and Fitness Resort in Tucson, Arizona. Plan your routine before you go to the gym and do your best to stick to it—unless circumstances or opportunities dictate otherwise.

"We ask our clients to focus on their fitness goals because they can be overwhelmed with all the choices or start talking to other people about fitness programs," Gorrell says.

4. **Be ready to adapt.** Darwin had it right: The animal that adapts to its surroundings can thrive; the animal that can't is destined to become a creaky old fossil. As it is in nature, so it is in the gym. Be flexible, be resourceful. Rather than waiting for one machine after another to become free—a process that can cost you 15 minutes or more per workout—be prepared to adapt your routine.

If there's no flat bench free to perform chest presses, for example, hit the incline bench—it will actually work your upper body muscles in a more efficient way, says Bob Lefavi, Ph.D., sports training specialist at Armstrong State College in Savannah, Georgia.

5. **Rev up your fat-burning furnace.** Treadmills are great for walking, jogging, or running, but doing a little of each can help kick your body's fat-burning ability into high gear, says Barroll. Start with 5 minutes of walking as a warmup. Then jog for 3 minutes and run at a higher level for 2 minutes, alternating back and forth. Continue alternating until you reach the 30- to 40-minute mark. Then allow yourself a 5-minute walk to cool down, Barroll says. "This routine always seems to go quickly, and it's a great fat burner," she notes.

6. **Bring a bottle.** We had to sneak a drink-your-water tip in here somewhere. You could take a hike to the water fountain every time your mouth screams for a drink. A better idea is to carry a plastic bottle filled with water, diluted juice, or a sports drink. And you won't just be saving time. Dehydration is also one of the main causes of cramping, which can really put a crimp in your exercise plans, says Barroll.

7. **Join the dawn patrol.** If you want to train for peak performance, avoid exercising at your club during peak hours—between 6:00 and 7:45 P.M. in most gyms. You'll wind up wasting time standing in line for machines. "It's really tough to get a good concise workout then because it's usually so crowded," explains Barroll. Most gyms have fewer patrons in the early-morning hours, she says.

8. **Bear down on a bench.** Lock onto a workout bench and make it your base of operations. A single bench can be your workout island in a sea of exercise chaos, allowing you to do chest and shoulder presses, triceps extensions, upright rows, pullovers, and other exercises—even crunches. This workout goes smoothest when you have an array of barbells and dumbbells nearby, but you can work out with either type of weight, says Barroll. "The only time that you'll have to move is to grab different weights."

9. **Warm up wisely.** It makes sense to warm up by walking on a treadmill—just 5 to 10 minutes raises your body temperature, helps get your blood flowing, and lubricates your leg joints. But you can also prepare for an upper-body workout by performing lateral and front arm raises and weightless shoulder presses while you walk, suggests Barroll. "Sometimes I'll do backward arm circles and then throw a few punches to break it up," she says.

10. **Visit Mr. Smith.** Increasingly popular with hotels and other facilities with limited space, the Smith Press Station, better known as the Smith machine, is a gym unto itself. In the confines of its ultra-sturdy frame, you can perform squats, calf raises, incline or flat bench presses, military presses, upright rows, and other exercises. And best of all, you don't need a spotter, since special hooks attached to the bar allow you to rest the weight safely when you get tired.

11. **Take the cardio cross-train.** If your gym enforces a 20-minute limit on all cardiovascular fitness machines, you can still get in a great workout simply by switching from treadmill to bike and rowing machine or stairclimber for 20 minutes each, Barroll says. "That way you can get in a full hour of work and never leave the cardio area."

12. **Beat the clock.** When you're crunched for time, try taking a 30-second rest between sets instead of a prolonged break, says Marc Goodman, a fitness instructor and personal trainer at Crunch, a gym in New York City. "Keep an eye on that second hand and then, boom, it's time for your next set," he says.

13. **Go to prep school.** You probably don't lay out your workout clothes the night before you wear them, but prepping for your next exercise between sets can help save time. If you're going to use dumbbells, for example, pull them from the rack and place them at the bench you're going to use. If you're going from squats to leg presses, load the machine with plates. And so on. This also alerts others to your interest in the equipment, says Wheelock.

14. **Gravitate toward a Gravitron.** If you need to get in a good arm and back workout fast, this combination pullup and dip machine can't be beat—unless of course you consider its unplugged cousin made by Cybex. Both machines are designed to provide enough assistance so that almost anyone—regardless of their fitness level—can do pullups, chinups, and dips at will, says Joe Ogilvie, a fitness leader at Chelsea Piers Sports and Entertainment Center in New York City.

15. **Put yourself on the rack.** Your gym buddies may not appreciate it, but you can cut training time dramatically by spending your time in front of the dumbbell rack instead of constantly moving from one machine to another. Consider the range of exercises within easy reach: shrugs, rows, incline and flat bench presses, flies, curls of all kinds, shoulder presses, lateral raises, lunges, triceps extensions, and many others, says Ogilvie.

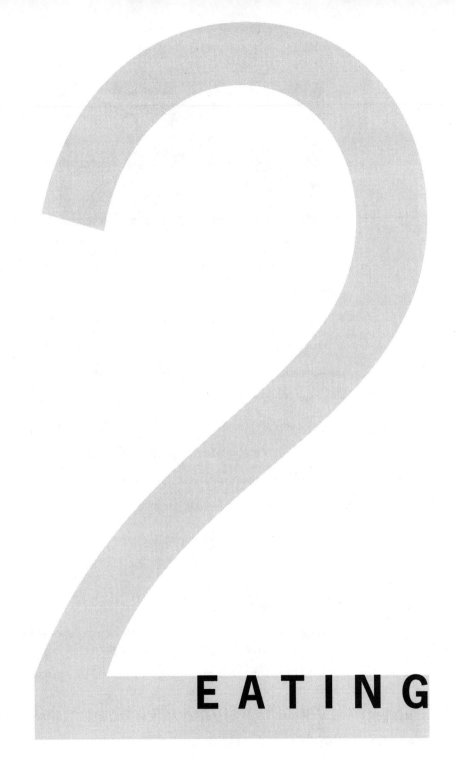

EATING

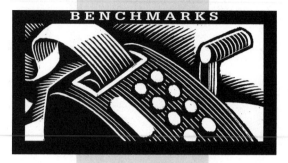

BENCHMARKS

AVERAGES

■ Favorite Ben & Jerry's Ice Cream flavor: Chocolate Chip Cookie Dough

■ Amount of ice cream an American eats annually: 6 gallons

■ Most popular candy in the United States: M&M's

■ Amount of meat consumed in the United States annually: 261 pounds per person

■ Number of times per week the average man eats out: 4.3

■ Number of rodent hairs allowed by law to be in a candy bar: 2

■ Percentage of Americans who twist their Oreo cookies open before eating: 35

■ Percentage of people who twist pasta around their fork: 55

■ Percentage who use a spoon to eat pasta: 13

■ Number of times per week the average person eats breakfast at home: 5.38

EXTREMES

■ Longest banana split ever created: 4.55 miles long, made in Selinsgrove, Pennsylvania, April 30, 1988

■ Oldest beer: circa 3500 B.C.

■ Strongest beer in the world: Baz's super brew, 23 percent alcohol by volume and sold at The Parish Brewery in Somersby, England

■ Strongest beer in the United States: Samuel Adams Triple Bock, 17.7 percent alcohol by volume

■ Largest cake ever created: 128,238 pounds, 8 ounces—including 16,209 pounds of icing

■ World's most expensive spice: wild ginseng, with prices reported as high as $23,000 per ounce

■ Largest hamburger: 5,520 pounds and 21 feet in diameter

■ Longest sausage: 28.77 miles

VITAL READING

A Plateful of Colors

For a balanced diet, pay attention to the color
of your food, not the calories.

At first glance, eating a diet of all the right foods looks like pretty hard work. You have grams to convert, Daily Values to memorize, and food groups to balance. It's like a little math quiz each time you go to the supermarket. Well, toss the calculator and forget about all those tables and charts. We've discovered an easier way to pack your diet with loads of nutrients and other important stuff you need: Make your meals as colorful as possible. Simply fill your plate with a variety of colors—especially reds, greens, and yellows—each time you sit down to eat, and you'll automatically be on your way to a healthful, complete diet.

Granted, if your idea of multicolored foods is maraschino cherries, jelly beans, and lime Popsicles, then we can't help you. On the other hand, follow the simple suggestions that we've provided on these pages, and you'll never have cause to regret the year that you spent sleeping through math class.

Blue

Blackberries have 7.2 grams of fiber per cup—more than twice the amount that blueberries have—and substantial amounts of vitamin C. They're a fair source of calcium and iron, too.

Blueberries and other blue and purple fruits and vegetables contain anthrocyanins, which may help prevent cancer.

Eggplant is filling, not fattening, and a great meat substitute. It's a source of potassium, which tends to flush excess sodium from the body, helping to lower blood pressure. (Potassium is also needed for healthy nerves and muscles.)

Prunes are a super source of fiber. They're full of magnesium and potassium, which may help maintain normal blood pressure.

Brown

Brown rice and cereals are good for complex carbohydrates and fiber.

Dried figs are fiber heavyweights and a good source of calcium and potassium.

Mushrooms supply respectable amounts of fiber and complex carbohydrates—and they're a superb choice for men watching their weight, since they contain almost no calories.

Nuts are high in fat, but most of it is monounsaturated, which can help control cholesterol. They're also good sources of the immunity-strengthening nutrients vitamin E, iron, and folate—plus zinc to maintain prostate health.

Pumpernickel contains thiamin, a B-complex vitamin essential for energy.

Green

Avocados are high in monounsaturated fat, the type that has been shown to lower cholesterol. Ounce for ounce, they're also higher in potassium than bananas.

Broccoli, spinach, and zucchini deliver blood-nurturing folate, vitamin C, and beta-carotene.

Grapes contain a substance called ellagic acid, which may kill certain cancer-causing compounds in the body.

Green cabbage is one of the best vegetable sources of vitamin E. It also contains magnesium and potassium.

Green peas contain vitamin C, folate, magnesium, iron, and zinc.

Kiwifruit is an excellent source of vitamin C, good for protection against certain cancers, and it contains some magnesium and fiber.

Leeks, chives, and parsley are underrated sources of vitamin C.

Lettuce, especially romaine, is high in folate, vitamin C, and beta-carotene.

Olive oil is high in monounsaturated fat and vitamin E, a natural immune-system booster.

Orange

Apricots, peaches, and nectarines provide fiber and vitamin C.

Carrots are about the best source of vitamin A you'll find, and they help protect against cancer and boost immunity. A carrot supplies enough fiber to help lower cholesterol, control diabetes, speed weight loss, and help fight digestive system cancers. And the extra fiber can reduce the risk of hemorrhoids.

Lentils are an extraordinary source of folate and provide potassium and magnesium—two minerals that combat weaknesses and fatigue and stave off high blood pressure.

Mangos contain vitamin B_6, essential for healthy blood. They are good sources of the antioxidant vitamins A, C, and E.

Oranges (fruit or juice) offer vitamin C, fiber, and folate.

Pumpkin and cantaloupe are excellent sources of vitamins C and A, which help heal wounds and enhance immunity.

Shrimp (and other shellfish) are a great low-fat source of protein and nerve-protecting vitamin B_{12}. They also carry a good amount of iron and niacin.

Red

Apples and strawberries, like many other red plant foods, contain cancer-fighting anthrocyanins. They also offer vitamin C, insoluble fiber (to help prevent constipation and protect against colon cancer), and pectin (a soluble fiber that fights high cholesterol).

Kidney beans are packed with fiber and folate. They are also good sources of potassium and magnesium.

Red peppers contain loads of vitamin C (a half-cup provides 158 percent of the Daily Value), and they're a good source of vitamin A, which speeds healing and helps boost immunity.

Red wine contains flavonoids, which may discourage formation of blood clots that bring on stroke and heart disease.

Salmon, beef, and pork are good sources of proteins and iron. (Choose lean meat.) Salmon is also high in omega-3 fatty acids, which can help reduce cholesterol and protect against heart disease.

Tomatoes (and ketchup) are high in the carotenoid lycopene, which may help lower your risk of colon and prostate cancers.

White

Cauliflower and other white cruciferous vegetables contain high levels of indole glucosinolates, compounds believed to have a variety of cancer-fighting effects.

French bread is a good source of blood-building iron and offers fair amounts of niacin, riboflavin, and thiamin, B-complex vitamins that are involved in the production of energy in the body.

Oatmeal provides fiber plus thiamin and magnesium for healthy blood, nerves, and muscles.

Onions and garlic contain vitamins and selenium and are blood thinners.

Tuna, oysters, and squid (calamari) contain loads of heart-healthy omega-3 fatty acids and, in many cases, zinc.

Yogurt, cottage cheese, sour cream, and milk all deliver proteins and calcium. Choose low-fat or nonfat varieties.

Yellow

Bananas are high in vitamin B_6, which helps fight infection. And their duo of high potassium and low sodium may protect against high blood pressure.

Beer contains carbohydrates, minerals, and B vitamins. Try to keep to no more than two drinks a day.

Cheese contains protein, potassium, and fat. Look for low-fat varieties.

Eggs contain protein, several B vitamins, and vitamin A. If you eat eggs often, try egg substitutes to cut cholesterol.

Pasta provides a healthy dose of iron and respectable servings of thiamin and niacin, nutrients that help produce energy. It also includes some magnesium, riboflavin, and folate.

Pineapple, lemons, and grapefruit deliver soluble fiber as well as vitamin C to help enhance immunity.

Potatoes have almost twice as much potassium as bananas, plus plenty of complex carbohydrates and fiber.

Eating for Every Occasion

When your dining prospects look bleak, try these simple, tasty foods.

Man's ideal eating environment is the restaurant buffet. It involves so little thinking. Our primal gathering instinct kicks in, and we fill our plates until the olives tumble onto the carpet.

Piece of cake. But real-life eating isn't a 30-item buffet. It's much tougher than that. It's filled with question marks: What's in the fridge? Can I microwave Pop-Tarts? Is that blue cheese or a new form of life? Where's the freakin' number for Shamansky's 24-hour kung-pao-chicken-and-pierogies delivery?

Think about it. How many times have you opened the refrigerator door and stood there bathed in pale light for 5 minutes, as if that empty pickle jar would turn into a grilled-chicken sandwich if you waited long enough?

We've been there. And we can help. We've contacted the chefs and the diet experts and waded through all the crapola you hear about good nutrition to give you a practical guide to healthful eating in all the confusing circumstances life throws your way.

Here, gentlemen, is what to eat when...

...you want to lose weight fast. Eat dinner for breakfast. Rather than having a big meal at night just before you plop down to watch *Frasier*, try having it for breakfast or at noon instead. "Sometimes all men need to do (to lose weight) is eat more in the first half of the day and less in the second half," says Cheryl

Hartsough, R.D., a nutritionist for the PGA National Resort and Spa in Palm Beach Gardens, Florida. This gives you most of your active day to burn off the fat and calories. Eat light at night, when you're less active.

...*you want to burn more calories.* Keep eating throughout the day. Depriving yourself of food slows your metabolism. The trick is to keep your body modestly stoked all day, starting with breakfast. Juice and high-fiber cereal with low-fat milk and a piece of toast with jam will help you burn calories faster the rest of the day.

...*you're sick of bland high-fiber cereal.* Go scrambled. You probably have five or six almost-empty cereal boxes in your cupboard. Mix them for a new taste. The best combos are Fiber One and Rice Krispies; Corn Chex and Raisin Bran; Kellogg's Corn Flakes and Frosted Mini-Wheats; and Cheerios and Nut & Honey Crunch.

...*you've just had an orgasm.* Make yourself a hamburger and baked beans. You'll want to replenish your zinc supply since you lose about 0.6 milligram of it with each ejaculation. Six top zinc sources: one oyster, 12.7 milligrams; 4 ounces of lean, broiled hamburger, 6 milligrams; 2 tablespoons of wheat germ, 2.1 milligrams; ½ cup of baked beans, 1.8 milligrams; ¼ cup of cashews or sun-flower seeds, 1.8 milligrams.

...*you need long-burning energy.* One word: oatmeal. Let's say that you're about to go one-on-one with that aerobics instructor you met at the grocery store. You need staying power. What will deliver it best? Oatmeal, say researchers at Pennsylvania State University in University Park. In an experiment, 18 students ate equal-calorie amounts of oatmeal, ready-to-eat oat rings, or ready-to-eat rice cereal. Then they cycled to exhaustion on stationary bikes. It turned out that the students who ate oatmeal kept going the longest—5 hours, compared with 4 hours for those fueled with the other foods. Because oatmeal is the highest in soluble fiber of the group of three foods, its energy is more slowly delivered into your body. You avoid a spike and dip in blood sugar that makes you feel weak, says William J. Evans, Ph.D., who heads Pennsylvania State University's renowned Noll Physiological Research Center. Other soluble fiber-rich foods, such as lentil-barley soup and beans, should have the same energizing effect. Dr. Evans recommends eating them 45 to 90 minutes before you exercise, to give your body time to absorb the slow-release energy.

...*all you have in the cupboard is white bread.* You have ketchup in the fridge, right? Good. Try this traditional Appalachian recipe: Spread ketchup on two halves of white bread. Voilà!—ketchup sandwich. This, you're asking, is nutritional advice? Well, you're mistaken if you think that white bread is a nutritional wasteland. Some fortified white breads have added calcium and fiber that give them as much as or more than the whole-grain varieties. For example, a two-slice serving of Wonder Light contains 15 percent of your Daily Value for calcium and 5 grams of fiber.

...you're training for a marathon. Carbohydrates, of course. But how many? Do this: Multiply your body weight by four. The product is the number of grams of carbohydrates (such as pasta) you should eat per day, says Owen Anderson, Ph.D., editor of *Running Research News.* Eat less and your leg muscles may become depleted of glycogen (a fancy way of saying muscle fuel), leading to lower-quality workouts and an increased risk of overtraining.

...you're prone to ulcers. Eat some onions. That's right. Dump them into soups and sauces. Eat them raw on sandwiches. Just eat 'em—about half an onion a day. Scientists think the pungent sulfur compounds in onions attack the bacterium *Helicobacter pylori,* which is believed to cause ulcers and maybe even stomach cancer.

...you don't want to overeat. Have an appetizer. Make it a fiber-rich salad or a bowl of vegetable soup. "Fiber is nature's appetite suppressant," says Stephen P. Gullo, Ph.D., president of the Institute for Health and Weight Sciences in New York City and author of *Thin Tastes Better.* "Take the edge off hunger with a bulky, low-calorie first course," he says. "Since it takes a while to eat, you'll start to feel full before you finish your main course." A glass of cold tomato juice works, too.

...you're hungry at 4:00 P.M. This is your dietary danger zone. "There's typically a blood sugar drop around 4:00, and this makes the body cry for food," Hartsough says. That's when most folks snack on high-fat cakes, chips, and other goodies from the lobby vending machine. The answer is to bring an orange for a snack. Researchers in Australia found that this fruit fills you up three times better than a candy bar and keeps you feeling that way for hours. Popcorn rated high, too.

...you're trying to lower your cholesterol. Eat almonds. You may think we're nuts, but a study by Gene A. Spiller, D.Sc., Ph.D., director of the Health Research and Studies Center in Los Altos, California, found that people on low-fat diets who started eating 3 ounces of raw almonds a day experienced an average 21-point drop in their low-density lipoprotein (LDL, the "bad") cholesterol levels. Other cholesterol-crushing foods include soy (found in tofu and soy burgers), avocados, apple cookies, bean burritos, low-fat yogurt and cheese, safflower and olive oils, and chili peppers.

...you haven't eaten your vegetables. Have a V-8. A V-8 Plus, that is. This new drink contains 70 percent of the Daily Value for antioxidant vitamins A, C, and E. A 5½-ounce can has only 40 calories and is lower in sodium than the original version, and it tastes virtually the same.

...you come back empty-handed on opening day of deer-hunting season. Mail-order venison. Call the Cervena Council (800-877-1187) for ordering information about Cervena farm-raised venison from New Zealand. At $15 to $24 a pound (depending on the cut), it's pricey meat, but worth it. It has the same juicy, tender consistency of a filet mignon steak, but with half the calories of beef.

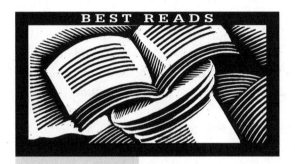

BEST READS

Smart Eating Habits

Most everyone knows that crash diets don't cause long-term weight loss. But why not? And what is the alternative? In their book Body Engineering: How to Reinvent the Way You Look and Feel *(Perigee Books, 1997), John Abdo and Kenneth A. Dachman, Ph.D., do a good, simple job explaining the physiology of calorie burning and also provide some guidelines on how to eat in a way that maximizes efficiency and weight loss. Here's a thin slice of their thinking.*

Contrary to popular belief, weight loss is not about deprivation. (Remember that when we talk about weight loss, we mean the loss of fat, not the diminishment of muscle or other vital tissues.) You can shed excess fat by building muscle and increasing your metabolic rate. You don't have to drastically reduce your caloric intake, although you may need to change the source of some of the calories you consume. Your internal systems crave good food. In fact, each time you eat, your metabolic rate increases. Combining exercise to build muscle with smart eating to stimulate your metabolism will enable you to lose fat quickly and easily.

When you drastically reduce your normal caloric intake, your body's operating systems downshift into a defensive mode, convinced that starvation is just over the horizon. Your metabolism slows to a careful crawl, intent on conserving fat stores. Most of the weight you lose under a strict lo-cal eating regimen is primarily muscle, not fat. And you lose muscle from all parts of your body, including vital areas within your respiratory, circulatory, and digestive systems. This is why we almost always regain the weight we lose in diet programs based on deprivation. By losing muscle we weaken and slow down our body's operational systems. Our metabolism becomes sluggish and inefficient. As soon as we resume anything close to a normal eating pattern, we quickly regain the weight we've lost (and, often, another dozen pounds as well).

Body Engineering's basic tenets forbid restrictive lo-cal diet regimens. Deprivation is of no value in the quest to lose fat and gain muscle. The work needed to renew and reshape your body must be fueled with calories. Activity and nutrition are inseparable factors in your renovation equations.

Instead of starving yourself, eat often and eat well. Eating balanced, reasonably sized meals several times a day stimulates metabolic activity and promotes efficient digestion. When you eat large heavy meals, you place unreasonable demands on your digestive system and slow all of your body's absorption, distribution, and waste-management functions. Even if you eat only healthful, nutritious food, gargantuan portions will lead to internal gridlock—and nasty fat backups at important metabolic intersections.

Eat smaller meals, and when you've finished, leave the table. Take a walk, do the dishes, read, play cards, surf the Internet, fold laundry, or telephone a friend. Do anything, just don't do dessert—until later. And when you do have dessert, go for something nutritious. This eating strategy will give your digestive system an opportunity to absorb and allocate the nutrients you've just consumed and create very little troublesome waste.

Eating smaller meals several times throughout the day will help you lose fat because the entire process of eating, digesting, and assimilation requires the expenditure of body energy and increased metabolic activity.

Eating Strategies

Eating wisely requires a little common sense, a little control, and every now and then, a little treat. Your main focus as a new body engineer should be to enjoy your new eating behavior. Don't agonize over food choices, and don't spend hours weighing food or counting calories. Make healthful eating a low-hassle, natural part of your daily routine.

Right now is a good time to begin developing a practical, realistic, and healthy attitude about food. Start by respecting yourself. Set standards for the quality and value of the food you will put into your body. Become aware of the impact of junk foods on the new machine you're building. Realize that your revised eating habits are not only the right thing to do now but also an excellent investment for your future. Come to terms with the fact that if you want to feel and look terrific when you're 70 years old, you'll need to begin now to prevent or postpone the deterioration that inevitably accompanies aging.

Healthful eating requires the development of a realistic, effective meal plan incorporating nutritional foods from several food categories in proper proportion. Eating a variety of foods is important to prevent boredom and to ensure complete attention to all your body's needs.

Healthful eating means investing the time, effort, and money necessary for the creation and maintenance of a sound eating program. Planning meals and snacks, selecting foods, storing foods at home to keep them fresh, and preparing foods properly must become routine tasks.

I guarantee that the rewards will justify the costs. Remember, you are investing in your body—and you can expect some extraordinary payoffs in the long run. Junk food has made America fat because too many of us won't spend the time and effort required to eat sensibly. It has become far too convenient to hop in the car, cruise the nearest drive-through, and inhale a burger and fries for dinner.

Healthful eating means creating and following a consumption routine that provides your body with constant nutrition in manageable doses. Your daily intake of food should deliver the benefits you are after—energy, increased strength, heightened mental acuity, physical competence, and a sleeker appearance. Instead of eating when you're hungry, it's a better idea to eat at specific times each day—and only at those times. Try to eat every 3 or 4 hours instead of waiting until hunger forces you to the table. The timing of your meals is important. Eat breakfast, lunch, and dinner at strategically scheduled times and plan a snack midway between lunch and dinner, and again between dinner and bedtime. In other words, eat all day. But never stuff yourself at any given meal or snack time. Overeating disrupts your digestive system. If you're tempted to binge, remind yourself that you've had enough for the moment and that you'll be eating again in a couple of hours.

Healthful eating means making a conscious effort to control sugar consumption. Eating too many sugar-laden foods will cause major (and erratic) swings in energy levels and moods and drive your internal fuel-management systems crazy.

Healthful eating means being realistic. There's no need to banish your favorite foods from your life. If chocolate cake or apple pie or Rocky Road ice cream makes your pulse race and your mouth water, feel free to indulge yourself once in a while.

Healthful eating doesn't mean *always* eating carefully. Never deny yourself any food you love. Instead, manage these necessary pleasures—create room for them in your renovation process.

Finally, **healthful eating means expecting and enduring a major cleanup inside your body.** It's possible that you may not see or feel immediate benefits when you implement your new eating plan. Toxins and other waste products will be broken down and eliminated from your body. During this process, toxic particles dislodged from comfortable havens often enter the bloodstream. Once in the circulatory system (which acts as a conduit for elimination), these waste particles can move to various body channels and cause discomfort. As unappealing as this chain of events sounds, a valuable purification is under way. Be patient; it doesn't take long.

Within 10 to 14 days from the time you implement the nutrition plan that you'll design as part of the Body Engineering process, significant changes in your physique and your mental state should become apparent.

Nutrients

There are six kinds of nutrients that the body needs for growth, development, operations, maintenance, and repair:

1. Proteins form the structural framework of living cells. Your body requires protein for the repair, replacement, and growth of all tissues.
2. Carbohydrates contain carbon, hydrogen, and oxygen and are useful energy sources. Many carbohydrate foods also include fiber—bulky plant materials that aid digestion and waste management and reduce cholesterol.
3. Fats (lipids) provide energy and insulation. The body also uses small amounts of fats to repair and enlarge some tissue.
4. Vitamins are complex chemicals that the body requires for sustenance and operations.
5. Minerals are vital to maintaining physiological processes, strengthening skeletal structures, preserving the vigor of the heart and brain, and strengthening the muscle and nervous systems.
6. Water increases blood volume, transports nutrients, comprises approximately two-thirds of muscular tissue, eliminates waste, and regulates body temperature. You lose about 4 pints a day via body functions such as respiration, perspiration, and elimination. It is essential, therefore, to drink at least 64 ounces of water each day to maintain a proper level of hydration.

Stone Age versus Phone Age

You aren't built any differently than your great-great-great-grandfather some 100,000 grandfathers back. But your world bears small resemblance to his. He killed his lunch with a stone; you can get it delivered by lifting a phone. Needless to say, he burned up more calories than you do. In this handy—and hilarious—chart from Banish Your Belly *(Rodale Press, 1997), author Kenton Robinson shows how many calories Grandpa might have burned in a Stone Age day, compared to you.*

Grandpa's Day		Calories	Your Day		Calories
7–8 A.M.	Hunt for breakfast	500	7–8 A.M.	Grab Egg McMuffin at drive-up window on way to work	166
8–9	Still hunting for breakfast	500	8–9	Eat Egg McMuffin at your desk and check e-mail	100
9–9:20	Run away from breakfast	901	9–10	Eat pineapple Danish. Read report on possible acquisition	100
9:20–11	Hunt for smaller, more docile breakfast	832	10–12	Attend 2-hr. meeting to discuss need for more meetings	210
11–12	Kill breakfast and carry it back home	435	12–1:30 P.M.	Hop in car for lunch at Fat Boys Bar-B-Q	149
12–1 P.M.	Skin breakfast and chop wood for fire to cook it	650	1:30–2	Conference call with Los Angeles	50
1–2	Cook breakfast and eat it	124	2–2:30	Flirt with secretary at accounts receivable	55
2–2:30	Regale your fellows with tale about killing your breakfast	67	2:30–4	Type up the Gorsky proposal	172
2:30–3	Beat up fellow who calls you a liar	437	4–4:10	Grab candy bar from vending machine, eat it	17
3–5	Sit around in dazed torpor	49	4:10–5	Talk to old college friend on 800 line	83
5–6	Eat more breakfast	100	5–5:15	Drive to health club	27
6–7	Do dance in honor of the spirit of breakfast	305	5:15–5:45	Jog on treadmill	378
7–11	Sleep	299	5:45–6	Shower and get dressed	56
			6–7	Drive home, open brewdog, order and eat small pizza	112
			7–11	Watch TV. Drink 2 more brewdogs. Eat tortilla chips dipped in salsa	338
Grandpa's Total Calories Burned:		**5,199**	**Your Total Calories Burned:**		**2,013**

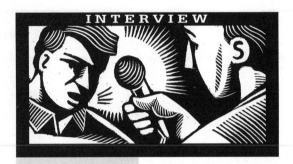

Louis Lanza on

Cooking Dinner Fast

Most of us love to eat, but if the cooking were left up to us, we'd starve. It's not that we can't cook—we just don't have hours to spend in the kitchen boiling and broiling up gourmet cuisine.

You don't need hours, according to Louis Lanza, executive chef and owner of Josie's and Josephina, two healthier-food restaurants in Manhattan. Like the rest of us, Lanza wants to eat good food without adding inches to his gut. Here he offers cooking tips for preparing healthful, tasty food in a flash.

Most of us have a few dishes that we do well, but beyond that we don't really have a clue about what to do in the kitchen. Is it possible for a regular guy to learn how to cook?

It's definitely possible. You can't get too elaborate, but you can definitely make good, healthy, quick food at home. You can make everything in one pan. It will taste good. Just keep basic supplies in the house.

What are the must-have items to help men whip up healthy meals in a hurry?

You need a really good quality 10-inch Teflon pan, not a cheap one, and a good stainless steel pot, like a 4-quart pot to make your grains and rice in. You also need a plastic cutting board—bacteria stays in the wooden cutting boards. By the way, always cut your vegetables on the board first and then put your meat on afterward. You don't want to pick up bacteria from raw chicken and throw the carrots or asparagus on there and start slicing them up.

In addition, you need a decent knife. That's a must. And a good steel to keep your knife sharp. And a colander. Everyone needs a colander. Plus a sturdy wooden spoon to stir. You don't want a plastic one because it will probably melt on you. A Crock-Pot would be handy, too. You don't need much else.

Guys are so busy these days. How difficult would it be to prepare several meals ahead of time, and which ones would be easiest?

Protein, which is meat, chicken, seafood, or tofu, would not be prepared ahead of time, necessarily, but you would prepare all of the other ingredients ahead of time. Say you're going to do your carbohydrates—brown rice, beans. You cook a potful of the brown rice, some quinoa grains, or a potful of beans— enough to last a couple of days. Or you can cook rice and beans twice as fast in a small pressure cooker or in a Crock-Pot. They're great things to have. You can put rice and beans in there in the morning, and when you come home, it's ready to go. You just have to cook your meat, chicken, or fish.

Then you have your vegetables. You can prep those ahead of time by cutting them and putting them into storage bags in your refrigerator for a few days.

I think the easiest, quickest way to get a healthy meal is to use a Teflon pan, in-stead of using a lot of oil. Put a little liquid in the bottom of the pan—like water, a soy marinade, chicken stock, apple juice. It all depends on what kind of flavor you're trying to get out of it. Bring it up to a simmer and add the protein first so that you don't really need any oil. I don't mind a little oil because I think it's good for you, but if you want real low-fat, then you just simmer the meat, fish, or chick-en right in the liquid. Cook one side and turn it over, then add the already-cooked brown rice, beans, or grains, and then you could add the diced vegetables. Cover for a few minutes. You could be eating within 15 minutes if you do that work ahead of time. It's almost like a stir-fry without any of the oil, and you could put different seasonings in it. You could put low-sodium soy sauce in there, you could put a little lemon juice or rice-wine vinegar. You could put balsamic vinegar in it sometimes, if you want to do a little Italian flair. Whatever flavor you put in is going to be absorbed into the meat or chicken or seafood or tofu.

A lot of guys are really into grilling. What are some quick and healthy meals that a man can make on his grill? Everybody knows how to do steaks, chicken, and burgers, but is there something different he could make?

You can cook a million things on a grill. Seafood is the best thing on the grill, to me. But most people tend to overcook it. The key to getting good flavor out of the grill is to marinate the fish or the meat first. What happens is that a lot of guys don't have the patience when they're grilling. You have to let the fire go down. Most people see the fire and, all of a sudden, they put the meat on. It flames up and gets so charred that it's almost unhealthy. Plus, it's raw on the inside. I think the biggest thing when it comes to grilling is to be patient, let the grill simmer down to a nice even heat. And then you can cook whatever you want, fast.

What kind of marinades do you suggest?

Tamari is an idiot-proof one. You take apple juice, some tamari (a type of soy sauce that has little or no added wheat), some lemon juice, a little curry powder, a little coriander, and a little cumin. Mix it together and, if it gets too strong, you can add water. You don't have to put oil in the marinade but you can take a rag or paper towel, put some oil on it, and rub it on the grill before you fire it up. Then the meat or fish won't stick to the surface. Invest in a good wire brush for your grill. You have to really scrape the grill in between each time you cook.

How long should you marinate your meat?

I'd say a half-hour at room temperature is good.

Say a guy who's completely lost in the kitchen wants to make dinner for his girlfriend. What's a great, easy meal he could make that would really impress her?

Chicken breast or salmon with a good honey-mustard sauce—that's the easiest sauce in the world to make. You can go out and buy any flavor mustard you want nowadays. Mix it with a little honey and set it aside. Sauté one side of the chicken or salmon in a no-stick pan. Instead of turning it to cook the other side, put it in a baking dish. Coat the top of the chicken or salmon with the mustard sauce. Put it under the broiler for 4 to 5 minutes. Not too long. As you're doing that, cook vegetables and rice in the pan that you used to cook the chicken or fish. Place the vegetables and rice on a plate, then set this nice piece of chicken or salmon on top.

You've mentioned different seasonings here. What are the two or three spices that a guy can't live without?

Make sure you have a pepper mill. If you like Middle Eastern, you can have curry and coriander powders in the house. You want a nice premium-quality soy sauce, like wheat-free tamari, and a chili-garlic paste—both of these give a nice Asian flavor. If you're going to use herbs in cooking, use fresh herbs—parsley, basil, and so on. If you're cooking meat, you can put a sprig of sage or rosemary on top; if it's fish, use a sprig of cilantro or dill. That makes such a difference.

Once we've cooked all this stuff, how can we clean up the kitchen—fast?

I always practice the clean-as-you-go method. That's the number one rule in any commercial kitchen. And if you practice that in your own home, you never have that big of a mess. Also, use only one pot and keep a sponge nearby.

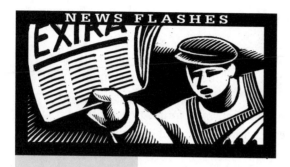

Vitamin C Cuts Heart Attack Risk

KUOPIO, Finland—Add vitamin C deficiency to the ingredient list in the recipe for coronary heart disease. Researchers at the University of Kuopio found that older men who lack vitamin C have a 2½ to 3½ times' greater risk of having a heart attack than men who get adequate levels of the nutrient in their diets.

The researchers recorded the incidence of fatal and nonfatal heart attacks in more than 1,600 middle-age Finnish men for eight years. They then compared those figures with the men's blood levels of vitamin C. Of those deficient in vitamin C, more than 13 percent had heart attacks during the course of the study. However, less than 4 percent of those with adequate amounts of the vitamin had heart attacks.

Those lacking in vitamin C have even more in common. "Men deficient in vitamin C were older, had smoked more in their lifetimes, and were in lower socioeconomic groups," the researchers wrote. And compared with the participants who had sufficient amounts of vitamin C, these men exercised less often, had lower iron intakes, and had higher alcohol and coffee consumption.

But don't think that popping a vitamin C supplement will solve the problem. The researchers found that supplements did not reduce the risk of heart attack. Rather, a healthy intake of foods naturally rich in vitamin C may be the best way to go, they say.

Fatty Foods Cloud Contact Lenses

NEW YORK CITY—Now people who eat high-fat diets can see the results of their excess for themselves. Or rather, they can't. That's because an unhealthy, fatty diet can cause deposits—known as jelly bumps—on contact lenses.

Researchers found that diets full of fat, protein, or alcohol reduce the human tear's ability to prevent certain fats from depositing and sticking to contact lenses. These deposits are painful and can lead to eye infections, says Dean E. Hart, O.D., associate research scientist at Columbia University and founder of the Contact Lens Research Foundation, which conducted the study. If a lousy diet destroys contacts, Dr. Hart cautions, imagine what it does to your body.

Rye Bread May Reduce Heart Disease Better Than Vegetables

HELSINKI, Finland—Rye and other whole-grain breads can help reduce the risk of heart disease better than other fiber-rich foods, including fruits and vegetables.

A study of more than 20,000 Finnish men found that those who ate 35 grams of fiber a day had a 31 percent lower chance of dying from heart disease than those who ate 17 grams a day (about American men's average). It seems that the fiber-loving Finns got most of their intake from rye bread, which researchers found reduced the risk of coronary heart death slightly better than other forms of fiber.

But, to get that fiber, look to other whole-grain breads besides American rye. Because it's made of refined wheat flour and only a little rye, American rye bread offers only about 1 gram of fiber per slice, which doesn't quite stack up to the Finnish version that packs 5 grams per piece. Finding Finnish rye bread may be difficult, but you can try rye crispbread (a form of cracker)—available in most supermarkets or health food stores. It carries a walloping 16 grams of fiber per serving (10 crackers).

Real Type A Men Eat Meat

SHEFFIELD, England—Touchy, impatient men already have the odds of dying of heart disease against them, just from their personality type. A study has found that these men further increase their risk by downing burgers, chips, and cheeses.

Men with type A personalities, a tendency to be hurried and easily angered, often reach for timesaving foods, which are usually snack foods and fast foods. Their power-seeking, controlling nature also makes them gravitate toward red meat, according to a study done at the University of Sheffield. Psychologists think that men subconsciously associate meat with power, maleness, and virility. Of course, foods like burgers, chips, and cheeses are also high in fat and protein—both causes of coronary heart disease.

By the way, female type A personalities are drawn to the wine and cookie diet. That wine, the researchers say, may even decrease women's risk of heart attacks.

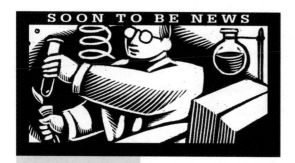

SOON TO BE NEWS

Making Fiber out of Flour?

Doctors keep telling men to eat more fiber to lower their colon cancer risk. But new research suggests that we might not have to eat fiber to get some of fiber's cancer-busting benefits.

Fiber helps fight cancer in two ways. First, since it's too complex to be properly digested, it passes through the digestive system without getting absorbed into the bloodstream. By doing so, fiber helps to keep bad stuff like fat, cholesterol, and toxins—which all contribute to cancer—from getting absorbed by the body as well.

Meanwhile, intestinal bacteria usually ferment fiber, producing quite a bit of gas. As the body manufactures the stuff that eventually makes you pass wind, it also produces a fatty acid called butyric acid, says Bruce German, Ph.D., professor of food science in the department of food science and technology at the University of California, Davis. It's this fatty acid that researchers say may provide some cancer-fighting benefits.

In the future, you may not have to eat bran muffins and dried prunes to get a good dose of butyric acid into your system. Dr. German says that scientists may be able to process other foods so that they, too, cause the body to manufacture butyric acid. Food manufacturers, for example, are working on ways to make starch less digestible—like fiber—so that it might generate cancer-fighting butyric acid. The National Institutes of Health has begun clinical trials to look at the possible benefits of butyric acid in other cells in the body as well.

Fresher Fruits and Vegetables?

A plan to feed astronauts in space may lead to fresher out-of-season produce for those of us stuck on planet Earth.

Because space shuttles don't have room to carry enough nutritious foods like tomatoes, carrots, and bananas to last a typical trip, NASA has been looking into ways to build an outer space greenhouse. Researchers from several New Jersey schools have been able to build an enclosed greenhouse that provides plants with artificial light and heat. In the greenhouse, growers don't need to worry about changing seasons, since fruits and vegetables can be grown inside. They're also trying to extract and recycle chemicals from the inedible portions of the plants, which can be sprayed back onto the plants as a fertilizer (since shuttles don't have room for that, either).

Using these methods, researchers have so far succeeded in growing the first "space-age" tomatoes. You may even have eaten one. In the New Jersey grocery stores that stock them, the first batches of tomatoes were such a hit that they didn't last an afternoon, says Harry W. Janes, a plant scientist and research coordinator at Rutgers University's Cook College in New Brunswick, where the greenhouses are being developed. The high prices didn't scare off consumers who wanted unseasonably fresh produce. Even when prices jumped to $3.49 a pound, the tomatoes still disappeared within two days.

Astronauts won't be the only ones to benefit from this research. Eventually, these enclosed greenhouses could pop up all over the country, growing unseasonably fresh produce like papayas, tomatoes, and corn year-round.

A Super Cucumber?

It's hard to hate cucumbers; there's nothing really bad about them. On the other hand, there's nothing really good about them. Cucumbers contain roughly the same amount of vitamins as you'll find in a glass of water—zilch. But not for much longer.

Thanks to plant breeding, cucumbers may soon have the same amount of beta-carotene as carrots and cantaloupe. Beta-carotene, an intermediate form of vitamin A, helps maintain vision and healthy skin. The only hitch: These cucumbers won't quite resemble the ones we've all come to know and love— they'll be orange on the inside.

Philip W. Simon, Ph.D., a plant geneticist at the U.S. Department of Agriculture–Agricultural Research Service Vegetable Crops Research Laboratory in Madison, Wisconsin, has crossed a U.S. pickling cucumber with one from the Orient. The result: a cucumber that provides a large amount of beta-carotene. For example, an 8-inch cucumber may provide 1.43 to 7.15 milligrams of beta-carotene. This amount could help men meet or exceed their need for this nutrient. Just for perspective: Adult men need 6 milligrams of beta-carotene a day. The cucumber should be able to hold onto this vast store of vitamin A even when peeled or pickled. The orange cucumber will especially be helpful in developing countries where vitamin A consumption is low.

Though the orange cucumber has already been invented, you won't see it in grocery stores just yet. Researchers are looking for ways to grow orange cucumbers that have more consistent levels of vitamin A. If all goes well, someday a single cucumber could be your sole source of vitamin A for the day.

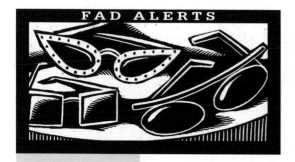

Fat-Free Diets

 Pick just about any product in the grocery store these days, and chances are that you'll find it sitting on the shelf next to a fat-free version of the same food. You might think that eating these leaner counterparts would turn you into a fat-free version of your former self, but you'd be wrong.

In fact, eating too many fat-free foods may actually make you fatter. In a recent study, people who replaced 20 percent of their fat intake with fat substitutes like olestra not only were ravenous by the end of the day but also devoured almost *twice* their normal quota of fatty foods the next day. So while those fat-free potato chips may satisfy you while you're munching away, a few hours later you'll be hungry again. That's because fat substitutes don't slow down digestion the way real fat does, says Stanley Segall, Ph.D., professor of nutrition at Drexel University in Philadelphia. As a result, you may end up bingeing on high-fat foods. So go ahead and skip those nonfat foods, and follow an eating plan that's just low in fat.

Stuffed-Crust Pizza

 Try to order a simple pizza these days and it seems like more and more pizzerias just tell you to get stuffed. Literally. At least two major pizza chains—Pizza Hut and Little Caesars—have added stuffed-crust pizza to their menus, and their customers seem to love the stuff. Pizza Hut's Stuffed-Crust Pizza accounts for one-fourth of its business, or $1 billion in sales, says Rob Doughty, Pizza Hut's vice president of public relations. But the pizza's crust, filled with string mozzarella cheese, isn't the only thing that's getting stuffed—so are your arteries.

How's this for a mouthful? One slice of Pizza Hut's Stuffed-Crust Meat-Lover's Pizza packs 500 calories, 23 grams of fat, and 1,510 milligrams of sodium. And who eats just one slice? Forgo the meat toppings and you're still getting 380 calories, 11 grams of fat, and 1,160 milligrams of sodium per slice. Our take on stuffed-crust pizza: Leave stuffing for the turkey.

Dessert Yogurts

Yogurt makers are pumping out new products faster than you can put away a cup of Milk Chocolate Cheesecake Yogurt. The problem is that many of these dessertlike products have made yogurt less healthful and more sugary by the mouthful.

First to hit the dessert yogurt scene was SnackWell's with its chocolate yogurts. We tried them. They taste good—more like pudding than yogurt, but that's no surprise when you check out the label. A 6-ounce serving of Snack-Well's Milk Chocolate Peanut Butter Yogurt packs about 30 more calories and 12 more grams of sugar than plain low-fat yogurt. But more important, Snack-Well's yogurts lack the live and active bacteria cultures that give yogurt many of its health benefits. SnackWell's purposely kills the bacteria during production to tone down the bitter taste of the chocolate.

Meanwhile, yogurt giant Dannon just released a new line called Double Delights. With flavors like Cherry Cheesecake, Lemon Meringue Pie, and Strawberries 'n Cream, they sound—and taste—a lot more like decadent desserts than healthy snacks. No wonder: They may have live and active cultures but they're also loaded with sugar and extra ingredients like whey protein concentrate, modified cornstarch, kosher gelatin, potassium sorbate, annatto, and xanthan gum. Compare that to plain low-fat yogurt's ingredients: cultured milk, skim milk, and pectin, a natural substance used to gel the yogurt.

The National Yogurt Association, a trade group whose members include several of the major brands, is trying to get SnackWell's products bumped off the yogurt shelf. The association has petitioned the Food and Drug Administration (FDA) to declare that a food cannot legally be called yogurt if it has been heat-treated after culturing. Heat-treating is the process that SnackWell's uses to kill the live and active cultures in its yogurt. The FDA has not yet made a decision. In the meantime, if you're eating yogurt for its health benefits, stick to flavors that don't resemble dessert.

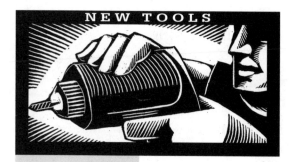

NEW TOOLS

Leaner Meat

Plevalean Cherry Burgers

Here's a healthy burger that doesn't taste like the pits: It's called Plevalean. Made with 91 percent lean beef, cherries (yes, the fruit), oat bran, and spices, this burger boasts a slew of benefits over regular beef burgers. And don't let the cherry part scare you; you don't taste them at all. But they do seal in the meat's juices and keep the burger from shrinking when it's cooked. Cherries also have a natural ingredient that more than doubles the burger's shelf life. And when you reheat a Plevalean burger, it tastes like it was just freshly made. But best of all, it's a lot lower in fat and calories than an all-beef burger. One 3-ounce Plevalean patty (about the size of a McDonald's regular burger) has 160 calories and 8 grams of fat, compared to a beef burger's 245 calories and 18 grams of fat. And the makers of Plevalean don't do just burgers. They also make ground meat, sausage, Canadian bacon, meatballs, pepperoni, and by the end of 1998, lamb burgers and buffalo burgers. Call (616) 228-5000. $15.50 plus shipping for eight 3.2-ounce Plevalean patties and three 1-ounce packages of Plevalean ground meat.

Zestier Food

Garlic Juice Spray

You probably don't think of garlic when you hear the words "fresh-squeezed," but now you can buy a garlic juice spray that lets you spritz rather than mince your garlic. Each bottle contains the juice from more than 150 cloves of garlic, cold-pressed to preserve the fresh garlic flavor. Your recipe calls for one clove of garlic? Use eight sprays of juice. And yes, the spray has all the cholesterol-lowering benefits of the regular cloves. Plus, the spray has no added fat, salt, artificial colors, flavors, or sweeteners. One bottle will stay fresh for a year and doesn't even have to be refrigerated. Look for Garlic Juice Spray at health food stores, gourmet shops, and supermarkets, or call Garlic Valley Farms at (800) 424-7990. An 8-ounce bottle costs $4.99.

Water to Wake You Up

Caffeinated Water

It looks like water. It tastes like water. But there's one thing added: caffeine. That's what you get when you take a jolt of Water Joe. Created by a college student who didn't like coffee or cola but still needed caffeine to pull all-nighters, Water Joe has no calories, sugars, preservatives, or carbonation. But one 16.9-ounce bottle gives you about the same caffeine hit as a cup of coffee or a can and a half of cola. For a double jolt, some people brew their coffee with Water Joe, or they use it to mix with their concentrated orange juice, says David Marcheschi, creator of the beverage. But if you're looking for a thirst quencher, remember that any beverage containing caffeine will act as a diuretic, causing you to lose fluids, not gain them. Look for Water Joe at supermarkets and convenience stores, where it sells for 89 cents a bottle, or call (800) 862-1066.

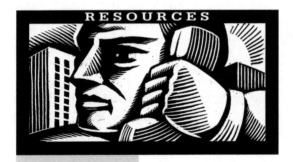

Cheesy Chart

American Institute for Cancer Research
(800) 843-8114, extension 52

Cream. Bleu. Swiss. Cottage. It's tough trying to keep the 20 or more varieties of popular cheeses straight nutrition-wise. Now it's easier to be cheesier, thanks to the American Institute for Cancer Research, which offers a handy slide chart with the nutritional breakdown of the cheeses you'll find in the supermarket. Call to get it and other useful information, such as grocery lists of cancer-fighting foods.

Healthy Eating Online

Virtual Nutrition Center Web Site
http://www-sci.lib.uci.edu/HSG/Nutrition.html

If you can chew it, suck it, sip it, or swallow it, you'll find it here. This comprehensive site from the University of California, Irvine, libraries has thousands of links to food references and health encyclopedias; information and recipes for your favorite foods and drinks (including beer, wine, and cocktails); plus, an assortment of online calculators that let you compute body fat, calories burned during a workout—even how long you have left to live.

Fast-Food Facts

Interactive Food Finder Web Site
http://www.olen.com/food/index.html

When the siren song of your favorite burger joint calls, you can't resist. But before you wend your way to the nearest drive-up window, you can at least make some smarter choices by checking out this nutrient-analysis database run by the Minnesota attorney general's office. It lists the most popular fast-food restaurants and their fattening (and not-so-fattening) fare. You can check out the fat, cholesterol, or sodium content of the food at your favorite eating emporium or search to find out who is serving pizza slices with sodium levels registering fewer than four digits.

Wine Finder

Wine Spectator Online Web Site
http://www.winespectator.com

By now, you certainly know that drinking a little wine is an act of good health. Now you can make your next glass an act of good taste by selecting the perfect type to go with what you're eating. This site, the online counterpart to the highly respected *Wine Spectator* magazine, makes it simple to choose a wine suited to your taste. Search more than 55,000 wine reviews by price, quality rating, or varietal. Survey retailers or restaurants near you to find the best selection and service in your area. Learn the theory behind food and wine pairings. Get inside information on what's hot now or what's aging in the world's wine cellars for future vintages.

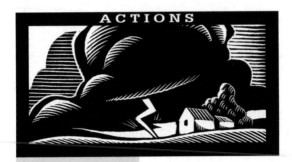

Tired of hearing that everything you like to eat is bad for you? Here's some good news. Lots of foods have healing powers—you just have to find out which foods are good for what. Here are 13 actions that will make you food-smart.

1. Break open the brew. Research has shown that drinking beer may actually be beneficial. A study of 632 men at the University of Washington School of Medicine in Seattle found that beer-drinkers were 53 percent less likely to form kidney or bladder stones than nondrinkers. Just one 8-ounce glass a week brought on the benefit, but drinking more than one beer a week didn't provide additional protection.

A study done by Harvard University researchers has shown that drinking one beer *a night* can help protect against heart disease and cancer. But those health benefits turn into health risks if you reach for a second brewski, says Charles H. Hennekens, M.D., professor of medicine at Harvard and lead researcher of the study.

2. Throw away the antacid. If the four-alarm chili you ate for lunch gave you heartburn, grab a guava instead of your regular antacid. Guava, a greenish-yellow, baseball-size fruit, may help relieve heartburn or acid indigestion. One cup of guava juice is all you need to get relief, says medical anthropologist John Heinerman, Ph.D., director of the Anthropological Research Center in Salt Lake City and author of *Heinerman's New Encyclopedia of Fruits and Vegetables.* Guavas are also supercharged with vitamin C—just one packs more than twice as much vitamin C as an orange.

3. Avoid the deep freeze. If you like your coffee strong, store your beans in the fridge, not the freezer. Beans that are frozen could lose some of their oils, and the coffee's zing along with it. An added bonus for your beans: Keeping them cold will also keep your coffee from tasting stale.

4. Stop a big fat headache. California researchers have found yet another reason to eat a low-fat diet—to take care of your headaches. A study by researchers at Loma Linda University School of Public Health in Loma Linda found that 54 migraine sufferers who cut their fat intakes to fewer than 20 grams per day for two months experienced fewer and less-intense headaches. The reason, researchers say, is that fat may release a chemical into the brain that triggers headaches.

5. Make your own menu. When you eat out, you don't have to put your healthy diet on the back burner. If there aren't any healthy choices on the menu, make your own healthy meal out of appetizers. Order shrimp cocktail with soup and a salad. Just stay away from cream soups and ask to have the salad without cheese and croutons.

6. Work in a sports drink after working out. Sports drinks may actually keep your immune system in shape. A study sponsored by the Gatorade Sports Science Institute in Barrington, Illinois, found that drinking carbohydrate-loaded sports drinks before, during, and after prolonged exercise may keep an athlete's immunity from taking a nosedive. The carbohydrates in most sports drinks seem to cancel out some of the stress that exercise places on the immune system, says David Nieman, Dr. P.H., lead researcher of the study and director of health degree promotion in the department of health, leisure, and exercise science at Appalachian State University in Boone, North Carolina. But be sure to drink your sports drink cold—and with a straw. The acid in sports drinks can damage your tooth enamel. The warmer the drink, the greater its enamel-eroding potential. Using a straw will also help reduce damage by getting it past your teeth quickly.

7. Swallow your C. Taking vitamin C supplements can help boost your immune system and protect against heart attacks. But vitamin C tablets can also be tough on your teeth. The American Dental Association (ADA) says that taking too many chewable vitamin C tablets could erode some of your tooth enamel. Taking just one chewable vitamin C a day should be okay, but if you take more than one, you should switch to a nonchewable form, according to the ADA.

8. Milk it. Drinking 2 cups of milk a day can cut your risk of the most common type of stroke in half. That's the word from the Honolulu Heart Program, which conducted a study of middle-age men and the effects of drinking milk. Researchers aren't sure what substance in the milk cuts the risk of stroke, but they theorize that it may be a combination of something in the milk and the healthful lifestyle that milk-drinkers tend to lead. But if you want to do your brain *and* your body good, stick to low-fat or skim milk.

9. **Keep it fresh.** Your fresh, frozen, or canned fruits and vegetables could be losing some of their nutrients before making their way to your plate. Here are some ways to keep those nutrients from jumping ship.

- If you're always tossing your lettuce before you can toss it in your salad, ask the produce clerk about buying just half a head of lettuce. Many supermarkets allow customers to buy smaller quantities of fresh produce— you just have to ask. We did, and almost all of the stores agreed to fill our request.
- Don't wash and cut your fresh fruits and vegetables immediately after bringing them home. Waiting to wash and chop until *just before* cooking or eating them will preserve their vitamins, says the American Institute for Cancer Research. You should also avoid cutting them into tiny pieces, which can reduce vitamin content.
- If you buy frozen fruits and vegetables, avoid buying bags that have turned into rock-solid chunks. When buying by the box, make sure the package has no colored stains and that no liquids are oozing out. These are all signs that thawing and refreezing have taken place, which could rob your veggies of some of their valuable nutrients.
- If you're a can man, store your canned fruits and vegetables in a cool, dry place away from your kitchen stove. Over time, heat can steal away the foods' nutrients.

10. **Don't believe everything you read.** Women aren't the only ones who lie about how much they weigh. Researchers at New York University found that the food labels on common snacks often fib about their weights, too. In some cases, single-serving muffins, brownies, or cookies weighed as much as 25 percent more than their labels promised. And that could make you weigh more, too. Researchers found some snacks to have as many as 175 more calories than their labels indicated.

11. **Lick your cravings.** Next time your sweet tooth screams for some sugar, tear open a Tootsie Pop. Or if you prefer, binge on a bubble gum–center Blow Pop. These candies on a stick will stick around for about 30 minutes, but they won't stick to your waistline, says Franca Alphin, R.D., director of nutrition at the Duke University Diet and Fitness Center in Durham, North Carolina. Tootsie Pops and Blow Pops pack a mere 60 and 80 calories, respectively. And as far as fat goes, these lickable goodies have a big fat zero. Bonus: Now you can find out once and for all just how many licks it takes to get to the center of a Tootsie Pop.

12. **Know which cork to pop.** You probably already know that having a glass of wine a day is good for your heart, but do you know which wine is good with lobster? Red or white? Sweet or dry? If you're going to be heart-healthy, do it with style and taste. To help you do just that, we consulted *The Wine Guide*, published by the Pennsylvania Liquor Control Board. Here's what they suggest.

Beef	Barbera, Barolo, Burgundy, Cabernet Sauvignon, Pinot Noir, Proprietary Red
Ham	Beaujolais, Blush, Gewürztraminer, Zinfandel
Lamb	Chianti, Pinot Noir, Rhone, Zinfandel
Pork	Alsatian White, Vin Rosé, Vouvray, Zinfandel
Veal	Cabernet Sauvignon, Chardonnay, Johannisberg Riesling, Pinot Noir, Zinfandel
Chicken	Chablis, Chardonnay, Chenin Blanc, Johannisberg Riesling, Loire, Sauvignon Blanc
Turkey	Chenin Blanc, Johannisberg Riesling, Loire, Sauvignon Blanc
Fish	Alsatian White, Chardonnay, Chenin Blanc, Johannisberg Riesling, Sauvignon Blanc
Clams, Oysters, Scallops	Chablis, Chardonnay
Lobster, Shrimp	Chardonnay, Gewürztraminer
Crab	Chablis, Nonvintage Champagne
Spaghetti	Barbera, Barolo, Chianti, Proprietary Red, Zinfandel

13. **Fish for your feelings.** The omega-3 fatty acids found in salmon and some other fish may keep you from feeling down in the dumps. Belgian researchers recently discovered that seriously depressed patients had lower omega-3 levels than those who were healthy or only mildly depressed. It's not clear what the connection is between omega-3 levels and depression, but we do know that the brain needs omega-3's to form healthy nerve cells. To keep your omega-3 levels—and your spirits—up, try eating one to two servings a week of salmon or some other omega-3 rich fish like tuna, mackerel, sardines, herring, or anchovies.

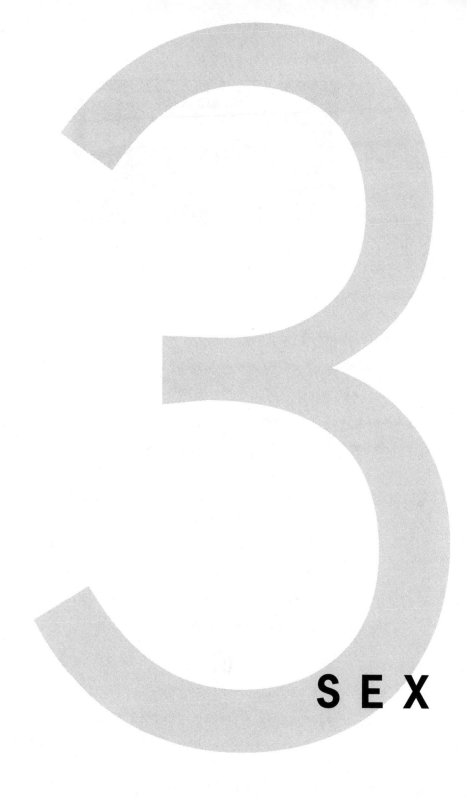

SEX

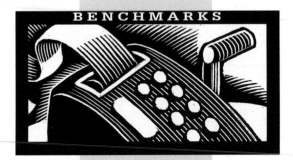

BENCHMARKS

AVERAGES

- Percentage of Americans who believe that pornography provides information about sex: 59

- Chances that an adolescent boy in America has been intentionally kicked or hit in the genitals: 1 in 10

- Average amount that a male buyer spent on women's lingerie in 1995: $50

- Average amount that a female buyer spent on lingerie in 1995: $23

- Percentage of sexually active women who carry condoms: 56

- Number of clients the average prostitute in a Nevada brothel sees in one day: 6

- Percentage of British men who report cross-dressing at least once: 25

- Percentage who report doing so weekly: 8

- Number of times the typical American has sex during the year: 135—26 times more than the international average

- Age at which the average American becomes sexually active: 16.2

- Average age for the rest of the world: 17.6

- Time of day people are most likely to have sex: 10:34 P.M.

- Total hours per night that a healthy man has an erection while sleeping: 1 to 3½

EXTREMES

- Cost of a sex change to go from a woman to a man: $20,000 to $25,000

- To change a man to a woman: $10,000 to $12,000

- Minimum length for condoms set by the European Committee for Standardization: 6.7 inches

- Length of the jail term to which a Pennsylvania man was sentenced for repeatedly oinking at his ex-wife: 30 days

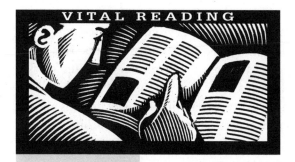

Straight Talk for Penile Injuries

Acrobatic sex may be fun, but sometimes it can scar
or bruise your equipment. Here's how to plot a
straight course away from "intimate injuries."

The walrus has it made: With a long, hard bone running the length of its re-
tractable penis, it rarely runs the risk of intimate injury. We humans, however,
are not so lucky. "Three to four million American men are impotent because of
injury to the penis during masturbation or intercourse," says Irwin Goldstein,
M.D., professor of urology at Boston University. And new research suggests that
many of those private wounds are so minor that as many as 45 percent of the
injured are unaware of a mishap—until they wake up six months later with
bent or narrowed penises.

Such penile alterations have been observed for more than a millennium.
Byzantine Emperor Heraclius, born in A.D. 610, was said to have a penile de-
formity that caused him to "urinate in his face." François de la Peyronie, a barber and surgeon, was the first to formally describe the problem. In 1747, he
observed that "rosary beads" of scar tissue extending the full length of the
penis were associated with curves and impairments of function. Physicians
now refer to bends and narrowings of the penis as Peyronie's disease and believe them to be the result of an impairment in wound healing following a penile injury.

The Not-So-Straight and Narrow

Here's what can happen: During sleep, intercourse, or masturbation, the
erect penis can be jolted up, down, or less commonly, to the side. If the stress on
the penis is severe, it may rupture one of two interior "balloons" that fill with
blood during erection (called corpora cavernosa). The result—a penile fracture—would cause immediate, severe pain and rapid bruising.

But such outright fractures are relatively rare. More common and more sub-tle may be the small penile stresses that lead to Peyronie's disease—things like straining to penetrate with a semi-erect penis or suffering minor hits. This penile roughhousing can tug the corpora cavernosa away from two sheaths of skin (called the septum) that anchor the penis to the body. In some men, the body's re-pair mechanism in response to these tears goes haywire. Think of the cells making up the anchoring penile tissue as pickets on a fence. Since they're all lined up, they can easily stretch to allow erection. But, in Peyronie's disease, the body lays down repair planks in a random manner—some diagonal, some horizontal.

This haphazard placement of tissue (known as a plaque) prevents the penis from expanding fully, creating either a bend or a narrowing around the scar. And often these alterations in form lead to significant impairments in function.

There's good reason why 75 percent of the 2 million men afflicted with Pey-ronie's disease are over 45. "As the collagen that makes up the structure of the penis ages, it changes character and becomes less elastic," says Gerald Jordan, M.D., professor of urology at the Eastern Virginia Medical School in Norfolk and director of the Devine Center for Genitourinary Reconstruction Surgery.

Think again of a balloon: In younger men, the rubber of the balloon is so elastic, it can be filled to a high pressure. If this fully filled balloon is hit, it re-bounds, deflecting damage. In older men with less elastic tissue, the balloon is slightly underinflated. When it's hit, it tends to absorb the blow, developing a small injury, thus initiating the potentially dangerous wound-healing cascade.

Who's at Risk?

Researchers have found a surprising link between Peyronie's disease and a disorder of the hands called Dupuytren's contracture. "As many as one out of three men we see with Peyronie's disease also have some sign of Dupuytren's," says Dr. Jordan.

Why the connection? Like Peyronie's, Dupuytren's appears to be a disease of wound healing—only in Dupuytren's, the tissues that become scarred and in-elastic are on the palm of the hand. The first signs of Dupuytren's (which usual-ly shows up in a man's forties or fifties) are small, painless bumps beneath the pinkie finger and dimpling of the skin on the palms. Sometimes nodules form on the knuckles, making it difficult to wear rings. Eventually, the fingers may contract permanently—pinkie first, followed by ring and index finger.

While Dupuytren's contracture afflicts only about 5 percent of most popu-lations, one out of four people of Celtic ancestry (usually fair-haired people with light skin) suffers from the disease.

But genes alone do not a curve make. It takes a triggering event. "We think the genetic component has to do with deficient tissue healing. The process that leads to a bend won't begin unless you suffer an injury," explains Laurence A. Levine, M.D., associate professor of urology and director of the Male Sexual Function and Fertility program at Rush–Presbyterian–St. Luke's Medical Center in Chicago.

So if you or any of your immediate relatives suffer from Peyronie's or Dupuytren's, don't panic. But do pay special heed to the following advice.

Scared Straight

We're used to hearing doctors attribute various maladies of the penis and prostate to sexual inactivity. That's why we were startled to hear that Peyronie's disease frequently affects sexually *active* middle-age men. "Many of these men freely volunteer that they often have acrobatic sex lives—and that's fairly unusual among men in their fifties and sixties," says Dr. Jordan.

Since having erections brings rejuvenating oxygen to the tiny muscles in the penis, and ejaculation clears built-up secretions from the prostate, we're not mandating less sex. But a few safety rules and precautions are definitely in order.

Enter with caution. "One of the most common means of injury is the penetrating thrust that misses," says Dr. Goldstein. If the penis misses the vagina while the man is on top, it will often bang against the woman's perineum (that hard, diamond-shaped area of skin between the vagina and anus), potentially causing considerable damage.

What can you do? Before your thrust, try an ancient Oriental technique: Take the shaft of the penis in your hand and run the glans along your partner's clitoris in long, upward movements. Then teasingly enter her partway before fully penetrating. You'll protect yourself and give her arousal a boost in the process.

Use a lubricant. As women age, their vaginal tissues can stiffen. That plus a postmenopausal decrease in lubrication equals a recipe for penile injury. "Lubrication is not only helpful; it's imperative, especially in prolonged sessions with varying positions," says Dr. Goldstein.

She can help by exercising and eating right. Both will increase the blood flow to her vaginal tissues (making them more sensitive and flexible). Also, she can take supplemental estrogen to increase her natural lubrication. You can help by keeping a high-quality lubricant by the bed.

Take care when she's on top. "The most common injury is what we call rodeo sex: the woman is on top and has pulled herself up and off the penis.

Then she comes down hard, moving the penis out of alignment," says Dr. Gold-stein. If she makes a sudden movement backward, forward, or sideways while you're inside, she can also cause injury.

To make woman-on-top sex safer, coat your penis with lubricant before she moves down on you. And have her very carefully maneuver into a position that respects the natural angle of her vagina and your penis. Instead of achieving extra stimulation by moving up and down your shaft, ask her to squeeze the pubococcygeal muscles that surround her vagina (as though she were doing a Kegel exercise) as she gyrates slowly around the penis. And caution her against any sudden movement.

Use a vacuum pump. As we mentioned before, the softer the penis, the more vulnerable it may be to small tears. If your erections are firm enough for penetration but softer than they used to be, ask your doctor about using a vacu-um pump. These devices, which use suction to firm and enlarge erections, were shown in a recent study to reverse some men's penile curves.

One caution: "In terms of major injury—tripping and falling on an erect penis, say—the harder the erection, the more severe will be the fracture," says Dr. Goldstein. So firming up with a vacuum pump may be an excellent idea for men with soft erections. But it's crucial to use the devices and the ensuing erec-tions with care.

Diagnosis: Curvature

"An absolutely straight penis probably doesn't exist," says Dr. Levine. "I wouldn't recommend treatment unless the penis were bent more than 30 de-grees in any direction or had a narrowing that created a 'hinge' effect, in which the tip of the penis swings."

To check for scarring, grip the head of your flaccid penis and pull gently until the shaft straightens out. With the other hand, feel up and down the shaft for any raised areas. Also think back over the past few months: Can you remem-ber any sexual move that caused pain?

If you discover scars, feel pain in your penis on erection, and notice a bend or a narrowing, see a urologist right away. "If medical treatment short of surgery is going to work, it needs to begin very early in the disease process," says Tom Lue, M.D., professor of urology at the University of California at San Francisco.

By the time you notice a curve, the scar has already begun to form, but it hasn't completely set. "It takes a year to a year-and-a-half for the tissue replace-ment to be completed," says Dr. Jordan. All of the nonsurgical therapies appear to work best if begun within six months of the onset of the curve, so it's important to act fast. Unfortunately, all of the following treatments are supported by purely anecdotal results. Only a handful of doctors are willing to try these three relatively unproven approaches. So it's imperative to see an expert in Peyronie's disease if you notice a curve.

Verapamil. As penile scars harden, one-fourth develop calcium deposits. Maybe that's one reason that Dr. Levine has had success injecting the scars with a calcium-blocking medication called verapamil, usually administered orally to lower high blood pressure. Researchers have found that people taking verapamil orally for several years appear to have less arteriosclerosis-forming plaque in their blood vessels than those who don't take it. "We've now treated 90 men, and 62 percent show measurable improvement, while 75 percent say that they feel improvements in their erections," says Dr. Levine.

Colchicine. Dr. Lue favors administering a drug called colchicine, which is used for gouty arthritis. When he gave 24 men 1.2 milligrams of the drug orally twice a day for three to five months, 78 percent reported a reduction in pain and 37 percent exhibited reduced curvature. "This approach works best when used within the first three to four months after the onset of the disease," says Dr. Lue.

Collagenase. Only one drug is currently in development specifically for Peyronie's disease. In a small study, 11 patients received an injection of collagenase in their scars, and 11 got no treatment. Although only 4 men receiving the drug showed improvement, none of the men in the other group improved.

Trick Questions

Here's what to do next time she asks a question
that always gets you in trouble.

It is Saturday afternoon, and you're exactly where you should be: stretched out on the couch in front of a televised sporting event, opening beer number two, relaxed in the knowledge that the pizza you ordered is even now on its way. Nothing could improve this moment, except maybe a bigger television. Suddenly your wife enters the room and says, "What exactly do you think you're doing?"

Is this a trick question or what?

Yes, it is. The trick is that no matter how you answer it, you'll find yourself driving to a home-improvement center, where you'll spend the rest of the afternoon trying to choose the type of curtain rod that's right for you.

How does this work?

It has as much to do with the nature of the question itself as with anything else. Women are expert at posing questions that seem to have no right answer. Here's a common example.

Do I look fat? There is no answer to this question that won't be interpreted "yes." "No" means yes. "Yes" means yes. "I don't know" means yes. "It doesn't matter" means yes. The briefest hint of a pause before speaking means yes, yes, yes. Most of us would rather take the SATs again than field this one, yet it may well come up several times a week.

Your only real choice is to say no, clearly and immediately, leaving no possibility for any subtext, and making it sound like a widely acknowledged fact and not simply your personal opinion. This doesn't work, but all the other options are even worse.

There are several other questions for which "no" is the only answer and several more that call for an emphatic and unqualified "yes." In all of these cases, elaboration, justification, or any attempt to be funny is unlikely to pay off. Consult this handy chart.

Just Say No	*Just Say Yes*
Is there someone else?	Do you still love me?
Do you still fantasize about her?	Do you ever fantasize about me?
Are you tired of me?	Do you like my hair this way?

Unfortunately, many female inquiries require more than a simple yes or no response. Some of them are more like riddles, such as this one.

Which shoes look better? Typically, you're already late for dinner when your wife confronts you, with one pair of shoes on and another alongside them. This is no ordinary choice. It's a devious chicken/egg puzzler. If you pick the shoes she already has on, she'll think you're trying to hurry her. If you pick the other pair, she'll think it's because you know you can't pick the ones she has on. Some men try a nonlinear approach and opt for a third, unoffered pair of shoes, but this is inevitably taken as either an attack on her judgment or an opportunity for her to attack yours. On no account should you suggest another dress. You might as well say, "You're fat."

This raises the question of why she's asking you at all. She knows you don't know which shoes look better, and she knows you don't care, so why is she trying to elicit your opinion? This is part of an ongoing campaign to domesticate you. As part of the same campaign, she will occasionally consult you about alternative table settings or new towels. In these two cases, a disdainful and dismissive "beats me" should do the trick, but don't try that with the shoe dilemma, or you'll miss your reservation. Instead, suggest that she try on the other shoes, then tell her the first ones look better. This lets you more or less off the hook, as long as you don't raise a fuss when she decides that the second pair are better after all.

How many people have you slept with? Hmmm.... Now, you can tell her the truth, unless the truth is more than 12, or you can have a guess at the number she's more or less expecting. Like most arithmetic problems, the answer is a lot easier once you have a formula. This one should work, as long as neither of you has sex for a living: Number of people she's slept with + Number of people she knows you've slept with + Number of people you actually have slept with. Add these up and divide by 2. If you round up to the nearest whole person, you should end up with a realistically healthy but not particularly shocking number. If the result is greater than 12, then say 12. Let's move on.

Why don't you lighten up? This rhetorical gem is used whenever you express your disapproval of shoplifting or speeding, or whenever you go to a nightclub and spend the whole time complaining because the music is too loud and there aren't any chairs.

There's no good answer to this one. You could draw attention to her inconsistency in this matter, noting that she doesn't like it when you act like a kid or when you act like your dad; then again, if you do that, she's liable to see your point and open a whole new can of worms.

Notice anything different about me? This question is of a piece with two others: "Have you forgotten what today is?" and "Have you been listening to a word I've said?" Apart from being questions that are easier to answer wrong than right, they're the kinds of things that women say in sitcoms. They are best treated in an ironic postmodern context, that is, just say what Ward Cleaver would say.

HER: Notice anything different about me?

YOU: New apron?

HER: Have you forgotten what today is?

YOU: Of course not. It's Thursday.

HER: Have you been listening to a word I've said?

YOU: That's nice, dear....

Funny, huh? Well, it's not your fault if she doesn't get it. If she wants a better answer, she's going to have to start asking better questions.

Have you taken a look at yourself lately? This question and its cousin, the almost-always-uncalled-for "Who do you think you are?" are ways of gently reminding you how much of a factor pity was in her original decision to go out with you and how that decision could be rescinded if you behave in any way that cannot be described as abject. You probably brought this rebuke on yourself by mentioning that you reckon Brad Pitt is getting a little chubby or by speculating that Jack Nicholson doesn't have to wait until *his* birthday for oral sex. You're not really supposed to answer either of these questions. You're just supposed to apologize for wantonly having self-esteem. Instead of apologizing, just smile. Your manifold inadequacies as a husband—nay, as a man—are a kind of revenge all by themselves. Next!

Do you believe in fidelity? Like most philosophical questions that seem to pop up out of the blue, this question doesn't pop up out of the blue. This general query about fidelity is in fact a coded inquiry about the extent of your fidelity on a specific occasion or occasions. Your response will also have to be coded. Consult this translation chart before giving your answer.

You Say	You Mean	She Thinks
Yes.	How much does she know?	He's hiding something.
It depends.	How much does she know?	I knew it!
Why do you ask?	How much does she know?	Jerk!
I dunno. Do you?	How much does she know?	How much does he know?

There are several more variations, but they're not worth going into. By the time she asks you this question, you're already in deep trouble. It doesn't really matter what you say, as long as you don't blush when you answer.

Let's look at an example that calls for more straightforward lying.

What are you looking at? She means, "You were looking at that girl, weren't you?" And you thought you'd perfected that trick of keeping your neck still and just letting your eyes swivel.

Obviously, the truth is not the best answer here. We all know that the truth can set you free, sometimes before you've found somewhere else to stay. It may seem easy enough to answer this question with a cunning lie, but when men are caught off guard, their ability to deceive is impaired.

Here are a few of the more common mistakes that men make when asked, "What are you looking at?"

Too specific: "The rust around the bolts on the handle of that mailbox on the northwest corner."

Not specific enough: "That thing."

Too good to be true: "A diamond necklace in that window back there that would be perfect on you."

Too true to be good: "A see-through nightie in that window back there that would be perfect on you."

Too obvious: "Nothing."

Way too obvious: "That blonde over there with the big...means nothing."

Here's one that requires a little interpretation.

What are we going to do now? This one often crops up whenever some kind of emergency or seemingly unsolvable problem arises. The part that requires interpretation is the mysterious "we" in the middle.

This means two things: In one sense, "we" clearly means "you," as in, "What are you going to do now?" but there is also a sense of "we're in this together," implying that you bear equal responsibility for the fact that she's just dropped her keys down a grate or that she stores her jack and spare tire in her garage so they won't get stolen.

In such situations, you'll probably find that the only answer to "What are we going to do now?" that you can think of is "We are going to get a divorce. Goodbye." Most likely, you'll decide not to say anything. After which she will probably let loose with the rather ill-advised:

Why don't you say something? Whether you answer this one is up to you. There is only one question that you should never, ever answer. Keep silent, cower behind your Fifth Amendment rights, pretend you didn't hear, run away, whatever, but don't say anything when she asks:

Should I get all of my hair cut off? If you say anything, then when she *does* get all her hair cut off (and let's face it, she's already made up her mind) and she hates it (and she will hate it), it will be your fault. Even if you say absolutely nothing, the best you can hope for is that she will come home with all her hair cut off, stare you straight in the eye, and say:

Does it make me look fat? You're on your own.

Recharge Your Sex Drive

There's more to raising desire than candlelight dinners.
Here's how you can boost the chemical responsible for it all.

Sure, we think ambience is an important factor in fantastic sex. And yeah, we know that if you're angry or frustrated with your partner, you're not going to feel a lot of sexual passion. But when it comes to libido, lovey-doveyness and candlelight are touted as cure-alls. You and I know better: There's a hard, biological reality to sex drive in men that has largely been ignored by researchers and the press alike. We asked a handful of experts to cut to the libido chase and tell us what we can do to keep ours going strong.

The first thing that the experts told us is something that we're sure you already know: The importance of a man's libido to his psyche cannot be underestimated. By libido, we don't just mean how often you have sex with your partner; we mean how often you fantasize, masturbate, or just want sex—regardless of whether you can have it. We're talking about desire as one of life's key forces, as that quality that lets us know we're still vitally, essentially, a male animal.

In a study of men ages 40 to 79, researchers found that sexual satisfaction is largely predicated on having a strong sex drive. Men in their seventies were just as happy with their sex lives as men in their forties—as long as their drives and erections were strong. "We were quite surprised at the impact the men's sex drive had on their overall contentment," says Joseph E. Oesterling, M.D., professor and urologist in chief at the University of Michigan Medical Center in Ann Arbor.

Now for the bad news: The percentage of men in the study who reported feeling sexual stirrings more than once a week dropped with each decade. Among men in their forties, 77 percent felt desire more than once a week, compared to only 10 percent of those in their seventies.

But it doesn't have to be that way. From getting more exercise to taking in more minerals to avoiding certain drugs, there are things you can do today to boost your desire and increase your overall sense of well-being.

While researchers have known for decades that testosterone is the libido's master switch, studies have uncovered a more specific relationship. After tracking 92 Greek army recruits, researchers concluded that the key to the male sex drive is a special type of testosterone manufactured in the testicles. It's called dihydrotestosterone. During the study, the recruits were asked to report the number of orgasms they had each week from sexual intercourse, masturbation, and spontaneous nighttime erections. While the average recruit reported 3.9 orgasms each week, those with higher dihydrotestosterone had as many as 11.

The key, then, to boosting sexual drive is encouraging the testicles to manufacture more dihydrotestosterone—something that testosterone supplementation (in the form of injections or patches) can't do. Taking in testosterone from outside sources increases the level of "free" testosterone in the blood but doesn't necessarily impact dihydrotestosterone. You may be able to jump-start your machinery in other ways, however. Here's how.

Choose meat. Lean chicken, beef, and fish are all excellent sources of zinc, a mineral that as many as 30 percent of us may be deficient in. And even a minor deficiency can have major effects on the body's manufacturing of testosterone. "We're finding that testosterone declines in men with relatively minor zinc deficiencies," says Ananda S. Prasad, M.D., professor of medicine at Wayne State

University in Detroit and author of an ongoing study. These declines, however, soon reverse as men consume more zinc.

Meeting the daily zinc requirement of 15 milligrams a day does take some doing. Shellfish and red meat are the best sources, and one serving (about the size of a deck of playing cards) of either will give you a full day's requirement. With chicken and fish, you need two servings to fill the bill. Unfortunately, most vegetables and grains contribute a form of zinc that is poorly used by the body.

If that much meat isn't in sync with how you eat, you have two options: First, you can munch on pumpkin seeds, a powerful source of zinc and a rumored aphrodisiac. Second, you can supplement. "We usually suggest 30 milligrams a day taken on an empty stomach," says Dr. Prasad. Any more than 50 milligrams may deplete your body's store of copper, which can cause decreased immunity. And combining zinc with other minerals (say, in the form of a multivitamin) may inhibit zinc absorption.

Get physical. Both exercise and sunlight have been shown to boost sex drive. In one study, men who exercised aerobically three times a week had sex more, masturbated more, and had more frequent orgasms than their couch-potato counterparts. Researchers speculate that exercise affects sex drive by boosting circulating levels of testosterone. In another study, testosterone was shown to rise significantly after men ran on treadmills for 30 minutes.

Peruse your pills. While many prescription or over-the-counter drugs may decrease libido by interfering with testosterone production, drugs used to treat hypertension, or high blood pressure, and depression are the biggest offenders.

Of the antihypertensives, most inhibitors have been associated with libido-lowering effects. "If you're taking an antihypertensive and feel great, there's no need to worry," says James Goldberg, Ph.D., research pharmacologist and co-author of *Sexual Pharmacology*. "But if you do notice an effect, talk to your doctor about switching medications." A good libido-preserving choice: captopril (Capoten).

A study comparing the sexual side effects of the antidepressant nefazodone (Serzone) with those of sertraline (Zoloft)—a drug similar to fluoxetine (Prozac)—found a striking difference. While 89 percent of the male nefazodone takers were satisfied with their sex lives, only 50 percent of sertraline users were. Trazodone (Desyrel), an antidepressant similar to nefazodone, has such significant libido- and erection-boosting side effects that it's sometimes used to treat impotence. Another good antidepressant choice is bupropion (Wellbutrin), which has also been shown to improve libido.

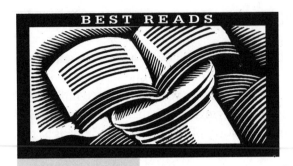

Waist Not, Want Not

What part of a woman turns you on? Shapely legs that never seem to end? A bust that doesn't need help from the Wonderbra to look stunning? How about a woman's waist-hip ratio? According to an evolutionary psychologist in Kate and Douglas Botting's Sex Appeal: The Art and Science of Sexual Attraction *(St. Martin's Press, 1995), eons of evolution have programmed the human male to unconsciously use this ratio to assess a female's sexual capability. And he has the statistics to back it up.*

Professor Devendra Singh, an Indian psychologist working at the University of Texas in Austin, has applied scientific analysis to the matter of the female figure.

As an evolutionary psychologist, Singh was looking for sexually attractive features that were common to every woman in every society and every epoch. He began by studying the so-called vital statistics of the women in *Playboy* centerfolds from 1955 to 1990 and the Miss America beauty contests between 1923 and 1987 and found that the measurements had changed during these periods.

Miss America's vital statistics, for example, had shrunk from 35-24½-35 in 1940 to 35-23½-34½ in 1987, while her weight had gone down by between 11 and 16 pounds. The ideal Western woman, it seemed, was becoming lighter and slenderer, with a smaller upper torso, especially around the bust.

But Singh's calculations showed that, though the female figure had been shifting from relatively full and heavy to relatively slim and light, the ratio of waist measurements to hip measurements (calculated by dividing the waist measurement by the hip size, counting the buttocks in with the hips) remained remarkably constant. It was this waist-hip ratio, in Singh's view, that was the crucial indicator of the sexual attractiveness of a woman's body.

Women who are perfectly healthy always have a waist-hip ratio below 0.80, regardless of their whole body weight. The ideal range for premenopausal women is between 0.67 and 0.80 (which works out at between 24- and 28-inch waists with 36-inch hips, and 27-inch to 31-inch waists with 40-inch hips). The lower the waist-hip ratio, the more sexually attractive the woman becomes.

Other features of a woman's body, such as bustline, physique, and body weight, have had their importance over the years in Western society. But none of them have displayed the same consistency. The ideals of feminine beauty in nineteenth-century Britain and America were big-bosomed and comfortably built. By contrast, the most sought-after fashion models of the 1960s took after Twiggy, and were slender and flat-chested. The one thing these two extremes of female attractiveness had in common was a low waist-hip ratio. At 31-24-33 in her flat-chested heyday, Twiggy still had a low average waist-hip ratio of 0.73.

But was it the waist-hip ratio that enabled Miss Americas to win the beauty titles or *Playboy* Playmates to secure coveted centerfolds? Or was it the shape of the breasts, the length of their legs, the promise of the smile, the pout of the lips?

To find out, Singh asked 580 men and women of different ethnic groups and educational backgrounds between the ages of 18 and 86 to rate drawings of 12 female figures on the basis of their good health, youthful looks, attractiveness, sexiness, and desire and capability for having children. The faces and breasts of the women in the drawings remained the same, only their weights and hip-waist ratios were different. So four of the women were normal weight, four were overweight, and four underweight, and in each group the waist-hip ratios ranged from low to high.

Among both the men and the women the favorite figure of all—the sexiest, most attractive woman with the best health and the greatest desire and capability for having children—was judged to be the normal weight woman with the low waist-hip ratio. Out of the overweight and underweight groups the favorite figure was invariably the woman with the narrowest waist.

The men did not appear to equate plumpness with fertility or thinness with beauty. This last finding (a by-product of the test) was a surprise, given the current shibboleth in America and the West that thin is beautiful.

Why do men react in this way? Singh believes that the male reaction amounts to an unconscious assessment of the female's sexual and reproductive capabilities, based on clues provided by the dimensions of the woman's waist, and that these clues have their origins in man's deep past.

Waist-hip ratio is to do with the distribution of body fat, a great signifier of a person's age and sex rather than the amount of fat. At 10 years old, for example, a girl has much the same figure as she will have around the age of 40. On reaching puberty, she will begin to deposit more fat on her hips, which gives her not only her classic female shape but also a waist-hip ratio that is much lower than the males'. This remains the case until the female menopause, when the female waist-hip ratio becomes similar to that of the male.

A recent report has found a direct link between waist-hip ratio and fertility. Married women who have a high waist-hip ratio experience greater difficulty in becoming pregnant and also have their first live birth at a later age.

The human male, concludes Singh, has learned to use the waist-hip ratio as the most important bodily clue to a woman's reproductive capability and health status.

Mature Games

When it comes to sexual variety, even the hottest couples sometimes find themselves blowing furiously on the embers, trying to keep things crackling. The problem isn't a lack of love or attraction—it's just the all-too-human desire for a little variety in your sex life. In this excerpt from A Lifetime of Sex *(Rodale Press, 1998), Stephen C. George and K. Winston Caine reveal how to eliminate sexual boredom by exposing it to the powers of creativity, imagination...and nude volleyball.*

According to many reports, the major sexual problem in our culture is sexual boredom. Same partner. Same place. Same time. Same way. Next stop: abstinence. If your diet were like that, you'd stop eating.

You don't accept a third straight day of tuna casserole. Instead, you book a table at some restaurant with an unpronounceable name and order up your first-ever portion of honey-lime salmon with black bean and mango sauce.

And for sexual boredom? The solution is just as obvious. Beckon your honey and challenge her to a rousing game of Nude Indoor Volleyball.

Still with us?

In fact, we're serious. Or rather *not* serious, and that's the point. Just listen to Gerald Schoenewolf, Ph.D., a psychoanalyst and director of The Living Center, a therapeutic cooperative in New York City. "All sex really is is adult play," he says. "The more you can be a child during sexual activity, the better. So a silly game like nude volleyball challenges you to let go of the tensions of middle-age life."

Dr. Schoenewolf should know. He literally wrote the book on adult sexual play. His *Erotic Games* is an adult compendium of dozens of mature diversions with names like "Reverse Headache," "Indecent Proposal," "Massage Poker," "The Last Person on Earth," and, of course, the aforementioned "Nude Indoor Volleyball."

There's a message to this mirthful approach. The games, many of them essentially scripted role-playing, are designed to address specific impasses in a relationship. Passive-aggressive couples, for instance, might try their hand at "The Master and the Maid," in which she seduces him in a deliberately provocative way designed to provoke active, rather than passive, aggression.

"The idea is to get stuff to the surface," Dr. Schoenewolf says. "Playing the games brings up the feelings and conflicts that led to the impasse."

Take Nude Indoor Volleyball. (Please.) As far as we know, there's no rules committee, but here's how you play: Blow up a balloon, tie a string across your bedroom or living room, close the shades (this is decidedly *not* a spectator sport), mark some out-of-bounds points, and take off your clothes. You each get three taps to get the balloon over the string. Play to 15. There's one key rule: You're allowed—in fact, encouraged—to distract your opponent by touching and fondling her. And she employs the same tactic. All erogenous zones are eligible for this diversionary touching.

"Of course, this leads to sexual play," Dr. Schoenewolf says. "If you give up the game entirely and fall to the floor in sexual passion, then you both win."

You may just as likely fall to the floor in hysterical laughter, but no matter. You can't say your sense of play wasn't stirred, if only for a few spikes and squeezes. One way or another, says Dr. Schoenewolf, sex games will shake things up in a stale marriage.

Role-playing games are particularly effective for middle-age couples, according to Dr. Schoenewolf. In "Seduction Surprise," you greet her at the door in a tuxedo with the lights low, the music wafting, the table set, the whole 9 yards. She's queen for the day, you're the sophisticated seducer, and you keep it up until she gets into the spirit of the thing and the seduction is consummated. Here you're doing an exaggerated version of the kind of romancing that you know you should have been doing all along. But because it's a role, a shtick, almost a caricature, you can do it. "And she'll be bowled over by it," promises Dr. Schoenewolf.

There are all kinds of fantasy scenarios you can create for good, clean fun— "The Nude Cleaning Lady," "The Prostitute and the John"—but Dr. Schoenewolf stresses that those back-of-the-classifieds, "Helga-the-Dominatrix" encounters aren't beneficial for couples. "Those games tend to maintain one's neurotic way of life," he says. "They prevent you from having a genuine relationship with somebody."

Getting Started

Whether it's because couples are more bored these days or more liberated, there's something of a cottage industry springing up in mature games. Dr.

Schoenewolf's book focuses on psychotherapy-derived games, but less thera-peutically minded titles such as Laura Corn's *101 Great Nights of Sex* or Michael and Barbara Jonas's *The Book of Love, Laughter, and Romance* are sourcebooks for the saucy. Or try some of the board and card games out on the market, rang-ing in raunchiness from the mild *Getting to Know You Better* to *Dirty Minds*. The Jonases' Games Partnership Limited (800-776-7662) has sold almost 800,000 boxes of *An Enchanted Evening*, which takes a suggestive, leave-it-up-to-you ap-proach ("Gently caress something your partner has two of"). And this is not just a mail-order phenomenon. You can buy your "foreplay in a box" at depart-ment stores—in the lingerie department, of course.

Want to play? Here's how to get started.

Take a chance. Even occasional bouts of "Gender Reversal" or "Erotic Cards" aren't something you can wander into casually. "You have to make a commitment to do it," says Dr. Schoenewolf. "You have to both say you're going to do this thing no matter how long it takes."

Bribe her. It may be the understatement of the decade to say that it could take some convincing to get her to play "One Night Stand" or "Politically Cor-rect Sex" with you. Do it the old-fashioned way: Bribe her. "You know by now what it will take," says Dr. Schoenewolf. "Everybody has her price."

You may have to go see *Cats* or sit through a Julio Iglesias concert. But a deal's a deal.

Stick with it. Let's face it. Playing "Deserted Island" doesn't come natu-rally. The temptation will be to say, "This is unbelievably idiotic," and chuck the whole project before you get to first base. Hang in there. Remember, you're doing this for your sex life, and the rewards can be big. "It may take several weeks," says Dr. Schoenewolf. "At first, you both may just take off your clothes and argue about how stupid it is. That's part of working through the process."

And if things never leave the ground, don't worry. Sometimes games just don't do it for a couple. The ultimate goal, of course, is fun and creative sex and intimacy, and there are many other roads to take to it.

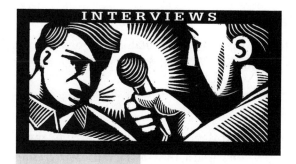

INTERVIEWS

Helen E. Fisher on
Monogamy versus Polygamy

Can men commit? Do we really want to sleep with every woman we see? These aren't exactly questions that philosophers debate, but anthropologists do. Especially Helen E. Fisher, Ph.D., a researcher in the department of anthropology at Rutgers University in New Brunswick, New Jersey. She's also the author of Anatomy of Love: The Natural History of Monogamy, Adultery, and Divorce. *Here she helps explain why we want to sleep around. She also tells why men can commit to one partner, and why we might value marriage more than our wives do.*

Monogamy is one of the core topics in your book, *Anatomy of Love,* **so we figured that you were the best person to answer this question: Is monogamy natural?**

I think monogamy is natural. The drive to pair up and rear your children as a team is natural. But the drive to cheat is also natural. The drive to have several partners is natural, and the drive to have one partner is natural. That's the problem with the human animal. We have a whole mix of drives that evolve together—and sometimes they're in conflict.

Like the urge to settle down and the urge to sleep around.

What I've maintained in my book is that we evolve to do both. This is why we have such troubles. At one point in our lives, we only want one partner. We want to be faithful to that partner, and we want that partner faithful to us. We want a particular kind of what they call a reproductive strategy. And at other times, we want to have several partners. I think men need to know that the human animal is built to want it all. But since we've developed a cerebral cortex, we are also able to make choices, think clearly about what our options are, and choose the option that is most suitable to us at the time.

So guys who cheat on their partners can't blame it entirely on genetics.

No. As a species, we are not totally driven by our genitals or by our ancestry. Although there are factors at work in the human brain that do play a significant role in our mating strategies.

For example?

I think the human animal has evolved three different brain circuits, three different emotional systems for mating. One is lust, the craving for sexual gratification. One is infatuation or attraction—that's the feeling of euphoria and giddiness that you feel with somebody you don't know too well. And the last is attachment, the feeling of calm and security and peace that you can feel with a long-term partner. So here we are, an animal that can feel really all three almost simultaneously. You can feel deep attachment toward a long-term partner. You can feel infatuation toward somebody in the office. And you can feel lust when you see a woman walking down the street whom you don't know at all. You can feel lust, infatuation, and attachment all for different people.

And you can juggle all three at once?

Sure. One of the things that most of us want is to have all three feelings for the same person. I think that's the reason that we so enjoy young lovers, or people who are in that state of being totally infatuated—deeply attached and still very sexually stimulated by each other. We're all looking for that, and during our lives, most of us get it at least once. But after a while in some long-term relationships, the sex drive goes down, infatuation disappears, and you're left actually with the very distinguished emotion, attachment. But it's not an exciting emotion.

So when we date around, we're really looking for the one person who elicits all of these responses in our brains.

Not always. There's something called short-term reproductive strategies and long-term reproductive strategies that can come into play. If you have no intention of marrying a person—because they're not your kind of person, whatever that is—you're pursuing a short-term strategy. If you are going for a short-term strategy, you may want your sex now and that's all you want to do. Or maybe you just want to show off with the person. There are some people who will work very hard just to be seen with a particular model a few times, for example. They don't even need to sleep with her. They just want to be seen. So the motives can be different, but the strategy is the same.

You say that we can feel monogamous or polygamous at different times in our lives, depending on the circumstances. Are we more likely to feel polygamous in our twenties or later, at midlife? And what about monogamy—more likely to happen in our thirties, maybe?

You can shift back and forth as you age, but these feelings are not entirely dependent on age. For example, there are a lot of men who marry in their twenties and are extremely serious about having families. But then when they get older and they've had their families, they break up those marriages and go find younger women. In society, it's frowned upon. But from a Darwinian perspective, it's adaptive under some circumstances. The younger woman has fresher eggs and is more likely to bear more viable young. Moreover, variety among your children is adaptive. So how you pursue love is not necessarily dependent on age; it can be a factor of circumstance and the choices you've made in life.

Such as the choice to be single or be married. But it seems like you're saying that if you are monogamous for a long enough time, eventually, you'll get sick of it and start wanting to be with several women. It seems like we'd just be better off if we had a society where it was acceptable to have more than one partner all the time.

Around 84 percent of cultures in the world permit a man to have several wives at the same time. What anthropologists are discovering is that there's a great deal of divorce in these societies, not to mention competition and treachery among the wives occasionally—they even poison each other's children. Because there's tremendous competition not only for the man but also for the man's resources. There's nowhere in the world where people share a mate nicely.

That's interesting. You hear about the ancient pharaohs having more than 100 wives, but you never hear about the wives...

...killing each other's children. The human animal is not built to share a mate. We want to sleep with more than one person, but we're not inclined to let our partners sleep with other people. The only way polygamy can be sustained over a long time is if the purposes of it outweigh the deficits—for example, if the man is very rich and none of the women can leave because they have no resources (and no way to get them) outside the marriage. You won't see that here because women don't have to stay in the marriage. Here, we have growing equality between the sexes. Women have more economic alternatives, and they can leave unhappy marriages.

So much for polygamy. But there are a lot of unhappy monogamous marriages out there, and you don't see people leaving them, even with the deeply rooted urge to couple with more than one partner. What's going on there?

Earlier, I talked about the emotional phase of attachment. That's what's going on there. Once you've reached the attachment phase with a partner, it's deep within the brain chemistry to stay put. We're beginning to know the brain physiology of attachment, and it's associated with chemicals in the brain. This is one of the reasons people don't leave unhappy marriages. You'll see a man or a woman who's in an awful marriage. Then they fall in love with the perfect person in the office or wherever. They have their affair. Finally, the moment comes when they promise that they will leave the wife and leave home.

But they don't.

No, because the attachment drugs in the brain are stronger than the infatuation drugs in the brain.

Does this happen more for men than for women?

It's my understanding that women complain much more about their marriages than men do. Men have fewer connections; men have fewer friends. They develop their friendships less. They put more focus on the marriages and depend more on the marriages than women do. Women definitely have more friends, more networks or connections than men do. I think that in many ways men value marriage more than women do.

Michael Cunningham on
What Women Really Seek in Men

You call it a bar; Michael Cunningham, Ph.D., calls it a laboratory. As a professor of psychology at the University of Louisville, Dr. Cunningham spent years in "labs" determining exactly what factors allow men to walk over to women they've never met and pick them up. Is it the right opening line? Good looks? A sense of humor? Flashing a wad of cash and talking about your new Porsche? Dr. Cunningham knows, and he has consented to share just a little bit of that knowledge with us.

We've heard that, on some level, women scope out the men who they think are most likely to provide well for potential offspring. Translation: Look like you have money and women will flock. But your work shows that the truth is much deeper.

Yes. There is well-documented evidence that women do look for good providers. But providers of what? There are other valuable resources beyond providing material goods. In fact, in our research, we find that money is the least important feature in females' dating choices. Aspects of personality come first, like being nice and agreeable and kind. Physical attractiveness comes second, and then wealth is influential only in third place.

So if you make a good living, you should hide that fact?

Not necessarily. We're finding that money on its own is less important. How you make that money, that's the key, that's the potential indicator of qualities that women will find attractive.

What qualities?

Let's look at an example: We have two men, equal in appearance and looks. Here's a guy who is a physician, and here's a guy who works at a burger joint. Which one does the woman want? Most will choose the doctor, but not because he makes more money. His occupation—and the salary he derives from it—are perceived as indicators of other attractive qualities. Compare a doctor to a burger flipper and women are going to intuit a variety of qualities within the doctor. They're going to see a guy who is intelligent and has social skills, dedication, ambition—as well as money—versus somebody who may or may not have any of those qualities.

But they don't know that the doctor has those qualities. The poor burger guy is getting the shaft based on superficial information.

Sure, but that's human nature. Like everyone, women make evaluations based on available evidence. But depending on how much information they have on a man, women won't always choose the doctor either. In one of the studies that we reported to the American Psychological Association, we gave women the choice between a guy who's a high school teacher making $20,000 a year—but with lots of time for family and kids—versus a physician making $500,000 a year. This guy was a successful surgeon but with no time for family or kids. The overwhelming trend was to choose the poor but generous teacher over the physician. Now when I say overwhelming choice, I'm talking 80 percent. Clearly, money was not the lure for the vast majority of women.

And according to your research, neither is looks.

Not to the degree you might think. Personality really is the first consideration. Are you nice? Kind? Funny?

Are you a conceited jackass?

Right. And sometimes women will make that kind of judgment based on someone's looks.

You mean: This man is gorgeous; he must know it; therefore, he must be full of himself.

Right. That's why it's important to let your personality show through so that it can counterbalance aspects of your personal appearance.

So if you have average looks or are an unattractive man, you need to really turn on the charm, the sensitivity, the humor.

Showing confidence, too, is not bad. Confidence in men of average looks seems to appeal to women, but it has the opposite effect if the man is very physically attractive.

So in the handsome man, confidence is seen as overconfidence or being egotistical? Gee, what's a good-looking guy to do?

Well, he can try self-deprecating humor. A good-looking guy who can make jokes at his own expense is typically seen as someone who's down-to-earth, not pompous.

Looks *and* humility.

Which make him more appealing to women. By contrast, men who aren't that attractive and who make fun of themselves tend to be less successful with that strategy. There's probably more of a perception of neediness, of feeling sorry for himself.

So you really have to take a good, honest look in the mirror before deciding how to play it with a woman. To get this information, you had assistants going into bars and trying out different pickup lines, giving different information to women to gauge their reaction. But we have to ask: In your opinion, are bars really such great places to meet women?

Well, I'll give you a flippant answer. They're great places to meet women who go to bars.

Or at least, women who go to bars that you like to go to, right? So if you like the atmosphere of a certain bar—if it reflects your character somehow— then that would increase the likelihood of meeting women in there who had similar tastes and interests?

That's true. But it's more than that. Bars actually serve a valid social function in our society. The advantages of bars—beyond being places where people with similar interests and backgrounds go—are that they are places where the norms are that one can be sociable with strangers. Most places are not like that. The basic norm in America is that you don't strike up a conversation with people on the train or in the mall or at the grocery store. It's just a little weird. It's crossing a line. Bars create the venue where this is able to happen.

So it really doesn't have to be a bar, per se. It could be a coffeehouse, a juice bar...

Any place where meeting and talking to strangers is the norm. Ideally, it also should be a place where you can sit somewhere and be comfortable, have a view of the room, be able to spot somebody, look at her, have her look at you, and then make your approach. It's kind of like a plane. You can land anywhere, but if you're not on a runway, the odds that you're going to crash and burn are that much higher.

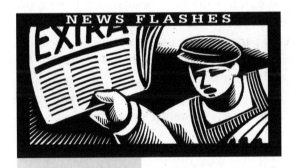

NEWS FLASHES

Radiation Treatment Cuts Impotence Risk

CALGARY, Canada—As far as some men diagnosed with prostate cancer are concerned, the cure may be worse than the disease. Many would rather chose a less effective form of treatment—or no treatment at all—than risk impotence, a possible side effect of prostate cancer treatment.

A new study from researchers at the University of Calgary and the Tom Baker Cancer Centre may help men face that decision with more confidence. The authors wanted to find out how many men who had normal erectile function before treatment maintained it afterward. Reviewing 40 studies that used two equally effective procedures, radiation therapy and radical prostatectomy (removal of the prostate gland), they found that 69 percent of the men who had radiation therapy retained normal erectile function. Only 42 percent of the men who had surgery remained potent.

The authors believe that their review—which represents the experiences of over 9,000 men—is stronger than results from a single study. Still, they suggest some caution in interpreting their results. For example, because they analyzed all the prostatectomy data as a single group, the researchers couldn't compare the standard radical prostatectomy with newer, less drastic techniques, such as "nerve-sparing" surgery, which leaves the nerves responsible for triggering an erection intact. Nevertheless, the authors say that their results can be useful in helping men make the decision between radiation and surgery.

Infidelity May Increase Cancer Risk for Wives

BARCELONA, Spain—Unfaithful husbands can put their wives at high risk for cervical cancer. Studies in Spain have shown that husbands can infect their wives with a strain of human papillomavirus (HPV), a sexually transmitted disease that is linked to cervical cancer.

Researchers tested the men for the presence of HPV—their infection rates and their wives' risks of cervical cancer were related to the number of female sexual partners the men had. Wives of men who were infected were at least five times more likely to have cervical cancer. A husband who visited 10 or more prostitutes while married increased his wife's chances of getting cervical cancer 11-fold. Because the number of sex partners before marriage does not seem to be as important as the number during marriage, the authors suggest that the men could only infect their wives for a short period after their own exposures. Previous studies have shown higher rates of cervical cancer in women whose husband's first wives died of cervical cancer and among wives of men who traveled frequently.

Vitamin E Increases Erections in Men with Diabetes

NEW ORLEANS—Between 35 percent and 75 percent of men with diabetes suffer from erectile problems. But new research suggests that vitamin E supplements may slow or stop the damage that causes those problems.

According to Suresh C. Sikka, Ph.D., associate professor of urology at Tulane University School of Medicine, diabetes damages blood cells, and through the generation of free radicals, can damage the corpora cavernosa, the twin chambers in the penis that fill up with blood to form an erection. To see how this damage might be reversed, Dr. Sikka compared blood samples from impotent men with diabetes, potent men with diabetes, and impotent men without diabetes with samples from normal, potent men. Impotent diabetic men had much lower levels of vitamin E (alpha-tocopherol). This is important because vitamin E has been shown to halt free radical damage. Dr. Sikka suggests that taking 400 international units of vitamin E in combination with 500 milligrams of vitamin C daily could delay the onset of the impotence.

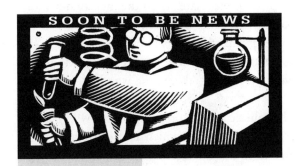

A Gel to Generate Erections?

So far, the most effective medication used to treat erection problems isn't exactly an item you can incorporate into foreplay. Known as alprostadil, this medication currently comes two ways—in a syringe that gets injected into the penis (Caverject) or in pellets that get squeezed into the urethra (Muse).

Thankfully, a more enjoyable treatment is in the works. Developed by MacroChem Corporation of Lexington, Massachusetts, the new method is a prostaglandin gel that, when rubbed on the penis, stimulates erections. The gel contains alprostadil, the same as Caverject and Muse. This hormone acts to expand arteries and allow greater blood flow into the penis, triggering erections. The gel contains an absorption enhancer that increases the passage of the drug through the skin into the bloodstream.

Based on promising early tests, the company plans to accelerate its development of the gel for public use and submit it for approval by the U.S. Food and Drug Administration (FDA). Given the lengthy FDA approval process, the gel probably won't be available until the turn of the millennium.

A Prostate Test You'll Enjoy?

If ever there was a necessary evil, it's prostate testing, especially the digital rectal exam. Just the snap of a rubber glove is enough to make most men tense up in apprehension. The other tests are no less torturous. The blood test for prostate-specific antigen (PSA), the marker for the presence of prostate cancer, involves getting stuck with a needle. The prostate biopsy combines the worst of both worlds—a needle is inserted into the prostate to collect cells for testing.

Thankfully, researchers from the University of Queensland and the Queensland Institute of Medical Research in Australia say that they've found an easier—even enjoyable—way to check for prostate cancer: by examining a man's ejaculate fluid.

In the study of 37 men suspected of having prostate cancer, researchers asked the volunteers for samples of their ejaculate. Then the men underwent a biopsy of the prostate, which would yield proof of whether cancer was present. In 75 percent of the cases, men with positive findings from the biopsy also had abnormal cells in their ejaculate. The researchers note that if more than one ejaculate sample was used, the ability to accurately predict who had cancer was even higher.

Study authors suggest that the muscle contractions that occur with ejaculation help separate cells from the prostate's surface, which are then carried in the seminal fluid and can be examined after ejaculation.

In the future, the authors say, the ejaculation test could free patients from unpleasant and possibly dangerous biopsies. Moreover, this noninvasive and, the authors readily point out, "easily repeated" test could help diagnose prostate cancer at an earlier, more curable stage.

No More Postsurgical Incontinence?

Undergoing prostate surgery is tough enough. To add insult to injury, anywhere from 5 to 40 percent of men have some degree of incontinence after the fact. That's more than many men are willing to accept; some even reconsider having prostate surgery for fear of incontinence—a decision that could cost them their lives.

A new procedure from researchers at Washington University Medical School in St. Louis may help reduce both the fear and the likelihood of postsurgical incontinence. By injecting collagen—a protein common in skin, tendons, and other connective tissue—into the bladders of surgical patients, doctors were able to narrow the necks of the bladders and prevent urine leakage. The principle is similar to using a washer to stop a leaky faucet.

Using collagen to narrow the bladder opening is not new, but the St. Louis approach is. Called an antegrade approach, doctors insert a needle through the skin above the pubic area and into the bladder. Then, using small scopes to view the surgery, the surgeons can place the collagen precisely where it's needed to narrow the bladder neck. After checking up on their patients an average of 8½ months later, the researchers found that 70 percent of their patients either regained total urinary control or had significant improvement after undergoing the antegrade operation.

Although the procedure is still experimental, further studies may well make the antegrade procedure the standard approach for curing postsurgical incontinence.

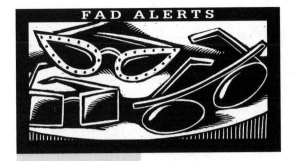

"Dry" Orgasms

We've heard of dry martinis, but dry orgasms? Yep. The idea is that a student of dry orgasm learns to strengthen certain pelvic muscles (the ones that control urination and that also contract during orgasm) to the point that, when orgasm approaches, he clenches those muscles, hard. This supposedly prevents ejaculation while still allowing orgasm.

The practice itself is nothing new. Conserving ejaculation and prolonging intercourse is one of the basic tenets of the ancient practice of Tantric sex, the ancient system of Hindu yoga, where the union of male and female principles are worshiped. We're all for prolonged intercourse. In fact, this ancient practice is really the first step to becoming a multiorgasmic man. If you can have an orgasm and prevent ejaculation, you'll likely maintain your erection and be able to keep going.

But the dry orgasm fad doesn't stop there. Practitioners go on to say that conserving your semen is supposed to preserve creative and psychic energy. We don't know about that, but it's on the strength of that assertion that at least one yoga center in California is teaching the practice of seminal conservation to certain misguided Hollywood types. What we want to know is this: If they're truly saving their creative forces, how come their movies aren't getting any better?

Other Erogenous Zones

For those of you who've spent enough time hunting for your partner's G-spot like a spelunker in a pitch-dark cave, we're sending you in search of new erogenous zones. There's a whole passel of trendy hot spots you can frequent—and we have it on good authority that they're just as knee-buckling as the G-spot or clitoris. Incidentally, there are similar such spots on your body, too. In his book *Secrets of Better Sex*, Joel Block, Ph.D., lays out the treasure map. "X" doesn't mark the spot, but just about every other letter in the alphabet does.

For Her
- The U-spot: This stands for the urethral canal, the opening of which is located about an inch behind the clitoris, directly in front of the vagina. Your partner can explore this herself first, gently stimulating the area around the urethral opening. If it feels good for her, she can teach you. Some women find the U-spot more sensitive with a nearly full bladder.
- The AFE: Otherwise known as the anterior fornix erogenous zone, this spot lies on the upper vaginal wall between the top of the G-spot (or where all those books tell you it's supposed to be) and the back of the vaginal barrel. Even if she doesn't experience intense pleasure, stimulating it should produce greater lubrication. Slide a finger up and down the area, then stroke the AFE in circles.

For You
- The F-spot: Also known as the frenulum, this is the loose bit of skin on the underside of the penis, between the head and the shaft. Stimulating it in an up-and-down fashion can quickly bring on orgasm (but you probably already knew that part).
- The R-spot: R is for raphe, the line in the center of the scrotum. Try gently running a finger up and down it (but not in public).

Couples Retreats

Call it sex camp, call it boot camp for couples, but these workshops—racier versions of the traditional marriage-encounter weekends offered by pastors and therapists—are growing fast. While most of these retreats all preach the same message of love, integrity, honesty, and open communication between partners, sexuality camps are quite a bit more X-rated. No, you don't have to sit naked in a room with 10 other couples, but you are expected to bare some of your thoughts, feelings, even fantasies about sex. For the average close-mouthed man, this sort of weekend could sound like a fair approximation of hell. We say, why the heck not? Any experience that wrenches sex from the darkened bedroom and positions it center stage for adult discussion is beneficial.

For more information, here's a partial list of some of the more popular and respected sex camps.
- Marriage and Family Health Center, Evergreen, Colorado: (303) 670-2630
- Canyon Ranch Health and Fitness Resort, Tucson, Arizona: (800) 726-9900
- Sacred Mountain Seminars, Scottsdale, Arizona: (800) 636-6780

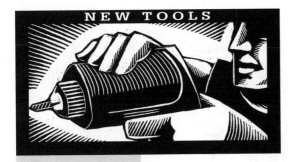

Premature Ejaculation Kit

Diagnostic Center for Men

If you suffer from premature ejaculation (defined as ejaculating sooner than you want to), this at-home kit from the Diagnostic Center for Men in Lenexa, Kansas, may be just the ticket. In an effort to treat those who are too embarrassed by their condition to seek professional help, the center created a home self-treatment program, which includes the books *How to Overcome Premature Ejaculation* by the late Helen Singer Kaplan, M.D., Ph.D., and *The New Male Sexuality* by Bernie Zilbergeld, Ph.D. The kit also includes a 38-minute instructive video entitled *You Can Last Longer*. Call (800) 462-1224 to order. Price: $79.95 plus shipping and handling.

Sperm Banking

University of Illinois at Chicago Sperm Bank
OverNite Male Delivery Service

For men who have health problems or are undergoing medical procedures that may leave them infertile, freezing samples of their own sperm for future use is science's contribution to preserving the family legacy. But sperm banks aren't exactly a friendly neighborhood institution. Most are situated in large cities, universities, or research institutions that are hundreds, sometimes thousands of miles out of reach for many men. But if you want to bank your sperm, and time, distance, travel costs, or health reasons prevent you from going to the nearest bank to make a deposit, a unique delivery service may be the perfect tool for you and future generations.

The service is called OverNite Male, but don't be fooled by the tongue-in-cheek name. This is a legitimate, serious service offered by the University of Illinois at Chicago's (UIC) Andrology Lab. For $350, the lab will send you an OverNite Male Kit via Federal Express—no matter where you live in the United

States or Canada. Inside, you'll find instructions and all the equipment you'll need to collect, store, and ship a sperm sample back to the lab for next-day delivery. From there, your sperm will be processed, analyzed, and preserved. The fee even includes the first year's storage fee of $175. For more information, contact the UIC Sperm Bank Coordinator at (312) 996-7713.

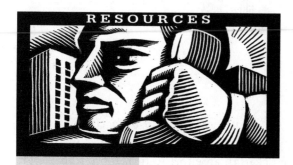

RESOURCES

Sizing Survey

The Definitive Penis Size Survey Web Site
http://www.connection.com/survey/result.htm

How do you really measure up? To get an idea without anyone ever knowing you asked, check here for the results of over 1,700 responses, correlated impressively and professionally into a detailed analysis of penile parameters. Besides the expected stats on length and circumference, the site, operated by the Canadian Cyber Communication Club, answers such burning questions as: Are gay or bisexual men more endowed than straight men? Is there any difference in size among the different races or between bodybuilders and couch potatoes? Is there any correlation between erect penis length and hand and foot measurements? Future editions of the survey will contain more in-depth information plus a discussion of the relationship of body fat and personality to penis size, but to get it, you'll have to pay a nominal fee to help the club defray the cost of maintaining the Web site.

A Man's Clinic

Male Health Center Internet Education Site
http://malehealthcenter.com

The Male Health Center is a real and highly respected place—in Dallas. Founded in 1989 by Kenneth Goldberg, M.D., the center is the first clinic in the

United States to specialize in men's health. This Web site serves as their "mobile clinic," and it's a real boon for those who don't happen to live in Dallas or are wary of the doctor's office. Ask a question that you'd rather keep private and then anonymously retrieve the answer. The subject matter covers more than just erections and other plumbing basics. This self-described "holistic" site takes on emotional issues such as masculinity, longevity, and addictions and tells you what your partner should know and can help you with.

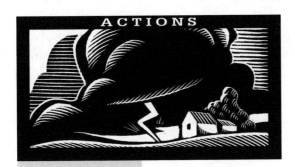

Just when you thought you'd learned everything there was to learn about sex, here are some new things you can try to make your sex life healthier and hotter. These 12 suggestions are culled from the latest research and writing about sex and relationships, and they're guaranteed to help keep things fresh.

1. Recognize the ruts. Complacency can be the death of sex. In the new book *A Lifetime of Sex*, authors Stephen C. George and K. Winston Caine offer these warning signs that your sex life may be taking a turn for the boring.

- You have sex in just one or two different positions, dismissing all the ones you used to use as "too much work."
- Like meat loaf on Tuesdays, you have sex on one night of the week, same place, same time.
- You actually believe that some things are more interesting than sex. Televised golf, for example.
- Sex? Hmmmm, come to think of it, you can't quite remember the last time you had sex.
- Two words: twin beds. Or its modern reincarnation—a king-size bed, which keeps the two of you far apart.

2. Stay married. Getting hitched and, more to the point, staying hitched, may increase your odds of living a long and happy life. According to research in the journal *Social Psychology Quarterly*, couples who stay married for 35 years report being just as happy as they were on their honeymoons. And in a separate study on survival rates among men with prostate cancer, researchers in Miami found that married men live almost three years longer than men who never married, or were separated, divorced, or widowed.

3. **Give and ye shall receive.** While Doreen Virtue, Ph.D., was compiling her book *In the Mood*, she polled hundreds of women to determine what their most romantic moments were. "Overwhelmingly, these moments all had a common denominator. Their lover was giving them something: a flower, a back rub, a glass of champagne, a compliment," says Dr. Virtue. So make some gesture of giving, especially if you're giving of yourself. "The act of giving is a sign of caring, of providing, of serving her needs. These are all important for a woman to feel intimate," says Dr. Virtue.

4. **Stand erect.** One simple way to boost your arousal level is to start foreplay standing up. According to Drogo K. Montague, M.D., director of the Center for Sexual Function at the Cleveland Clinic Foundation in Ohio, blood flow to the penis is strongest when you're standing. Thus, standing up during foreplay can give you a faster and stronger erection.

5. **Get those jewels appraised.** If a chance blow to the crotch leaves you gasping and clutching like a man drowning in a sea of pain, don't just take a deep breath and shake it off. When you take a hit below the belt, see a doctor. Even minor swelling can cut blood flow to the testicles, says Thomas J. Barloon, M.D., associate professor of radiology at the University of Iowa College of Medicine in Iowa City. If that happens, you only have 4 to 6 hours before tissue death sets in. So don't waste time trying to walk it off.

6. **Don't be a boron moron.** According to some studies, people who are deficient in the trace mineral boron have decreased blood levels of testosterone. How can you keep your levels high? There's no need to buy supplements. Just make sure that you eat five to nine servings of fruits and vegetables every day. Peanuts, prunes, dates, and raisins are especially good sources of this mineral.

7. **Help keep her on tract.** If your chosen method of birth control includes the spermicide nonoxynol-9, think twice before using it. Katherine Forrest, M.D., medical consultant with Forrest Associates in Portola Valley, California, says that women whose lovers use condoms with nonoxynol-9 have greater risks of getting urinary tract infections. If you want to hedge your bets against this, Dr. Forrest suggests using a type of birth control that doesn't have spermicide. Better yet, put nonoxynol-9 cream or gel inside the condom, keeping it on your side, not hers, adds Dr. Forrest.

8. **Take her on a roller coaster.** If you want to arouse your partner (who doesn't?), give her a good scare. Due to a cagey bit of mental wiring, the human brain tends to confuse fear for passion, says Perry Buffington, Ph.D., author of *Cheap Psychological Tricks*. Take her on a roller coaster or other scary ride and she's likely to attach lovingly to the person who weathered the horror with her (that is, you). Other scary experiences (watching a horror movie, visiting the in-laws) may have a similar effect.

9. **If it feels corny, do it.** Another gem of wisdom from Dr. Virtue. Her point: What feels corny to one gender is often quite arousing to the other. "For women, it feels corny to dress up in lingerie or erotic costumes, but men find it highly stimulating," she points out.

By the same token, the things that men feel corny doing—lavishing compliments on their women, snuggling and cuddling, waiting on them hand and foot—are highly effective forms of foreplay. "Many men say that they don't know what to do to make their wives happy. Well, they really do; they just can't imagine doing it or saying it. If you feel embarrassed or corny saying something, you now know that it's probably going to make her day," says Dr. Virtue.

10. **Rub those boys.** Okay, it's not exactly new—in fact, it's a centuries-old practice for boosting sexual energy. But testicular massage was new to us, so we thought we'd pass it along. Although there is no scientific evidence that this will do any good, we don't think that it will do any harm. According to Jack W. McAninch, M.D., chief of urology at San Francisco General Hospital, if the massage causes any discomfort, stop or decrease the pressure. Gentle massage is the key word. Also, he recommends doing it only once or twice a day.

- Warm your hands, then hold each testicle between the thumb and fingers of each hand.
- Firmly but gently massage your testicles for a minute or two by rolling them between finger and thumb.
- Now hold your penis up away from your testicles and tap them—lightly—for a minute or two.
- Now hold your penis and scrotum with your thumb and forefinger and lightly pull them forward. As you do this, clench your pelvic muscles (the ones that control urination). Repeat, this time pulling to the right with your hand and squeezing to the left with your pelvic muscles. Finally, pull to the left and squeeze to the right.

11. **Sleep in the guest room.** Everyone knows that vacation sex is some of the best sex around. Why? Pure and simple: Having sex somewhere new and different is exciting. But you can't always go on vacation to get great sex. Or can you? Sometimes, a break from the same old bed is all you need. Ellen Kreidman, Ph.D., lecturer and author of *Light Her Fire*, recommends checking into a hotel once in a while with your partner—enjoy a weekender or even a quickie. If you're pressed for time and resources, though, head for the guest room or the sleeper sofa in the basement.

12. **Take a cruise.** For a sexy, steamy vacation this year, skip the Civil War battlefield tour or even the beach house at the shore. Instead, get out on the water. According to a survey by *Cosmopolitan* and Royal Caribbean Cruises, 80 percent of cruise passengers said that they felt more amorous at sea. Nearly 60 percent were unable to wait more than 10 hours before rocking the boat.

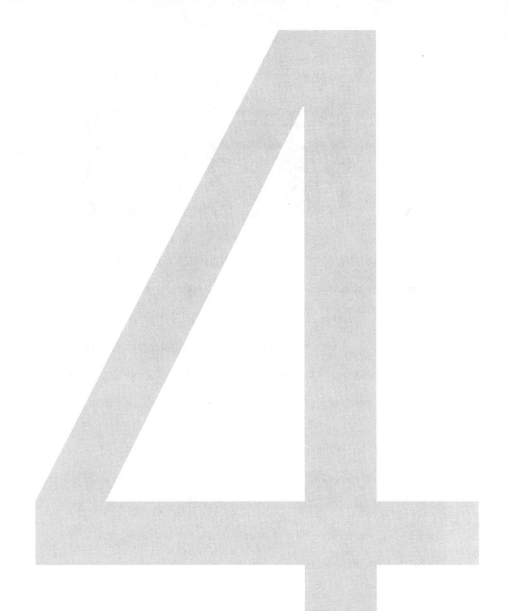

WEIGHT LOSS

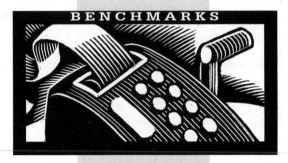

BENCHMARKS

AVERAGES

■ Number of doctors who are dissatisfied with their weight: 2 out of 5

■ Number of slang words in the American English language for the word "fat": 41

■ Percentage of U.S. men who are overweight: 31.9

■ Percentage increase of that number since 1960: 9

■ Average weight for a man between the ages of 18 and 74: 172.2 pounds

■ Pounds of caloric sweeteners available for consumption per person
in the United States: 143

■ Percentage of men who use diet supplements: 5

■ Percentage of men who undergo surgery in order to lose weight: 3

■ Percentage of men who think they need to lose weight: 43

■ Percentage of men who are trying to lose weight: 23

■ Average amount spent per person in the United States on restaurant dining in one year:
$463.82

■ Average grams of dietary fat consumed in one day by a man living in the United States: 96

■ Average grams of dietary fat consumed in one year by a man living in the
United States: 35,040

EXTREMES

■ Heaviest living person: weighs 891 pounds and has a 29½-inch neck

■ U.S. male age group that has experienced the greatest weight gain in the past 30 years:
65- to 74-year-olds, whose weight has increased by 20.4 percent

No More Diets

Use this simple man's plan to lose fat and build muscle for a lifetime.

The American diet industry is a gluttonous beast. It likes nothing better than to belly up to the table of opportunity and feast. And until a few years ago, it was doing just that—growing in total revenue by more than 10 percent a year on the fears and desires of overweight Americans, most of them women. But the 1990s have been relatively lean times for commercial diet companies, so they're looking for a new market: you.

Although such weight loss giants as Weight Watchers and Jenny Craig have yet to schedule a support group meeting at the local VFW, they are spotlighting more men in their advertisements. "It's a natural area of growth," says Karen Miller-Kovach, general manager of program development for Weight Watchers International.

The diet companies' rise to power has, perhaps not so coincidentally, been paralleled by the rise in obesity rates in America. In the early 1960s, 24 percent of adults were overweight. Today, the figure is 33 percent. Commercial diet plans have an overwhelming failure rate—nearly everyone who loses weight regains it within five years.

Diet plans simply don't work. So we decided instead to find a plan that would help men remake their lives and waistlines so the results would be permanent, not temporary. And that's how we found Jack Groppel, Ph.D., a licensed nutritionist and sports scientist with LGE Sport Science, in Orlando, Florida. He also thinks that it's time we start fighting fat a new way.

Dr. Groppel has spent the last 15 years studying, lecturing, and advising people about nutrition, performance, and weight loss. An admitted skeptic, he has devised a no-nonsense, decidedly male approach that he calls the Anti-Diet. The plan is so effective, yet so ingeniously simple, that it might make you forget that "potbelly" ever referred to anything other than stoves. Although it lacks the marketing polish of Nutri/Systems and the pungent scent of the cabbage-soup diet fad, it's the closest thing we've found to a simple, sane strategy for staying lean for life. According to Dr. Groppel, who has been a nutrition advisor to tennis stars Michael Chang and Monica Seles, "diet is a four-letter word." Once you go on a diet, you must eventually come off it, which guarantees a yo-yo existence that research suggests may be even more detrimental to health than staying consistently overweight. Plus, the entire concept of dieting to lose weight is flawed, says Dr. Groppel. Your body, he explains, can't tell the difference between dieting and starvation. Thus, when you skip a meal or cut calories, your body lowers its metabolic rate (the rate at which it burns energy) in order to conserve the fuel that's left. What's more, studies show that sedentary people who start dieting lose muscle before they lose fat. And since muscle is denser than fat, it's possible to lose weight while having your body-fat percentage increase. "You will become less healthy even though your weight will have gone down," Dr. Groppel adds.

What follows is a simple program that Dr. Groppel designed. While you may not see results as dramatic as those you would see on a short-term crash diet, keep in mind that this is a life plan that will ultimately make you leaner and keep you there. According to Dr. Groppel, someone who is significantly overweight can expect to lose about 16 pounds of pure body fat on this eight-week program. Others, who are just looking to trim down, can expect to shave off about 8 pounds of blubber.

Before you can decide what needs to be done, you must know where you're starting from. But don't step on that bathroom scale. In fact, take it outside, imagine that it's your TV during a Best of Barbara Walters Special, and smash it to bits. Then, never think in terms of "pounds" again. Not only was that scale a needless source of stress in your life, says Dr. Groppel, but it's also an inexact method of gauging health and fitness. In his plan, weight doesn't matter.

Dr. Groppel says that it's better to think in terms of body fat and lean muscle mass. In order to reshape your physique, you have to first reorganize these components. You do this by exercising to build muscle. Besides gaining more body tone and definition, you'll raise your metabolism and burn an extra 30 to 50 calories a day for every pound of muscle you add. Since you can expect to build 3 to 5 pounds of new muscle on this eight-week program, you'll be combusting up to 250 additional calories a day.

Here's a simple test to see if you can benefit from the Anti-Diet: Strip naked and stand in front of a mirror. Jump up and down. If you see any flab flapping, hop on the bus.

Audit Your Diet and Body

What did you have for lunch yesterday? Can't recall? How about snacks? Did you munch anything between meals? If you're having trouble remembering, then you've stumbled across a prime reason that you're out of belt holes. Most men just aren't aware of what or how much they eat. And that's why auditing your diet is so important.

The most uncomplicated way to do this is to keep a food diary in which you write, in intimate detail, everything you eat and drink for three days. We're talking astute label reading here, as in total calories per serving and individual grams of carbohydrate, fat, and protein. (If you're a moderately active 35-year-old man of average height and weight, you're aiming for about 2,500 total calories a day, divvied up as 55 percent carbohydrates, 25 percent protein, and 20 percent fat.) Although time-consuming, this exercise will give you a startling new awareness of your dietary habits and yet another baseline from which to measure improvement.

Grab a cloth tape measure and wrap it around a few body parts. Start with your chest, then do your biceps, and finally, measure your waist (just below the navel) and your thighs (at their midsection). The male tendency is to deposit fat in these last two places. Then measure again after the fourth and eighth weeks of the program. What you can expect to see, if you've stuck with the program, is that your shape is becoming more like a V and less like the letter b. It's another way to gauge progress without the bathroom scale.

The Eating Rules

Dr. Groppel doesn't like meal plans. They're constrictive, demoralizing, and often a hassle for busy men to organize and follow. So rather than tell you to eat skinless chicken for dinner every Monday and a baked potato for lunch on Tuesdays, he prefers to supply general nutritional guidelines and let you determine the specifics. Here's what you need to keep in mind.

Don't go hungry. Society has conditioned us to eat three meals a day, but this is unnatural and even unhealthy. If you have kids in your house, you know how difficult it is to get them to eat "normally." They're always looking in the refrigerator, sneaking a snack, or refusing to finish all that food you put on their dinner plates. That's because their natural tendency is to eat when they're hungry, not to postpone their appetite until some predetermined time or stuff themselves because "there will be nothing else for the rest of the night." Instead of chastising them, Dr. Groppel says that adults should follow their lead. Rather than three big meals, he advocates five or six smaller ones. The trick, however, is to not eat any more calories than usual but to spread them more evenly throughout the day.

Eat earlier in the day. Most men swallow the bulk of their calories after 5:00 P.M. This promotes fat storage and falling asleep on the couch during *Wheel of Fortune*. Try doing the opposite. Do most of your eating prior to 1:00 P.M. This will better fuel you for the day and keep your metabolic rate high.

Teach yourself to like low-fat food. Most American men grew up on high-fat diets. Our fathers and coaches advised us to eat red meat to grow big and strong. Our mothers kept a can of reusable frying grease under the kitchen sink. We've simply become accustomed to the taste of fat.

It is possible, however, to retrain your taste buds to stop craving and enjoying fatty food and start appreciating and savoring more healthful fare. Since just about every food product has a reduced-fat or nonfat version nowadays, it's relatively easy to wean yourself.

If you love potato chips, for instance, switch to a reduced-fat version for the first four weeks of the program and then to a nonfat brand or, better yet, pretzels. Take the same approach with dips, cream cheese, mayonnaise, cold cuts, cookies, and salad dressings. For foods that don't have healthful versions, such as candy and beer, simply reduce the portions. "It's really just the taste you're craving," explains Dr. Groppel. "If you give yourself a little, you'll be satisfied."

Exercising Options

These seven words—eat less fat and be more active—are the key to a long, lean life. But they're often misunderstood. To be most effective, the two must always be wed. Exercise without prudent eating won't bring results as quickly or dramatically, nor will a low-fat diet without regular workouts. Think of each as a separate blade on a pair of scissors. You'll trim body fat only if both are razor-sharp.

The minimum requirement to make this part of the program work is 4½ hours of exercise a week. If this sounds like a lot, consider that it's just 2 percent of the total hours available to you during that time. Plus, those 270 minutes can be divided among just three workout sessions.

There are two parts to Dr. Groppel's exercise plan:

Aerobic training. This is any type of vigorous activity that significantly elevates your heart rate for 25 minutes or more. Some of the best heart-pumping, calorie-combusting aerobic sports are tennis, cycling, swimming, running, rowing, and cross-country skiing. There's a difference, however, between what Dr.

Groppel prescribes and the way most people do these sports. Instead of holding a steady pace for the entire workout, he wants you to vary it. For instance, a typical half-hour run might start with a slow 5-minute jog, then progress through a series of intervals before ending with a 5-minute cooldown. These intervals, or bursts of speed, should be spontaneous rather than structured. For example, a ¼-mile sprint followed by a ⅛-mile jog; or a ½-mile brisk run followed by a few minutes of fast walking. The idea is to have your heart rate go for a roller-coaster training ride. This not only builds speed and endurance but also promotes quick recovery and helps burn fat.

"This type of workout covers all the bases," says Dr. Groppel. "When you're at lower heart rates, you're burning fat, and when you're at higher heart rates, you're strengthening your cardiorespiratory system and increasing your metabolic rate. Plus, it's a lot more fun."

Strength training. In order to build muscle and fight fat, Dr. Groppel recommends a total-body workout consisting of 9 exercises: bench press, leg extension/leg curl, seated pulley row, leg press, shoulder press, lat pulldown, biceps curl, crunch, and triceps pushdown. If you don't have access to a gym, you can get the same full-body workout by doing the following 10 exercises with dumbbells: bench press, concentration curl, deadlift, seated triceps extension, standing upright row, pullover, shoulder press, wrist curl, side bend, and calf raise.

For each exercise, start with a moderate weight that'll cause a fair amount of muscle fatigue after 10 to 12 repetitions (one set). Do two sets of each exercise with a brief rest in between. As you get into the program and start building strength, work up to three sets of 10 to 12 repetitions. Consult with a trainer if you're unsure of proper technique.

Burn, Baby, Burn

Teach your body to incinerate fat up to nine times faster.

Like Tim Allen's character on *Home Improvement*, constantly looking to turbocharge the vacuum, lawn mower, and toaster oven, guys naturally believe that more power is always better. Well, that's not always so, especially when it comes to fitness. Sometimes making like an Ironman isn't the best course of action, especially if your goal is to burn fat.

According to the latest research, working harder might actually leave you fatter. "One study found that walking at about 3.8 miles per hour for a half-hour burned 240 calories, 40 percent of which was fat," says Wayne Westcott, Ph.D., strength-training consultant to the YMCA in Quincy, Massachusetts.

"Running at 6.5 miles an hour for that same half-hour burned 450 calories; however, only 25 percent of them were from fat." Slow, easy, relaxed—effective.

The reason is that the harder you exercise, the faster you need energy. And the high-carbohydrate snack you ate before exercising is far more easily metabolized than the layers of greaseburgers and lager you've been carrying around for years. To burn this off, you have to retrofit your fat incinerator.

The key is *interval training*. Consider a study conducted at Laval University in Sainte-Foy, Quebec, where researchers measured differences in fat loss between two groups of exercisers following two different workout programs. The first group pedaled stationary bikes four or five times a week for a moderate burn of 300 to 400 calories per 30- to 45-minute session. The second group did the same, but only one or two times a week, and they filled in the rest of their sessions with short intervals of high-intensity cycling: They hopped on their stationary bikes and pedaled as quickly as they could for 30 to 90 seconds, rested, and then repeated the process several times per exercise session. As a result, these slackers burned only about 225 to 250 calories while cycling. But they also burned more fat by the end of the study than the hard workers in group one. In fact, their fat loss was nine times greater.

Researchers offer a theory about what happened to the second group: "It's true that during the actual workout, the harder you exercise, the more likely it is that your body will preferentially burn carbohydrates over fat," says study leader Angelo Tremblay, Ph.D., professor of physiology and nutrition at Laval University. "But eventually, after the workout is over, your body has to replace the calories it used. We think the fat-reduction effect occurs after the exercise."

While the jury is still out pending additional research, Dr. Tremblay suggests that short-term, high-intensity training may encourage the body to find lost calories by pillaging fat stores to a greater degree than it would after moderate exercise. And your body does it long after the last wind sprint is over.

"There are studies that show that the metabolism stays elevated for 15 hours after high-intensity strength training," says Dr. Westcott. So if you open your throttle for several 60- to 90-second intervals over the course of your workout, your fat burners may be turned up for two-thirds of the day. And this is an exchange rate we can all live with.

But before we get started, we'll need to agree on a definition of *high-intensity*. Exercise is really intense if you're pedaling, running, or stairclimbing fast enough to make conversation difficult. To test yourself, try chanting the first three lines of your favorite song at about the 60-second mark. If you can't make it to line two, you're in the target zone. If you can get through the first verse of "Layla" (acoustic version), you need to work harder. And you have to go hard for as long as you can, with 90 seconds as the goal. If you lower the intensity to last longer, your fat-burning inferno will die down to Zippo-lighter strength.

Okay, now we're going to up the ante. We want you to train using the interval method. And we want you to do it at the same time you're weight training.

There are two reasons: First, while the high-intensity interval trainers in the Laval study did rest between their short bursts of activity, their heart rates never dropped below 120 to 130 beats per minute. Some light resistance training will make sure that yours doesn't either. Second, you'll add muscle, another fat burner. "Muscle is more metabolically active than fat, so each pound of lean tissue you add means that you burn an extra 35 calories a day whether you are sitting, sleeping, or watching TV," says Dr. Westcott. Add 3 pounds of muscle to your frame and you can figure in about an extra pound of fat burned each month, without even trying.

To make the principle of interval training work for you, all you need is several pairs of dumbbells—say, in 10-, 15- and 25-pound denominations. Take whatever kind of aerobic-exercise machine you have—a treadmill, stairclimber, stationary bike—and stick it in one room. Now pick up your dumbbells and put them in an adjoining room. The idea here is to move back and forth between the two rooms and between the two forms of exercise so you get a brief—maybe 10-second—cooling-off period between each activity.

Here's the program.

Warm up. This is a strenuous workout, and the worst way to go about it is to explode from the starting block at top speed. Spend 3 to 5 minutes on a treadmill, bike, or steps, moving at a slow to moderate pace. And the same advice applies when you're cooling down at the end of your workout.

Go like hell. After you've warmed up, continue treading, pedaling, or stepping. But pick up the pace to heart-pounding levels. You've just started the workout proper. Do this for either 30, 60, or 90 seconds (whatever you can manage initially).

Bring it down. Now stop, walk down the hall (permission to pant granted) and pick up the dumbbells for a round of resistance exercise.

Lift weights. Do one set of one resistance exercise. Now drop the weights, head back up the hall, and do the aerobics for another 90 seconds. Then back down the hall. Get the picture?

Do a circuit of seven resistance exercises and eight aerobic bouts. This should take you about 20 minutes. Try to work up to twice around for a 40-minute workout. But be prudent. Do what you can. If 20 minutes seems to be your limit, use the remaining 20 for moderate aerobic activity—light walking, comfortable stationary biking. Eventually, you'll find yourself extending the heavy-duty workout and cutting back on the light to moderate. And as you do, watch the fat fly...fly away, that is.

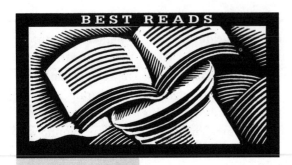

Quick-Start Your Morning Metabolism

Turning on your body's natural fat-burning switches is easy once you know how. In Low-Fat Living (Rodale Press, 1996), Robert K. Cooper, Ph.D., and Leslie L. Cooper offer dozens of ways to melt off excess pounds while staying away from the "fat makers" in life, too. In this excerpt, the Coopers tell you exactly how to throw Fat-Burner Switch #1—and you can do it as early as tomorrow morning.

Stop for a moment to reflect: What are your mornings like? Are you rushing around, feeling frantic? Or is it more your style to get up feeling draggy and lethargic?

This morning when the alarm went off, did you switch on one dim light as you climbed out of bed? Did you skip breakfast—or gulp down a cup of coffee as you flew out the door?

There are as many ways to get out of bed in the morning as there are people in the world who get out of bed. You have your own style; we all do. And since it has probably been a pattern with you for many years, it's not something you often reconsider.

Maybe you should, because research has shown that you can turn on a Fat-Burner Switch the moment you get up in the morning.

Lights—Action!

From the moment you get out of bed, your brain begins cueing your body to match current and anticipated physical demands. If your morning ritual takes place in low light and in slow motion, your brain gets a low signal. With that signal trudging through your nervous system on leaden paws, your body has little incentive to push your metabolism much higher than what seems near-hibernation rate.

Now suppose you extend this "sleepwalk" activity level into the morning— that is, your mind is moaning, "I wish, I wish, I wish I were back in bed." And suppose you decide to skip breakfast while you're trudging around trying to get things together.

In the process, you unwittingly fail to turn on your Fat-Burner Switch #1. And you may even stimulate fat-preserving and fat-storing processes instead.

Cock-a-Doodle Do's—And Don'ts

With the Low-Fat Living Program, you can reverse this trend. There are three key elements of giving an effective wake-up call to your metabolism.

1. Turn up the lights.
2. Get at least 5 minutes of easy physical activity.
3. Enjoy a great-tasting, low-fat breakfast.

These three simple actions combine to turn on your body's "thermic switch" and move your natural biological rhythms into higher revs.

If these three steps already make up your morning routine, congratulations. You don't have to give a second thought to this switch—though maybe I can suggest a few variations that may help speed your metabolism even more.

If, on the other hand, you're from the I-wish-I-were-hibernating school of morning rituals, you'll need to consider what you can do differently—beginning tomorrow morning—to put these methods in motion.

Let's consider the morning strategies one by one.

Turn Up the Lights

On sunny mornings, do you step outside for a breath of fresh air and soak in the brightness? Many of us do embrace this roosterlike routine on vacations but somehow neglect it the rest of the year.

Of all the signals the human brain responds to, one of the most powerful is light. The body has hundreds of biochemical and hormonal rhythms, all keyed to light and dark. Here are some ways to brighten your morning.

Get your good lux. Research has demonstrated that there's a direct link between the retina of the eye—where the light-receptor nerves are located—and a small portion of the brain that focuses our attention. In a study, a Harvard medical team took some volunteers through a series of light-exposure tests, experimenting with intensities ranging from 7,000 to 12,000 lux. This was comparable to the amount of light you'd get if you stepped outside the door into full daylight just after dawn.

By measuring the change in brain-wave patterns immediately following this exposure, scientists established the link between the retina and an area of the brain known as the suprachiasmatic nuclei. What this means, according to professors Richard Kronhauer, Ph.D., and Charles Czeisler, M.D., the two scientists who headed the three-year Harvard study, is that there is a direct connection between light exposure and the part of the brain that is thought to play a key role in attention focus and energy production.

Blaze away in the morning. When your alarm sounds tomorrow, flick on the light that you usually turn on, then look around for other light switches. The hall light? The extra lights in the bathroom? The lamp on the bureau?

That's right—they should all go on in the morning. For many people, the added light triggers an instantaneous alertness booster in the brain that shifts physiology away from sleep and toward a new day filled with more energy and higher metabolism.

Get at Least 5 Minutes of Easy Physical Activity

I don't know about you, but a rigorous, marine-style morning situp routine has never seemed like much fun to me.

Fortunately, it's not necessary, either. All you need is 5 minutes of activity, and it doesn't have to be the kind of effort that builds abs or pecs—or tests the limits of human endurance.

Easy activity should be just that—easy. Studies show that most of us are quite sedentary in the morning hours, and this keeps our metabolism sluggish. But if you can just squeeze in $\frac{1}{12}$ hour of morning physical activity—either before or after breakfast—you'll definitely increase your morning metabolism.

Get in the exer-habit. If you're just starting to do morning activities, don't worry about whether you'll be able to continue the routine. In all probability, you will. A study by the Southwestern Health Institute in Phoenix found that three out of four people who did some morning exercise continued the exercise habit one year later.

In fact, the morning exercise routine is easier to make habit-forming than a later-in-the-day routine. When researchers at the health institute contrasted a morning exercise pattern with the behavior of people who usually wait until midday or evening to get their exercise, they found that only half of the midday-exercise crowd continued their routine for more than a year. And only one in four of the evening exercisers kept it up that long.

If you rev up your metabolism and energy early in the day, you're establishing a pattern without even thinking about it. If you leave exercise until later in the day, you'll probably find it's easier to make up excuses like "I'm too tired" or simply "Whoops—I ran out of time."

Move on out. Should you exercise before breakfast or after?

It's up to you. There's some evidence, however, that moderate exercise in the morning before breakfast may give you a head start in burning off excess body fat. After a full night's sleep, you don't have as much stored carbohydrate (glycogen) in your muscles. So when you get up to exercise, the fuel that's pulled from your cells is more likely to be fat than glycogen.

Whether or not this applies to all kinds of exercise, it's certainly true for runners who work out regularly before breakfast. For regular runners, two-thirds of the calories burned in prebreakfast workouts come from fat, according to a study directed by Anthony Wilcox, Ph.D., at Kansas State University in Manhattan. By contrast, in the runners' afternoon workouts, less than half the calories they burned came from fat.

Respect your pace. If you're a slow riser, someone who simply doesn't like early-morning exercise, be honest with yourself. Make it a daily habit to get out of bed slowly, get dressed at a leisurely pace, and gradually increase your activity level.

Before or after eating breakfast, go through a gentle warmup period and then do a few minutes of light physical activity. Take 5 minutes to stroll around the yard or neighborhood.

Equip yourself. For a good morning start, an exercise bicycle, cross-country ski machine, or rowing machine comes in very handy. You can watch the morning news as you pedal at a relaxed, moderate pace on the stationary cycle; pull out some smooth, balanced oar strokes on your rowing machine; or go on an imaginary cross-country ski loop.

For variety, you might do some moderate strengthening or abdominal toning exercises. You may soon enjoy this "active time" so much that on some days it will stretch into 10 or 15 or even 20 minutes. That's even better, of course—but don't push yourself.

Enjoy a Great-Tasting, Low-Fat Breakfast

Breakfast is the meal that matters most. Even when you're in a hurry, there are ways to grab a great-tasting morning meal on the run. What you do eat or don't eat first thing in the morning can throw on the Fat-Maker Switches and throw *off* the Fat-Burner Switches for your entire day.

Here's why: When you eat even a small serving of a low-fat breakfast, you switch on your energy and fat-burning power. At the same time, you turn off a Fat-Maker Switch that kicks into high gear every time you miss a meal.

"Always remember that skipping a meal leads to bingeing," explains Kathy Stone, R.D., author of *Snack Attack*. "Eating breakfast is also essential to help control eating after dinner. Surprising, but true. What you eat in the morning affects how full you feel at the end of the day. If you think that breakfast makes you hungrier, that you are actually better off on the days when you go as long as possible without eating, think again. What happens when you finally start eating? Most times you lose control."

Researchers call the fat-burning process a thermic switch, and they've found that it's the key to the right start. When you wake up and get started on a new day, you must have breakfast to turn on your thermic switch, moving your body's rhythm from low ebb to high tide.

Don't skip out. Even though you know you should have breakfast in the morning to switch off one of the Fat-Maker Switches, it's easy to get into the habit of skipping. And you may feel as if you just don't have the appetite for breakfast.

If you've long avoided morning meals, you might simply begin with a piece of just-ripe fruit—an apple, a banana, an orange, or half a grapefruit, for example. Then have some 100 percent whole-grain toast or a bagel with nonfat cream cheese on it and a cup of tea or coffee. On some mornings, you may enjoy mixing whole-grain cereal with a 4-ounce serving of nonfat or low-fat yogurt. You'll reap the benefits all day long.

Go for the classics—plus. One of the best combinations for breakfast is the classic "health food special"—a bowl of old-fashioned oatmeal with low-fat or skim milk and a piece of fruit.

The food you get in the morning should provide both protein and carbohydrate, in part because of the overnight activity of your liver. "In the morning, your liver will be about 75 percent depleted of glycogen," notes Lawrence E. Lamb, M.D., medical consultant to the President's Council on Physical Fitness and Sports and author of *Stay Youthful and Fit.*

As I've noted, glycogen is the energy fuel that the liver makes out of blood sugar, or glucose. "If you want to protect your body protein, you had better provide some carbohydrate food early in the morning to replace that glucose," adds Dr. Lamb. "Your brain will function better, too, as it needs that glucose to maintain its ability to do all the complex tasks required of it."

But there's another reason to get protein and carbohydrate in this first meal of the day, and it has to do with the processes in your autonomic nervous system. That's the network that activates body parts that you never have to consciously think about, such as the lungs, heart, liver, intestines, and brain. When you feed this system an early-morning start-up breakfast of carbohydrate, protein, and fiber, you tend to automatically rev up hormones and neurotransmitters that prime you for an active day. So the right kind of low-fat breakfast actually helps set the fat-burning rate for the whole day.

Protein and carbohydrate are easy to get in this first meal. The protein can come from such low-fat dairy products as skim milk, low-fat cottage cheese, nonfat yogurt, or nonfat cream cheese. Since fiber-rich complex carbohydrates are found in any whole-grain foods, be sure to have whole-grain bread, a whole-grain boxed cereal, or old-fashioned oatmeal.

Eat on the drive in. If you drive any distance to work, you've got more than enough time for breakfast.

True, a bowl of cereal is a bit difficult to handle when you're obliged to steer, shift, and change lanes. But a number of low-fat breakfasts lend themselves to the morning commute.

Before you leave home, add some frozen berries and a handful of nonfat whole-oats granola to a cup of nonfat plain yogurt. Mix it all together in a pint container with a screw-on lid, and you're ready to go.

Another idea: Slice a whole-grain, rye, or pumpernickel bagel in two and spread it with nonfat cream cheese. Put the halves together and slip the bagel into a sandwich bag; you can have your breakfast break anywhere along the morning route.

Meet to eat. Make the first meal of the day more fun and interesting. Begin a breakfast partnership with your spouse, your child, a friend, or a co-worker.

If you eat with someone at home, take turns making the low-fat breakfast for each other. When you're meeting with a friend or co-worker, remember that you don't have to go to the local diner or gourmet-muffin breakfast shop, especially in good weather. Instead meet in a nearby park, where you can combine breakfast with a walk and a bit of sunlight. You can also meet a few minutes early at work or drop by a fellow commuter's house first thing in the morning and share a low-fat breakfast before starting out.

Steer clear of country specials. Stay away from the kinds of food that Ma and Pa Kettle used to have before hitching up Nelly and working in the fields. A high-fat breakfast of scrambled eggs and sausage is an invitation for fat to come right in and make itself at home—in your cells, that is.

Don't think you have to go to a greasy spoon to get more than your share of morning fat. You're also getting an overload of fat if you microwave some instant oatmeal, cover it with whole milk, and butter up a couple of slices of toasted white bread.

With any kind of high-fat breakfast, your blood sugar rises fast. Fat with breakfast sends your blood sugar up at twice the rate of lunchtime fat. And the fat-forming processes after breakfast are double what they are after lunch.

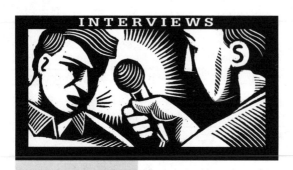

Diane Grabowski-Nepa on
Building a Balanced Breakfast

Breakfast is the most important meal of the day. You've heard this statement so often it could hardly be called food for thought. And still you race out of the house without so much as a slice of toast between your teeth. Maybe you won't anymore, once you hear what Diane Grabowski-Nepa, R.D., has to say. As the nutrition educator at Pritikin Longevity Center in Malibu, California, Grabowski-Nepa makes breakfast a habit for the people who go there—a habit that sticks around well after they leave. But you don't have to check into a health center to make breakfast work for you. All you have to do is check out the next couple of pages.

When it comes to weight loss, why is breakfast so important? If you skip it, you're saving yourself something like 400 or so calories, not to mention 10 to 15 minutes, right?

When you skip breakfast, you tend to eat tons of food at the end of the day. You actually gain more weight by skipping breakfast and stuffing yourself at dinner than you do by eating a sensible breakfast and avoiding hunger pains.

You may think you are going to save 300 to 400 calories, but in reality, when your body gets hungry later—as a result of not eating for a good 15 hours—you end up eating double the quantity of food. You overeat, which then makes your body store more calories in the form of fat. If you eat too much at one meal, you do tend to gain weight.

How can a guy start eating breakfast even if he has a gazillion reasons why he can't—like having no time or no appetite?

Often people just get out of the habit of eating breakfast. So then it becomes their new way of life to skip breakfast, eat a bigger lunch, and an even greater dinner. Also, it's a vicious cycle. Most of the time, you're not hungry in the morning as a result of eating a lot at the end of the day. So if you force yourself to start with breakfast and continue through the day by having meals on a regular basis—and even a couple of snacks—by the time you do have dinner, you are not gorging.

Some people really don't have appetites early in the morning—no matter how little they ate the night before. For them, it takes a while for their digestive systems to start sending hunger messages to their brains. But there is no rule that says such men have to eat as soon as they roll out of bed. They can wait an hour and then have breakfast. They can even keep it to something quite small. They just need to get their bodies used to eating.

Can guys who are used to snacking before bedtime and skipping breakfast the next day slowly incorporate breakfast into their lives so that it doesn't feel like such a huge change? For instance, could the first week of breakfast just consist of orange juice?

That's not a bad idea. It's better to get something into your system than to go without anything. So having only a glass of juice or a piece of fruit at first can work. There are also a lot of convenience foods for men who don't have a lot of time. For instance, they can eat yogurt or low-fat muffins. They just need to start that routine of reaching for some food.

And once they get used to their juice or fruit, they can graduate from beginner breakfasts to intermediate. They can add some whole-wheat toast or whole-wheat bagels. Then they can move on to advanced breakfasts, the ultimate goal. That's incorporating more than one food group. Once they are into the breakfast routine, they can start thinking about choices that can round out that meal. For example, a dairy choice would be yogurt or skim milk, fat-free cream cheese, or cottage cheese. Then, a complex carbohydrate would be hot or cold cereal, whole-wheat toast, or a bagel or a muffin. Rounding out the meal makes you feel more satisfied. It also works more nutrients into your diet.

You keep saying to eat whole-wheat items. What's wrong with plain old white bread?

I'm recommending whole-grain breads because they have more vitamins, minerals, and fiber. The fiber helps your body to keep insulin levels steady, which in turn controls food cravings and hunger.

What's the absolute best breakfast a guy can have?

A bowl of oatmeal. People who don't have time may automatically think that oatmeal is too much work. But you can microwave it. It's really as simple as a couple of minutes of preparation. Oatmeal is very filling. Actually, all hot cereals tend to be quite filling. The ones high in fiber, like oatmeal, also tend to keep your insulin levels stable. And they tend to be more satisfying.

And for those of us whose mothers made us OD on oatmeal when we were kids?

A bowl of whole-grain cereal like Shredded Wheat or Nutri-Grain. After that, whole-wheat toast or English muffins. Throw them in a toaster, and put a little fat-free cream cheese on them or a little jam. Something that's very fast—and I eat this when I'm in a hurry—is low-fat bran muffins. You just have to make sure that they are truly low-fat. Often, when we see bran muffins, we automatically think they are healthy. But some are loaded with fat. You can also put nonfat yogurt in the runner-up category.

What should you look for in a cold cereal?

The more fiber, the better. Aim for 4 to 5 grams per serving. Most cold cereals don't have a lot of fiber in them. They do have a lot of sugar and salt. So look at the list of ingredients on the box and make sure that sugar is not listed first. The less sugar in a cereal, the better. Sugar tends to make us hungry. A lot of people eat real sugary cereal at 8:00 in the morning and by 9:00, they're ravenous.

You mentioned putting a little jelly on some toast before. In the grocery store, you see things called "all-fruit" spreads. What's the deal with those? Are they better than using plain old jam or jelly?

In "all-fruit," the manufacturers do start with real fruit. But they also add in fruit juice, which is just a natural sweetener that is the equivalent of sugar. Your body can't tell the difference between fruit juice and sugar. All-fruit may be slightly more nutritious, but it still has the same—or only a slightly lower—number of calories as jam or jelly. So I would only use any of those options lightly—you know, just to give the bread some taste.

You also mentioned having yogurt. Which are the best kinds?

Get either nonfat or 1 percent fat (99 percent fat-free). Many yogurts are loaded with sugar. So look for one that is also either sugar-free or sweetened with fruit juice, which tends to have fewer calories than the kind sweetened with real sugar.

It has been said that if you're going to stuff yourself, breakfast is the best time to do it. Is this true?

Yeah, some people say that it's better to eat a lot of food earlier in the day because you have all of that time to burn it off. Well, logically that makes sense. If you overeat at dinner, you will be sleeping on it. But anytime you overeat, you do put more calories into your body, and your body is going to be more prone to store those extra calories as fat. If you exercise in the morning, you can get away with overeating at breakfast probably more often than the guy who stuffs himself and then sits at a desk for a few hours. If you are out walking and running around, then you are going to be burning a lot of calories.

What do you do when you are out for breakfast at a diner? Everything on the menu looks like a heart attack waiting to happen or like it'll take days to burn off, at least. But with the smell of bacon sizzling, who's going to order oatmeal? We wouldn't. What can we do?

Get an egg-white omelet filled with vegetables and maybe whole-grain toast on the side. That's actually a great option to have at home. But most people don't have enough time to make it for themselves. So it's a good treat to have at a restaurant.

Do you have to have traditional breakfast foods at breakfast? Is there anything wrong with leftover spaghetti or cold pizza? Or even a turkey sandwich?

Good point. Anything can be eaten at breakfast. No one says it has to be a cereal. For instance, there's nothing wrong with a bowl of soup—it's very European to have soup. You could have beans and rice wrapped in a corn tortilla with some nonfat cheese or sour cream. Or you could have leftovers. Why not?

Beth Bussey on
Eating to Lose Weight

As coordinator of the University of Alabama at Birmingham's EatRight program, nutritionist Beth Bussey, R.D., helps guys as large as 400 pounds—and sometimes larger—slim down to healthier proportions. The big boys that Bussey sees have to lose weight quickly to avoid life-threatening problems. But on the EatRight plan, they don't need to resort to extreme measures like stomach stapling or liquid foods to get the job done. Instead, they rely on an eating strategy developed during the past 20 years, based on research conducted by Roland Weinsier, M.D., Dr. P.H., professor and chair in the department of nutrition sciences at the university. A strategy, by the way, that makes space for burgers, steaks, and other delights. We figure that what's good for the big boys is good for us, too. Here's how it works.

What exactly is the EatRight program?

It is a weight-management program. We teach healthy eating, healthy living, healthy thinking, and healthy activity. Hopefully, as a result of that, people will become leaner and have fewer risk factors for disease.

The name of the program—"EatRight"—has a double meaning. We want people to eat right. And we have a food chart listing various food groups. We teach people to eat to the right side of our food chart.

So you don't rely on the government's Food Guide Pyramid? Instead, you've devised your own food groups and servings?

Correct. In our chart, foods are divided into five food groups: fats, meats and dairy, starches, fruits, and vegetables—in that order. The fats are over on the far left and the fruits and vegetables are on the right. Each group is divided into preferred and occasional foods. So, for instance, preferred fats are the "good" ones like monounsaturated, and occasional fats are saturated or hydrogenated, which aren't as healthy.

What makes some foods more preferred over others?

If you can eat it too quickly, consume too many calories, or take in the wrong kind of fat, then the food falls into the occasional category. So the preferred starches are high in fiber, like beans. The occasional are low in fiber, like mashed potatoes. The meats and dairy foods higher in fat, like beef and whole milk, fall into the occasional category. The preferred meats are lower-fat—fish, poultry, and low-fat dairy products.

So you also have occasional fruits and occasional vegetables? I thought we should be trying to eat as many fruits and vegetables as possible.

Yes, even fruits and vegetables have occasional eats. For fruits, you're looking mostly at canned fruit, which often loses some of its fiber. And the liquid is usually sweetened with sugar, making it higher in calories. Also, fruit juices fall on the occasional list because you can drink a lot of calories quickly without getting any fiber. And dried fruits fall on the occasional list because they are calorie-dense. For vegetables, the occasional ones are either canned or pickled. So if it is high in sodium, it's an occasional vegetable.

The preferred fruits and vegetables are unlimited. You can eat as many of them as you want. The goal is to average a minimum of three fruits and four vegetables a day, depending on how many calories you are eating. But you can always go above those numbers and are encouraged to do so.

So where do doughnuts, cookies, and potato chips fit in? They are fatty but don't really belong in the fats and oils category. And they don't fall into the starch category.

Those are special-occasion foods. Fatty foods that are either sweet or salty usually fall into this category. We ask people to keep their special-occasion calories below 200 a week.

Okay, so you can have 200 calories of special-occasion foods. What are the servings for the other foods? Are they similar to the government's serving sizes?

Yes. But we've lumped meats and dairy together into one category where 110 calories equals a serving. Fats are 45 calories a serving. Starch is 80 calories a serving, fruits are 60 calories, and vegetables are 25 calories. The amount of allotted servings depends on whether we have them eating 1,000 calories or 1,550 calories. Someone on the lower-calorie diet gets 2½ servings of meats and dairy and 4 servings of starch. Someone on the higher-calorie diet gets 4 servings of meats and dairy and 7 starches. The fats stay at 3 servings for both calorie levels. And fruits and vegetables are unlimited—as long as they fall in the preferred category. So really, the diet is not as low-calorie as it seems. It's 1,000 or 1,550, not including the additional fruits and vegetables, as desired. Most people eat a couple hundred more calories than that a day and continue to lose a half-pound to 3 pounds a week.

Where did this program come from?

It's based on research that Dr. Weinsier did more than 20 years ago called the time-calorie displacement diet. He actually had people come in for two years. The subjects were only aware that they were being asked to rate the desirability of the food. Basically, what he observed is that when foods were high in fruit and vegetable content and whole grains were offered freely, people automatically ate up to 1,000 calories less per day. Foods that generally don't require much chewing, don't take much time to eat, and have a lot of calories made people eat more total calories a day. So he concluded that if you rely on foods that take a long time to eat and don't have many calories, you are going to be walking around well-nourished and satisfied and spontaneously will take in a lot fewer calories and therefore better resist weight gain.

So how do you motivate people to eat this way?

We have a points system. If they eat less than their allotted fats, they earn 20 points. If they fall within a half-serving of their allotted meats and dairy foods, they earn 20 points. They also earn 20 points if they fall within a half-serving of their starches. And if they eat more than the minimum in the fruit and the vegetable targets, they can earn 20 points in each of those categories. That would add up to a perfect score of 100. But even if they ate all the right foods, they could lose points in the special-occasion category. As long as they keep their special-occasion foods below 200 calories a week, they don't lose points. But most people eat closer to 600 special-occasion calories a week. So they would lose 20 points off their scores.

So 100 is a perfect score?

Yes. What we do is have them add up the foods they ate for the week and then take an average. That way there's not so much emphasis on any one day. So someone could actually have a bad day—run out of fruit, not make it to the store, eat a lot of meat—and easily make it up by eating better on the other days. Or they could go beyond the 200 calories for special-occasion foods but make up for it by eating better in the other categories. For instance, someone who eats 600 special-occasion calories a week can still easily lose weight. So people get a new appreciation for food. They realize that they can have a buffalo wing as long as they are aware of how they eat.

We consider 95 and above excellent. That means that they are going to lose weight. Between 85 and 90 is good. If they score 75 to 80—which is fairly good—we ask them to analyze where points were lost and try to correct those areas the following week to bring up the score. If they score between 65 and 70, we ask them to take a close look at their food intake. And 50 to 60 is just considered a bad week. Try harder next time.

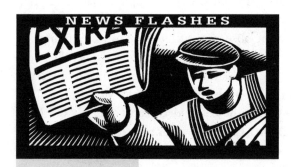

Single Living Is Slimming

BETHESDA, Md.—Well, there's one bright side to being divorced or single: You're likely to stay thinner than your coupled counterparts. A study conducted by the National Institutes of Diabetes and Digestive and Kidney Diseases found that men who are divorced, separated, or have never been married are twice as likely to lose weight successfully than married men.

What gives? It seems, oddly enough, that bachelors have better diets.

"Although it's speculative, there's a different lifestyle of men who are single than men who are married in terms of eating habits. It's possible that single men have more control over their diets than men who are married and eating in the traditional manner," says James E. Everhart, director of epidemiology in the clinical trials branch within the division of digestive diseases and nutrition at the National Institute of Diabetes and Digestive and Kidney Diseases. Also, there's more social pressure on single guys to drop pounds, says Everhart. They want to look slim and trim to attract a mate, he says.

Other than being single, men lose weight more successfully if they have a weight-related health problem to worry about, such as diabetes or high blood pressure. The study also found that men, in general, have an easier time losing weight than women.

Slim Men Eat Salads

OXFORD, England—Forget about that high-protein diet you were just reading about in that best-seller. Researchers at the University of Oxford have concluded that it's a meat-free diet that works best at fighting fat.

The researchers split 3,947 men into four categories: guys who ate any kind of animal they could get their hands on, guys who ate no red meat or poultry but would eat fish, guys who didn't eat meat but consumed animal products like milk and eggs, and vegans, who ate no animals or animal products whatsoever.

On the average, meat-eaters were 13 pounds heavier than their vegan counterparts. Vegans who have followed their diet for at least 5 years were the leanest group of all. Fish-eaters and vegetarians, in that order, were the next leanest. About 6 percent of the meat-eaters were heavy enough to be considered obese.

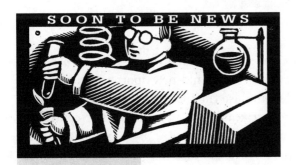

A Pill That Works Up a Sweat?

We already have our choice of weight-loss drugs that are supposed to help us eat less. But if we wanted to boost the number of calories we burn, there was only one way—exercise. That may not be true for much longer.

Researchers at the University of California, Davis; Duke University in Durham, North Carolina; and in Paris say that they've discovered the protein in the body that's responsible for calorie burning. Low levels of the protein—called Uncoupling Protein 2 (UCP2)—have been shown to hamper the body's ability to burn calories.

Evidence from studies conducted at the University of California, Davis, suggests that animals who are thin make more of this protein, while animals who are fat make less. It stands to reason, say the researchers, that the human body works the same way. "Just like people who are shorter or taller make less or more of a particular substance, people who are overweight or of normal weight make less or more UCP2," says Craig Warden, Ph.D., assistant professor in the department of pediatrics at the university.

Eventually this discovery may lead to the development of a pill that increases a person's production of UCP2, helping the body to burn fat, says Dr. Warden. However, he adds, it will take years before you'll be able to get your hands on this potential weight-loss wonder drug.

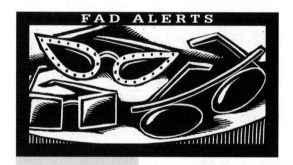

FAD ALERTS

Gut Barging

 Well, this is more of a weight-gain fad than a weight-loss fad, but it deserves mention. Opponents in this brand-new sport rub their ample stomachs with engine oil (some also rub margarine or lard on their nipples for extra protection). The referee yells, "Guts up," and the two contestants bump bellies in an attempt to knock each other off a 12- by 8-foot mat. A World Gut Barging Association has been formed and reportedly has designs on making it an Olympic sport. It sure beats figure skating. While you might be tempted to use this sport as a creative new excuse ("Honey, I can't start watching my weight now—I have a gut-barging match to fatten up for."), in this arena you're better off being a spectator, not a participant.

Macarena Exercising

Yeah, yeah. The dance itself is old news. But now, the dance is merging with aerobics and getting turned into exercise. We nearly chartered the next shuttle off the planet when a Macarena workout video hit the shelves of our local video den. Honestly, a half-hour of that chafing song or its hybrids would make us give up civil-defense secrets in a heartbeat. We recommend that you discourage any sick souls who may actually want to give you this tape by staying in shape.

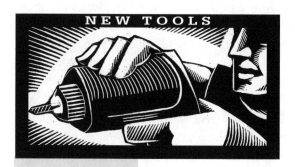

Better Peanut Spreads

Reduced-Fat Peanut Butter

Peanut butter is a potent source of protein, potassium, fiber, and carbohydrates. And it contains very little cholesterol. Unfortunately, with 16 grams of fat and 190 calories in every 2-tablespoon serving, peanut butter sticks to more than the roof of your mouth. Old chums like Peter Pan, Skippy, and Jif are trying to lure us back with healthier versions. But do they taste good? We tested them. Here are our picks.

- Peter Pan Smart Choice. We give it the major thumbs up. Tastes just like the real thing, even though it only has 180 calories and 11 fat grams.
- Reduced-Fat Skippy. Yum. The thing is, it has more salt and fat than Peter Pan, which is probably why it tastes so good.
- Reduced-Fat Jif. *Caution:* Take sandwich with a glass of water. This peanut butter is too salty.
- Polaner Natural Smooth Peanut Butter with no salt. You can tell natural peanut butter by the oil floating on top of the heavier peanut mash. You have to mix it with a spoon before you can spread it. It smells and tastes good. But it's a pain in the wrist to make a sandwich with.

• Smucker's Reduced-Fat Peanut Butter. At 12 grams of fat, 120 milligrams of salt, and 90 percent peanuts, this stuff is probably the healthiest real peanut butter on store shelves. But it tastes like—well—nothing. And it's runny.

Healthier Chewing

Ahi Jerky

Some guys pride themselves on doing things that other folks consider disgusting. Like entering belching contests. Appearing on the Ricki Lake show. Or eating pieces of tough, smoke-flavored beef known as jerky. Next time those weird urges strike, reach for Ahi Jerky. Instead of ordinary beef jerky—which has up to 4 grams of fat—Ahi is a naturally smoked tuna jerky that's fat- and nitrate-free. And, yes, like the beef jerky you're used to, it's dolphin safe. While we could do without the fishy smell (and the 520 milligrams of salt—though the beefy kind has more than 800 milligrams per ounce), we found that its texture and spiciness were very close to the real thing. These tuna jerks last a while, too—rest assured that as you read these words, one member of our editorial staff is still trying to dislodge a morsel from his molars. Our favorite is teriyaki. Suggested retail price: $4.95. Call Cascade Designs at (800) 531-9531 for a jerky dealer near you.

Lighter Chocolate Snacking

Low-Fat Chocolate Bars

When you eat chocolate, you're looking for a treat, not a low-fat label. But since there's a whole slew of "light" candy bars out there, we thought we'd give 'em a try. Since most candy bars pack 10 grams of fat and 280 calories—nearly 50 percent of which come from fat—it's good to have an alternative. Here are the choices that passed our bar examination.

• Hershey's Sweet Escapes Chocolate Wafer Bar: Tastes like an Oreo cookie, though not as crisp. No sacrifice here—we would eat these bars any chance we had.

• Milky Way Lite: Just as creamy, airy, and delicious as the original, but with half the fat and considerably fewer calories. Of course, it's also a tad bit smaller than the original candy bar (about three fewer bites).

• 3 Musketeers: Here's a low-fat candy bar that you may have eaten your whole life. We included the regular 3 Musketeers because it has 45 percent less fat than most candy bars, and it beats most low-fat candy bars in taste.

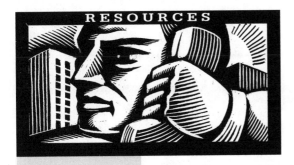

Trailblazing

American Hiking Society Volunteer Vacations
P.O. Box 20160
Washington, DC 20041

Talk about time management. You can get in a good calorie-burning work-out, you get a one- or two-week scenic vacation that makes for good bragging rights, and you end up feeling pretty darn good about yourself. The best part is that it won't even seem like work. Just volunteer to clean up trails for the American Hiking Society (AHS). This not-for-profit organization sends out hundreds of volunteers into America's national parks, forests, and rangelands to restore damaged hiking trails and build new ones. To be a part of the effort, send a stamped, self-addressed business-size envelope to AHS and request an annual Volunteer Vacations project schedule.

Cyber Fat Loss

Shape Up America! Web Site
http://www2.shapeup.org/sua/index.html

True, you won't burn many calories by using your index finger to click and type your way to the Shape Up America! Web site. But if you take the time to surf over, you'll be able to get the advice equivalent of consulting a doctor, di-etitian, and personal trainer—for free. Started by former surgeon general C. Everett Koop, M.D., the site aims to change the way people think about weight management. By visiting the site's "cyberkitchen," you can type in your height, weight, age, sex, and physical activity level, then have the computer calculate how many calories and fat grams you should be eating to drop pounds. The kitchen even will suggest meal plans and provide recipes. You can also visit the "Health & Fitness Center" and take an 11-question quiz to discover how much you really know about the benefits of exercise.

Fitness Time Management

American College of Sports Medicine
c/o Fitting Fitness In
P.O. Box 1440
Indianapolis, IN 46206-1440

Most of us really do have good intentions about exercise, but we just can't seem to find the time to fit it in (honest!). Now, help has arrived. The American College of Sports Medicine (ACSM), the largest sports medicine and exercise science organization in the world, has developed a new booklet to provide helpful tips on physical activity and healthy eating. The suggestions work because they're both practical and fun. For a free copy of the booklet "Fitting Fitness In, Even When You're Pressed for Time" send a self-addressed, 9" by 12" envelope, stamped with 55 cents in postage, to the address above.

Running

Road Runners Club of America Web Site
http://www.rrca.org/org/howsite.html

Jogging is one of the best ways to lose weight and shape up fast. Whether you are just beginning or already have a lot of experience, you'll find a ton of information from the Road Runners Club of America, a not-for-profit organization. The club's Web site includes information on where to find races, a product guide, and a list of even more running resources. You can even talk with fellow runners electronically by typing questions and comments onto the site's forum page.

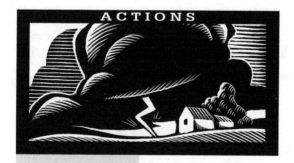

Seems simple enough: Eat less, weigh less. Around here, we call that tactic "starving yourself," and it works—in the short term. But then we just gain it back. Who wants to work that hard fighting fat when we're just going to see it again in a few months? Not us.

Here, then, are 10 enlightening, longer-lasting ways to declare war on body fat without suffering from diet deprivation.

1. **Enjoy your alcohol.** A lot of experts would have you skip out on alcohol if you're trying to lose weight. They tell you that it's too fattening to handle. But we know that's not realistic. So, instead, we've listed ways recommended by the Distilled Spirits Council of the United States by which you can minimize the damage inflicted by some typically high-calorie drinks.

- Cocktails made with club soda, seltzer, or diet soda, served over a tall glass of ice, are lower in calories. For instance, try a highball: 2 ounces of bourbon, gin, or vodka mixed with diet ginger ale or club soda.
- Cream cocktails such as grasshoppers, white Russians, and sombreros have considerably less fat and calories when you ask for skim milk instead of cream.
- Drink hot beverages such as Irish coffee, whiskey and tea, hot toddies, grog, or mulled cider slowly. Same deal for highly flavored beverages like Manhattans and martinis. The goal is to nurse these cocktails so that you spend more time on the one drink, instead of, say, chugging four or five beers in the same amount of time.

2. **Compare your width to your height.** Here's a quick trick for finding your ideal weight: Start with 106 pounds and add 6 pounds for every inch of height over 5 feet. Then add or subtract 10 percent depending on whether you have a large or small bone-muscle structure. (For example, a 5-foot-10 man should weigh about 150 to 182 pounds.) The problem is that almost every man claims he's a bit toward the "big-boned" side, even if he has arms like No. 2 pencils. That little white lie lets men carry extra baggage without guilt, but their heart and lungs suffer the consequences. "Envision your family reunion," says Nancy Clark, R.D., nutritionist at Sports Medicine Brookline in Boston. If your relatives look like linebackers, okay, give yourself the 10 percent. Otherwise, be real. Allow a little more if you work out a lot, because the muscles that make you strong are also pretty heavy.

3. **Drink yourself thin.** Want to burn 123 calories using only your throat muscles? Drink eight glasses (8 ounces each) of ice-cold water. Your body will use that much energy heating the fluid to 98.6°F.

4. **Beware of the graveyard.** A recent study of 31 security guards and 62 nurses and nurses aides at St. Luke's–Roosevelt Hospital Center in New York

City found that those who worked at night had gained an average of 8 pounds since being hired, while those who worked in the day had lost a few pounds. The causes are predictable. It's difficult to eat healthfully when your choices consist of vending machine snacks and all-night fast-food restaurants, and you may opt for sleep instead of exercise when you have time off. So how can you work at night and still fit into your clothes by day? "Eat your heaviest meal in the afternoon or soon after you wake up, not later in your shift," suggests Nancy Aronoff, R.D., research nutritionist at the hospital. Also, take some low-calorie beverages and snacks to every shift, and learn to whistle past the Snickers machine.

5. **Eat bacon.** No, that wasn't a typo, nor a literary mirage. True, bacon is one of the fattiest foods on a breakfast menu. But if you're going to have meat in the morning, bacon beats ham. Bacon is so flavorful, one slice should satisfy your craving for morning meat. Since that one slice is so thin, most of the time you'll be getting less fat than by eating a link of sausage. You can pat the bacon with a napkin to remove more of the fat.

6. **Go slow.** Maybe you could stand to lose a few pounds, but you aren't ready to go running with your greyhoundlike pals who enjoy racing commuter trains at lunch. Relax. Long, easy workouts may be the best fat-burning method for guys with higher-than-average body fat. Researchers evaluated the fat-burning rates in men with either optimal (less than 15 percent) body fat or high (21 to 25 percent) body fat. When the leaner men increased the intensity of their exercise, their fat-burning rates rose. But when the guys with high body fat increased workout intensity, fat-burning rates remained constant. "That means that they could exercise at a mild pace—just enough to work up a sweat—and still get the same fat-burning rate as if they had worked much harder," says Nancy L. Keim, Ph.D., of Western Human Nutrition Research Center in San Francisco.

7. **Spike your burn.** They say the average man needs about 2,500 calories a day to maintain a healthy body weight. That's fine. But what if you play beach volleyball (or watch TV) from dawn to dusk seven days a week? The point is that you may have different caloric needs from your peers, but how do you find out what those needs are? Simple—calculate your personal energy needs with this formula. All you need to know is your body weight (or the weight you'd like to be) and your activity level. Then do the math.

• Very sedentary (you rarely break a sweat)
  Current or ideal weight × 11 = daily calorie needs

- Moderately active (you play golf, do yard work, or walk—for at least 20 minutes three times a week)
Current or ideal weight $\times$ 13 = daily calorie needs
- Active (you exercise—cycle, stairclimb, swim, run—for at least 20 minutes, three times a week)
Current or ideal weight $\times$ 15 = daily calorie needs
- Very active (you exercise vigorously—rock climb, ski, row, play beach volleyball—for at least 1½ hours four times a week, or your job demands heavy manual labor.)
Current or ideal weight $\times$ 18 = daily calorie needs

8. **Don't break from breakfast.** Set the alarm 15 minutes earlier so that you can eat a decent breakfast. While you already know it's the most important meal of the day, now researchers say that it's the one that could keep your weight down, too. In a Spanish study comparing the eating habits of obese people with those of normal weight, researchers found that eating a big breakfast may keep you from becoming fat. In the study, the more obese subjects ate smaller breakfasts with minimal nutritional value, then followed with larger portions of heavier foods later in the day, causing the weight gain. Subjects who ate large quantities of several different breakfast foods—a variety of breads, fruits, and juices—ate less later in the day and maintained more normal weights.

9. **Deflate your spare tire.** Your stomach is like a balloon. Fill it to the brim with food (or beer) and it'll stretch. Abstain, and it will shrink. Now a study has found that you might be able to use the elasticity of the stomach to help keep weight off. Researchers from St. Luke's–Roosevelt Hospital Center in New York City found that obese people who traded their Henry VIII helpings for a semi-liquid diet for four weeks needed much less volume to feel full, as measured by an inserted, then inflated, latex balloon. Also, stomach capacity decreased by 36 percent. You don't have to slurp liquid food to see those benefits. Simply breaking down your three squares into six smaller meals may do the job. After a few weeks, you may feel well-stuffed throughout the day and, without nighttime bingeing, you may begin to lose pounds.

10. **Check your glands.** Feeling fatigued or depressed as well as fat? For as many as 10 percent of men over 50, the culprit's not what you're eating. It's a butterfly-shaped gland located just below the Adam's apple. The thyroid is in charge of producing hormones that regulate your body's metabolism. A deficiency in these hormones, a condition known as hypothyroidism, not only makes you sluggish but may also contribute to increased cholesterol levels.

The key to detecting the often-misdiagnosed disorder is a simple blood test know as a thyroid-stimulating hormone (TSH) test. "This is a safe, relatively inexpensive test that often leads to a diagnosis of a condition that can be very effectively treated," says Paul W. Ladenson, M.D., director of the division of endocrinology and metabolism at Johns Hopkins University in Baltimore and co-author of a recent study that found that such screenings are as beneficial to a man's health as tests for hypertension. Dr. Ladenson recommends routine screenings every five years for any man over 35.

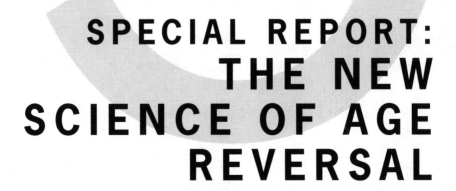

**SPECIAL REPORT:
THE NEW
SCIENCE OF AGE
REVERSAL**

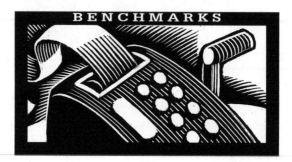

AVERAGES

■ Percentage of married couples in their sixties who report having sex outdoors: 20

■ Number of unmarried people 65 and over who live with their romantic partners: 324,000

■ Amount of weight in fat that a man gains unless he increases his exercise as he ages: 2.2 pounds a year

■ Number of times a 40-year-old man with average upper-body strength should be able to curl a 5-pound dumbbell in 30 seconds: 30 times

■ Number of times a 70-year-old should be able to curl the same dumbbell in the same time frame: 24 times

■ Amount a man's ears continue to grow throughout his life: 0.22 millimeter a year, or roughly 1 centimeter over 50 years

■ Number of years that listening to loud music regularly can prematurely age your hearing: 25 years

■ Life expectancy for the average guy: 72.8 years

■ Percentage of male baby boomers who are concerned about facial wrinkles: 44

EXTREMES

■ Oldest baseball player: Satchel Paige pitched for the Kansas City A's at 59 in September 1965

■ Oldest bridegroom: Harry Stevens, who at age 103 married Thelma Lucas, 84, in Beloit, Wisconsin, in 1984

■ Oldest man to swim the English Channel: Bertram Clifford Batt of Australia swam from France to England in 1987 when he was 67 years old

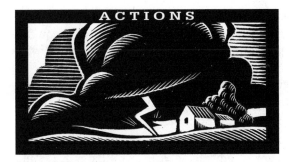

Today

Age reversal isn't instantaneous. To turn back the clock, you have to start doing little things right now—today—that are going to yield youthful dividends over the long haul. To get you started off right, here are six easy actions you can take to start feeling younger and better before the day is out.

1. Laugh it up. Skip the police drama tonight and channel-surf over to a sitcom instead. People who live past age 100 may have many differences—race, religion, national origin, socioeconomic status, education, and other characteristics. But one study has found that they do tend to have one thing in common: a fantastic sense of humor.

"Keep laughing," advises Ben Douglas, Ph.D., former assistant vice-chancellor for graduate students and professor of anatomy at the University of Mississippi Medical Center in Jackson and author of *AgeLess: Living Younger Longer.* "It gives you an internal chemical high. Don't take things or yourself too seriously. And stay around cheerful people—it's catching."

2. Speak slowly, live longer. Next time you open your mouth, make a special effort to slow down. According to a study in the *Journal of Cardiovascular Nursing,* talking fast may put you at greater risk for heart disease, which will certainly shorten your life. In the study, researchers measured cardiac patients' blood pressures and heart rates as they read the U.S. Constitution rapidly for 2 minutes, then slowly for 2 minutes. Blood pressures and heart rates rose during the rapid reading.

3. Don't watch your watch. An overwhelming sense of time urgency can age you and cause premature death, says Logan Wright, Ph.D., a psychologist and professor emeritus at the University of Oklahoma College of Medicine in Oklahoma City.

So, take off your watch right now. We're serious. Stop wearing a watch at least one day a week, suggests Ralph Keyes, author of *Timelock: How Life Got So*

Hectic and What You Can Do about It. Learn to rely on natural phenomena like sunrise and shadows to keep track of your day. Banish as many clocks as you can from your life and you won't be losing time—you'll be gaining it.

4. **Use a spot remover.** Age spots are likely to start appearing in your forties, especially if you've spent a lot of time in the sun. If you're worried that they make you look old, you can remove them. But you'll have to raid your wife's vanity table to do it. Over-the-counter fade creams that contain hydroquinone, like Porcelana, can ditch those signs of advancing years, says Barry I. Resnik, M.D., clinical instructor of dermatology and cutaneous surgery at the University of Miami School of Medicine. Dab the stuff on with a cotton swab. If this doesn't work, you may need a stronger, prescription solution of hydroquinone (Melanex or Eldoquin) or tretinoin (Retin-A), which gradually return the skin to its normal condition.

5. **Boost your brain with vitamin E.** Taking vitamin E every day may help protect your brain from deteriorating as you get older, according to a study done at the University of Arizona College of Medicine in Tucson. The brains of elderly mice that were given about 400 international units of vitamin E each day showed much less deterioration from free radicals (damaging oxygen molecules) than the brains of mice that weren't given the supplement.

"The brain tissue protein in mice is very similar to our own, so these results are definitely applicable to humans," says lead researcher Marguerite M. B. Kay, M.D., professor of microbiology, immunology, and medicine. Though vitamin E may not reverse damage, as little as 200 international units a day may stave off some of time's degenerative effects, says Dr. Kay.

6. **Flex your mental muscle.** Stopping by the store on your way home from work? When you go, leave the list in the car, says Michael Chafetz, Ph.D., a clinical psychologist in New Orleans and author of *Smart for Life.* Take a minute to memorize six or eight items that you need. Once you're in the store, get a cart and pick a starting point. Go get your first item, then return to the starting point. Then get the rest of the items, one at a time, returning to the starting point each time. That's all. This simple exercise will help strengthen your working and rote memory while at the same time improving the mind's ability to create a mental map of where things are. When you do this regularly, you'll find that you can remember more and more things—not only groceries but also tasks that you need to do at work or home—all at one time.

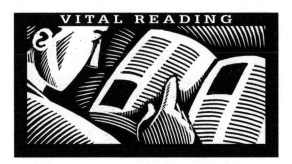

The Fountain of Youth

Here's how to hold on to your looks
and keep your edge through the years.

For most of us, our twenties are a time of figuring out who we are, struggling through identity crises while working menial jobs to pay for our hovels and suffering fools who think they're wiser than we are because they're older. But hit your thirties, and everything begins to make sense. You have that delicate balance of youth and gravitas (not to mention a little extra cash). Everything looks and feels just as it should.

Of course, that's also when you have to make a decision: Is age going to be your friend or your enemy? Up to this point, your youthful looks have held you back. Now that you're in full flower, you want to extend your heyday as long as possible. And that's a lot easier for men to accomplish than women. Guys like Sean Connery and Michael Douglas can go on playing the romantic lead into their fifties and beyond, while actresses have to abandon ingenue roles after age 25. Why? Men gain character as they age; it can actually make them look better.

While the typical guy starts to show signs of aging not long after reaching full maturity, there's no reason why further decline can't be halted indefinitely. "The human body is designed to live 110 years," says Ben Douglas, Ph.D., former assistant vice-chancellor for graduate students and professor of anatomy at the University of Mississippi Medical Center in Jackson and author of *AgeLess: Living Younger Longer*. "It's possible to look young and vital well into old age."

The science is simple. While you can coast with good genetics through the first few decades of life, lifestyle factors take over from there, becoming much more significant when it comes to staying, and looking, young. "You can be healthier in your forties and beyond than you are in your twenties, if you're smart about it," says James Webster, M.D., director of the Buehler Center of

Aging at Northwestern University in Evanston, Illinois.

Here are 14 ways to prevent, slow, or reverse the signs of aging—and keep your splendid looks.

Rub wrinkles out. If wrinkles start emerging, ask your doctor about Renova, a prescription cream that helps smooth them out. Developed by Johnson & Johnson, it contains a form of vitamin A called tretinoin. Unlike Retin-A and over-the-counter alpha hydroxy acids—which work on the skin's surface—Renova is said to work deeper in the skin, where pigment changes occur and fine wrinkling begins. In studies, 65 percent of patients showed a reduction of wrinkling and brown spots with Renova.

Use moisturizer correctly. Even the best moisturizer won't work on dry skin. These products are designed to trap moisture in damp skin, says Seth Matarasso, M.D., dermatologist and assistant professor with the University of California, San Francisco, School of Medicine. Wet your face, then put on a moisturizer. The water helps the moisturizer penetrate below the surface and into the pores, where it seals in water and temporarily smoothes fine wrinkles.

Eat like an Italian. Garlic may prolong the life of human skin. According to a study in Denmark, skin cells treated with garlic had seven times the life span of cell lines grown in a standard culture medium. Garlic-treated cells also tended to look healthier and more "youthful" than untreated cells. And garlic extract drastically inhibited the growth of cancerous cells. Now, we're not recommending that you concoct a garlic facial cream. But adding a few cloves to your meals, or taking a garlic supplement, couldn't hurt.

Blast your teeth. A new cosmetic-dentistry device can remove tooth stains in minutes, restoring the white of your youth. It uses a video camera that spots cracks and hidden decay, which can then be sprayed away with air/abrasive technology. The procedure removes stains in seconds with a concentrated blast of aluminum oxide, a safe gas. "If under the stain there's healthy tooth, you just stop and seal it," says Ronald Goldstein, D.D.S., author of *Change Your Smile*, who reported his findings in the *Journal of the American Dental Association*. "It's a new way of finding and stopping decay long before invasive surgery is needed." The procedure costs a few hundred to a few thousand dollars.

Clip your brows. Eyebrows that once stayed where they belonged can start growing out in all directions once we reach our thirties. Every few days, take a minute to seek out and clip off wayward hairs, says John Romano, M.D., *Men's Health* advisor and assistant clinical professor of dermatology at New York Hospital–Cornell Medical Center in New York City.

Cover your head. If you're concerned with premature graying, wear a hat when you're in the sun. One theory holds that the sun's ultraviolet rays cause pigment cells on your scalp to work overtime. That could make them burn out early.

Breathe deeply. Lung capacity starts to diminish in your late twenties, and this—besides sapping your energy—can cause your lungs to shrink by one-third of current capacity by the time you're in your seventies. But something as simple as taking deep breaths several times a day—anything that helps you breathe in and out as deeply as possible—can minimize the lung damage dramatically. "If you do this every day and don't smoke, by age 70, you'll have the lungs of a 45-year-old," says Dr. Douglas.

Stand straight. "You can take a 70-year-old who stands straight, looks alert, and walks with a steady gait and he'll look decades younger," says Dr. Douglas. "And a 40-year-old who slumps and shuffles looks like he's on his way out." To maintain a perfect posture, try this exercise. Stand against a wall, making sure that your shoulders and buttocks touch the wall. Slip your arm into the space between your lower back and the wall, and tilt your hips so that the extra space is eliminated. Hold the position for a count of 20. Do that exercise once a day for three weeks to ensure that good posture becomes a habit.

Stay hydrated. With age, the disks in the back begin to lose fluid, which is part of the reason why old guys have bowed backs. Drink 8 to 10 glasses (8 ounces each) of water a day to keep fluid stores replenished.

Make like the Man of Steel. The following exercise strengthens the back, abdominal, and gluteal (or butt) muscles—essential muscles for maintaining good posture. And it does so all in one move. First, lie facedown, hands at shoulder level—as you would for a pushup. Keeping your hips against the floor, straighten your arms to lift your upper body. Return slowly to the starting position. If you can do this 10 times easily, try doing the exercise with no hands, arms held against your sides. Once you've mastered 10 repetitions, you're ready to try it with your hands beneath your chin and your elbows out. Finally, work up to 10 repetitions in the "Superman" position: hips against the floor, chest up, arms extended directly in front of you.

Strengthen your shoulders. Aside from the knees and back, nothing is injured more often than the shoulders, says Allan M. Levy, M.D., team physician for the NFL's New York Giants and, formerly, the NBA's New Jersey Nets and NHL's New York Islanders. "As you age, your shoulders are likely to narrow as you lose muscle mass there quickly," he says. Countering these effects is simple. Strengthen the shoulders with shoulder presses, but also target your rotator-cuff muscles. Here's how. Grasp a light dumbbell with your right hand and hold it straight in front of you. Slowly rotate the entire arm inward (as if you're pouring a beer), then outward. Do 10 repetitions. Then try the same movement with your arm held out at different angles in order to work the entire muscle. Repeat the exercise, using your left arm.

Get plenty of sack time. Chronic sleep deprivation can permanently age you. Just look at our last few presidents. "Four years in that office does a 10-year job on their looks," says Dr. Douglas. That's because your body releases its greatest concentration of growth hormone—the substance that helps build strength and repairs damaged tissue—during sleep.

"When you get enough rest, you're more likely to perform at optimal levels and to maintain other healthy behaviors, such as exercise and a good diet," says Michael Vitiello, Ph.D., associate director of the Sleep and Aging Research Program at the University of Washington in Seattle. "Combine sleep with these other behaviors, and all those things we associate with youth—appearance, energy, and attitude—will ultimately improve."

Stretch these muscles. Okay, so you really dislike stretching. But preventing a loss in flexibility is crucial since it tapers at about the same rate as other major measures of aging—about 1 percent a year. For many men, that decline can start during the twenties. Do this simple two-step stretch to work both your back and hamstrings—the two muscle groups most likely to be stiffened by sitting at your desk all day.

Lie on your back and draw your knees to your chest. Hold for 30 seconds. This stretches the lower back. Now put both feet flat on the floor, knees bent, and raise your left leg straight up. Hold for 30 seconds, then repeat with the right leg. This stretches the hamstrings without putting strain on your back the way similar sitting stretches do.

Let someone do your nails. As you age, your nails start to get brittle, and ridges develop from the tip of the nail to the cuticle. Nails also become less flexible and more prone to snags and breaks. Once past a certain age, you ought to be secure enough in your masculinity to consult a manicurist once in a while, especially if you're in sales or another "meet and greet" profession. A manicurist can remove ridges and retard peeling by buffing and polishing the nail. Just tell her not to push back the cuticles—they protect the growth center of the nail.

Three Age Erasers

Keep these hormones' levels up for bigger muscles,
better sex, and a decent night's sleep.

Gentlemen, if you would like to keep your waistline thin, your muscles toned, and your mood upbeat, if you would generally like to postpone your middle age and preserve your youthful good looks, we have good news for you: There are not one but two ways to do it. One is free, natural, safe, and effective. The other, however, is expensive, painful, medically unproven, and potentially harmful.

Both methods have the same goal: to bolster your levels of certain key hormones—testosterone, melatonin, and human growth hormone—that play a significant role in fighting the aging process. Studies suggest that they can help promote muscle growth, jump-start your libido, and rejigger your sleep-wake patterns. Keeping them at optimal levels throughout your life may mean keeping your youth and vigor, too.

Sounds promising, doesn't it? And it's this promise that's the basis for a treatment called hormone replacement therapy, or HRT. The treatment involves supplementing your natural supply of hormones by pill, patch, or injectable pellet.

HRT does work—if you're one of the small group of men with clinically diagnosed hormone deficiency. But for the rest of us, men whose hormone levels will remain in the "normal" range into our later years, the therapy is still unproven and, some say, fraught with potential dangers.

There are, however, ways to go about preserving your hormone levels as you age—ways that may actually help stem the aging process. Here's what we know about the key hormones that decline with age and how you can help keep them, and yourself, up and running.

Testosterone

This is the hormone that we worry about the most because it plays a central role in sex drive and performance. But it may also be critical in helping to keep bones and muscles strong, body fat in check, and the mind agile. So it's good news that, in terms of age-related hormone declines, testosterone's isn't dramatic, says Marc R. Blackman, M.D., chief of the division of endocrinology and metabolism at Johns Hopkins Bayview Medical Center in Baltimore.

On the other hand, as we age, our testosterone receptors become less, well, receptive, while the amount of "free" testosterone in our bodies decreases, as a result of an increase in a blood protein that binds with the hormone, rendering it useless.

But supplementing testosterone can be downright harmful to men with average hormone levels. Side effects can include shrunken testicles, liver damage, and enlarged breasts. And even for men whose levels fall on the low end of normal, there's little proof that supplementing can provide any benefit. So to boost your testosterone naturally, without pulling a Pamela Lee in the T-shirt department, you might want to try these tips.

Pump some iron. In one study, testosterone and growth hormone levels rose in weight lifters following a workout. "Strength training is good for your muscle—and bone—health and also your endocrine and metabolic well-being," Dr. Blackman says.

Make sure that you rest enough. Overexercise, especially in conjunction with sleep deprivation, causes testosterone to plummet. Boot-camp recruits, for example, are wimps in the hormone department.

Be competitive. Serious competition of any kind—whether it's football or chess—seems to boost testosterone levels, researchers have found. Contenders demonstrated increases in testosterone that lasted a day or longer after competition, in a study by Alan Booth, Ph.D., a sociologist at Pennsylvania State University in University Park. Dr. Booth theorizes that long-term testosterone elevation may contribute to winning streaks, and the testosterone boost that comes with victory may help to sharpen mental acuity and reaction time.

Savor a steak. Whatever the other health consequences, meat-eaters churn out more testosterone than vegetarians. Those who eschew all meat in favor of tofu are particularly lacking in the hormone.

Melatonin

The subject of not one but two *Newsweek* cover stories and best-selling books recently, this pineal-gland hormone has been touted as the elixir of immortality. Some preliminary studies indicate that melatonin may help ward off cancer, heart disease, high blood pressure, ulcers, migraines, Alzheimer's disease, and just about anything else you might develop.

Now, however, the hoopla has died down a bit—a reflection, no doubt, of the millions who tried taking melatonin in pill form and said they saw no benefit or reported such side effects as nightmares, stomach cramps, and low sex drive. "We have yet to see a critical study that demonstrates that anything other than sleep is really affected by melatonin supplements," says Richard Spark, M.D., director of the Steroid Research Lab at Boston's Beth Israel Hospital and associate clinical professor of medicine at Harvard. Controversy has also arisen over the best way to take melatonin. To derive its full benefit, one researcher has suggested, you need to drink your morning urine. You may or may not live longer, but you'll be an interesting presence at breakfast, a glass of urine alongside your cereal.

There are, fortunately, less drastic ways to boost your melatonin level. And most of the following steps will also raise your level of serotonin (a feel-good brain chemical).

Seek out light. Mounting evidence suggests that exposure to bright light during the day can increase the amount of melatonin generated at night (to help you sleep) and the amount of serotonin created during the day (to make you feel chipper). Try to build "light breaks" into your day: Take a walk in the morning, or eat lunch outside when you can. Even choosing the window seat on the bus can help.

Keep the lights low. Less light exposure at nighttime has many of the same effects as increased light exposure during the day. Between 9:00 P.M. and midnight, the pineal gland cranks up its melatonin production. Research suggests that you can help it function more efficiently by turning down the lights at about 9:00 P.M. and keeping them dim until bedtime. Sounds like an excuse for candlelight to us.

Nosh at night. Many foods contain considerable amounts of melatonin; eating them before bedtime may help you get more and better sleep. Top choices include oatmeal, sweet corn, rice, ginger, tomatoes, and bananas. Other foods may help your body manufacture melatonin by providing one of its key building blocks, a compound called tryptophan. These foods include milk and cottage cheese as well as chicken, tofu, and pumpkin seeds.

Monitor your medicine. Taking aspirin or other pain relievers before bed can cut your melatonin production by as much as 75 percent. Two types of high blood pressure drugs, calcium channel blockers and beta-blockers, can also hinder melatonin production. If you're taking one of these drugs, ask your doctor to switch you to a once-a-day version that you can take with breakfast.

Growth Hormone

In 1990, a study in the *New England Journal of Medicine* created a stir by showing increased lean body mass, decreased fat, and increased skin thickness in healthy men older than age 60 who had taken growth hormone for six months. Supplementation of this pituitary gland hormone appeared to cancel 10 to 20 years of some age-related changes.

A more recent study, however, brought to light some of the downsides of growth hormone supplements. Researchers at the University of California, San Francisco, reported that, although men older than age 70 given growth hormone for six months did show a 13 percent decrease in body fat, no improvements in muscle strength, endurance, or mental ability were noted. In addition, patients "had swelling in their ankles and lower legs, their joints ached, and their hands were stiff." Human growth hormone supplements may also raise your risk of diabetes, and, like testosterone, they may also promote the growth of prostate cancers.

The National Institutes of Health are funding several major studies investigating growth hormone supplementation. The results should be in by the end of the decade. But in the interim, there are several steps you can take to stem the decline of growth hormone with time.

Look to aerobic exercise. "We know that short-term aerobic exercise increases growth hormone release," Dr. Blackman says. And one study suggests that long-term training leads to sustained increases.

Snack all day. High levels of insulin, the hormone that regulates blood sugar, can block growth hormone production. To keep insulin levels steady, snack throughout the day. And have a before-bed snack that includes a little protein (some cottage cheese or turkey, perhaps) and a little carbohydrate (some fruit or whole-grain bread).

Revitalize Your Body and Mind

Beat stress, fight fat, and generally feel terrific with this at-home plan.

Congratulations! You have just won an all-expenses-paid, deluxe spa vacation. The catch is that you're not going anywhere. Instead, we're bringing the spa to you. After speaking with experts at some of the most popular relaxation resorts in the country, we've designed for you the ultimate day of rest and rejuvenation. That's right, you're about to become Jell-O in a sport coat and khakis.

All we ask is 8 hours of your time and an open mind. You may initially regard this entire day (or at least some of its components) with skepticism, but we guarantee that if you stick with the program, you'll feel better than you have in years—almost as good as if you'd just emerged from one of those fancy (and expensive) spas. If you can't sacrifice a whole day—go ahead, you deserve it—any of the tips featured here can be used individually whenever you need something extra to keep yourself calm and collected.

Preliminary Plans

Disconnect the telephone and answering machine, and have someone hide the TV remote, just in case you're tempted to watch those transsexual midgets on Montel. Put a piece of duct tape over the doorbell, forget about the mail, and don't even boot up your computer. If the world should end today, then at least you'll die an ignorant and contented man.

Most important, take every timepiece and wristwatch in the place and either stuff it in a drawer or obscure its face. "When you take clocks away, you're inviting yourself to pay attention to your body and your experience," says David Tate, Ph.D., an instructor at Miraval, Life in Balance Resort in Tucson, Arizona. "Your body will tell you what it needs as long as you learn to listen to it."

Go to bed at a reasonable hour the night before, if only to ensure that your day spa doesn't become a daylong snore. Spend 5 to 10 minutes lingering in bed after you open your eyes, recommends Rubin Naiman, Ph.D., a clinical health psychologist at Canyon Ranch Health and Fitness Resort in Tucson, Arizona.

Tai Chi Relief

You've probably seen people doing tai chi in the park at dawn. It looks like some bizarre exercise for fitness-conscious mimes. Actually, tai chi is an ancient meditative practice, also known as Chinese moving yoga. According to William Phillips, president of the Patience Tai Chi Association in New York City, it's a great way to release stress, enhance balance, and develop speed. Plus, one study showed that 20 minutes of tai chi boosts the number of disease-fighting T cells in your body by 13 percent. That's why it's a staple activity in many spa programs.

What we could never figure out, though, is how something so slow and meditative could ever teach you to be faster and sharper. Phillips explains: "Take your hand and move it very slowly from left to right in front of your body. See all those little breaks—the stops and starts? Tai chi helps the muscles fire more smoothly; those breaks will diminish and eventually go away. Plus, it builds hand-eye coordination. So when you have to move, you can do it faster."

Here's a basic tai chi routine that Phillips recommends for beginners. It consists of three simple exercises that take all of 5 minutes in the morning. It's better than stretching at this early hour, because your muscles are still cold and susceptible to straining. Do the exercises slowly and in a flowing progression.

1. Stand with your feet flat on the ground, legs shoulder-width apart, hands comfortably at your sides. Raise both arms straight out in front of you, keeping your elbows and wrists relaxed. Stop when your arms are parallel to the ground, then raise your fingers until they make a straight line with your forearms. Next, relax your shoulders, letting your elbows fall back naturally toward the body and your wrists bend. Your position will resemble that of a begging dog. Straighten the wrists once again, reestablishing the straight line from your elbows to your fingertips. Then lower your hands to your sides.

2. Hold your hands in front of you, as if they were loosely gripping the back of an imaginary chair. Letting your body move naturally, shift all your weight to your left foot. Slowly raise your right arm almost as if a balloon were inflating beneath it. Then raise the toes of your right foot and pivot 90 degrees to the right. As you turn, envision your right arm draping over that balloon—palm at the top of the arc, wrist slightly bent. Turn your left palm up, about an inch below your navel, as if you were holding the bottom of that balloon. Finish the move by putting your toes back on the ground and shifting your body forward. Return to the starting position and repeat for the other side.

3. With hands grasping the imaginary chair, step forward with your left foot. Pick the heel off the ground first, followed by the toes; then put the toes down first, followed by the heel. As you shift your weight onto your left foot, raise your left arm from the shoulder and lower your right arm from the elbow. Turn your waist to the left, while rotating your right foot 45 degrees in the same direction. As you finish the turn, bend your left knee. Return to the starting position and repeat for the other side.

Breakfast

The recipes in this chapter were developed by Erich Striegel, executive chef at the Hilton Head Health Institute in South Carolina. Following his meal plan will give you a taste for nutritious eating. In fact, we think you'll be surprised at how good you'll feel after just one day on such a diet. There's no tofu quiche or beet juice to choke down either—just simple, good-tasting food that won't leave you with a gnawing hunger at the end of the day, as spa cuisine often does. Most important, you can make all this stuff yourself in less time than it takes to peel back the foil and heat up a Hungry Man. We know, we did it. If you eat what Striegel suggests, you'll consume a carbohydrate-rich diet of about 2,200 calories and 25 grams of fat. Here's breakfast.

French Toast

½	cup egg substitute
2	tablespoons skim milk
1	teaspoon ground cinnamon
½	teaspoon vanilla extract
3	slices whole-wheat bread

Combine the egg substitute, milk, cinnamon, and vanilla in a bowl. Beat with a whisk.

Heat a no-stick pan over medium heat and coat it with nonstick cooking spray.

Coat bread with egg mixture. Add bread to pan and lightly brown on both sides.

Focus on the Present

Remember when you were 10 years old and summer seemed so enjoyably endless? That's because you didn't have much of a past (at least not one you could vividly recall) and there was essentially no future (school wasn't something to anticipate). You lived in the present, fascinated by its every turn—and time crawled. Now it rushes by like traffic on the Autobahn, and you can't seem to find an exit.

One way to slow things is to master a mental technique called mindfulness. "It's the opposite of the 'been there, done that' attitude," explains Dr. Tate. "The idea is that each moment is a new moment that we can be fully aware of."

Dr. Tate explains that although we all live this way as children, we gradually "numb out" with age, fall into "the trance of everyday life," and end up existing on mindless autopilot. We're either worrying about the future or rehashing the past, while the present speeds by. One of the reasons that vacationing in an exotic locale is so invigorating and relaxing is that we're mindful of our new surroundings. We pay attention to everything, we sightsee, and we're energized and soothed by that.

To bring a little mindfulness into your day, Dr. Tate says there's one simple rule you should follow: Don't try to focus on more than one thing at a time. Our advice—don't eat while perusing the newspaper, don't wear headphones while exercising, and don't look in the mirror while having sex. By focusing your attention, you'll concentrate better on the task at hand and thereby enhance the experience. Food will taste better, exercise will be more enjoyable, and sex, if you can believe it, will be more intense.

Work Your Muscles

Exercise is vital for rejuvenation and relaxation. David Beck, director of the National Institute of Fitness, a resort in St. George, Utah, recommends an after-breakfast hike. This is best done on a woodland trail, even if you have to drive a short distance to find one. If you live in a city, head for a park, a golf course, or some particularly pastoral part of the suburbs.

"Don't just go to the gym, if that's what you normally do," says Beck. "Get out in nature and do some different kind of movement. The body is a master at finding its comfort zone. You need to break out of the box you live in."

Hiking is a great change of pace because it's something we all enjoy but rarely do. Plus, it's more physical (and manly) than walking and, because it's done outdoors, it makes us more aware of our surroundings. Depending on your fitness level, Beck suggests a hike lasting about 2 hours (including drive time). Start by walking at a comfortable pace for 15 to 20 minutes to warm your muscles, then find a rock, stump, or forest gnome and do some stretching. Once you're loose, hike vigorously for about 45 more minutes, using hills and hungry-looking animals to get your heart pumping. If the terrain allows it, head for an overlook or vista and spend a few minutes gazing across the miles. End the hike by walking comfortably for another 15 or 20 minutes to cool down.

Don't worry about measuring heart rate or calories burned, and since you won't be wearing a watch, just try to estimate your trail time. Make an effort to notice what's around you. Whenever your mind wanders, pull your attention back to the present by feeling the soles of your boots striking the earth. Working out in this way will exercise both body and mind.

Lunch and a Wash Down

After a peaceful and invigorating morning, it's time to refuel your body with a healthy yet tasty lunch.

Pita Pizza

4	ounces low-sodium tomato sauce
2	8" wheat pita breads
1	cup mixed vegetables (onions, peppers, mushrooms, broccoli)
2	ounces part-skim mozzarella cheese, shredded
	Pinch of Italian seasoning

Preheat the oven to 350°F.
Spread tomato sauce on pitas.
Place vegetables on a plate and microwave for 1 minute.
Sprinkle vegetables, cheese, and seasoning on pitas.
Bake for 10 minutes or until cheese melts.
Serve with 2 cups tossed salad with 1 ounce low-fat dressing and 1 cup of decaffeinated iced tea, for a total of 450 calories and 7 grams of fat.
Timesaving tip: Buy the vegetables and salad greens prechopped at a supermarket salad bar.

After a morning of strenuous activity, you deserve an afternoon of immobility. And there's no better way to reward tired muscles than with a hot shower.

First, apply a hot mentholated towel to your face, recommends Jossie Feria, director of The Spa at Doral in Miami. Hire a geisha to prepare one, or make it yourself by heating a pot of water and adding some eucalyptus oil, camphor, or a capful of mentholated aftershave. Let the towel soak for a few minutes, then test the water: It should be hot, not scalding. Wring the towel and lay it over your face. This will open your pores and soften your beard. If you want to shave, do so after this, then apply another hot towel to soothe your skin.

Once your face feels as if it belongs to someone else, look in the mirror to remind yourself of cruel reality, then get in the shower. With a soft, natural-bristle brush, clean and exfoliate your body. If you don't have a brush, use a washcloth.

One of the most popular spa treatments for men is a scalp massage. "It's probably because the scalp holds so much tension," says Feria. You can give yourself one in the shower. After shampooing, run your fingertips lightly across your scalp like a comb. Then apply a bit more fingertip pressure and move the skin of the scalp in small circles. Cover the entire head.

Although you may be tempted to spend the rest of the afternoon in the shower, keep it to about 20 minutes, then towel off.

A Rubdown and a Snooze

With your skin and muscles still warm from the shower, now is the time for a full-body rubdown. Karen Rutschmann, a massage therapist at Canyon Ranch Health and Fitness Resort in Lenox, Massachusetts, devised the following 20-minute self-massage program. All that's required is a pillow, a sock, two tennis balls, and baby powder or lotion.

1. Sit in a chair and place a tennis ball under each foot. Slowly roll the balls up and down your soles, applying pressure as desired.

2. While seated, cross an ankle over one knee and use both hands to rub lotion or powder on the foot. Then press into the bottom of the foot with both thumbs and make small circles. Start at the heel and work toward the toes. Finish by squeezing each toe, then gently bending it back and forth. Repeat on the other foot.

3. Lie back on the floor with a pillow beneath your knees. Put one tennis ball under the center of your left buttock and roll around on it. Use your body weight to apply pressure as needed. Work the entire area, then repeat on the right side.

4. Stuff two tennis balls into a sock and knot the end. Leave 4 to 5 inches between them. Lie back on the floor with the pillow beneath your knees. Lift your hips and slide the balls beneath you so they're resting on each side of your spine just above the buttocks. Then, using your body weight to apply pressure, gradually squirm them up your backbone to the base of your neck.

5. Sit up and clasp your hands behind your skull, with palms cradling your head and thumbs pointing toward your feet. Press into the base of your head with your thumbs and make small circles. Work from behind the ears until your thumbs meet above the vertebrae. Then work your thumbs back toward the ears along a different line. Cover the entire back of the neck.

6. Lie back down and place your hands at the base of your skull. Take a deep breath, then exhale while using your hands to lift your head off the floor. Gently pull your chin toward your chest, and hold for 10 to 15 seconds.

7. Sit up and, using a circular fingertip motion, lightly massage your temples and the muscles on each side of the jaw where it hinges. (If you clench your teeth, you'll feel these muscles pop.)

8. Yawn luxuriously and stretch your jaws for 10 seconds.

9. Sigh very, very deeply.

If you've done the massage correctly, you'll be feeling pretty languid. Don't fight it. Now's the time to do something you could never get away with at the office: Wrap yourself in a sheet and retire for a nap.

"Men think that they get tired in the afternoon because they eat lunch, but that's not true," says Dr. Naiman. "It's our nature to have a long period of sleep at night and a shorter period during midafternoon. Most cultures realize this, but ours doesn't. A nap is the best thing for keeping your energy and creativity levels high.

"Just listen to that inner voice, the heaviness that comes," Dr. Naiman adds. "To yield to it can be wonderful, if only for 20 or 30 minutes."

Dinner Is Served

You can't end a day this great by calling Domino's. Although the following meal may sound like a test of your culinary skill, it's not. If you prepare the salmon and potatoes a day beforehand, we promise it won't take more than a half-hour to deliver everything from fridge to table. In fact, why not invite your wife or a special friend to dinner? Light a few candles, put on some romantic music, and introduce the new you. (With this possibility in mind, all recipes are for two.)

Baked Salmon in a Garlic Crust

    1   cup bran-flake cereal
    2   teaspoons paprika
    1   teaspoon minced dill
    2   5-ounce salmon fillets, minus skin
    2   teaspoons fresh minced garlic

Preheat the oven to 350°F.

Mash the cereal in your hands.

Combine the crushed bran flakes, paprika, and dill in a bowl. Spray lightly with nonstick cooking spray so it sticks together.

Rub both sides of salmon with garlic.

Press the salmon into the bran-flake mix, coating both sides.

Coat a baking pan with nonstick spray, lay in the salmon, and bake for 15 to 20 minutes, or until bran flakes are brown.

Baked Stuffed Potatoes with Tomato and Basil

    2   8-ounce Idaho potatoes
    1   cup low-fat cottage cheese
    1   tablespoon chopped basil
    1   tablespoon chopped chives
    1   teaspoon tomato paste
    ⅛   teaspoon ground black pepper

Preheat the oven to 400°F.

Bake the potatoes for 40 minutes, or until soft.

Cut the potatoes in half lengthwise, scoop out the insides, and set the skins aside.

Mix the cottage cheese in a blender until smooth.

Combine the cottage cheese in a bowl with the potatoes, basil, chives, tomato paste, and pepper. Mix thoroughly.

Restuff the potato skins with the mixture and return to the oven for 20 to 30 minutes, or until the tops turn brown.

Serve each dinner with steamed green vegetables, 1 whole-grain roll, ¼ tablespoon margarine, a 5-ounce glass of wine or a 12-ounce beer, and 1 cup of decaffeinated coffee, for a total of 635 calories and 13 grams of fat apiece.

Sex You Won't Believe

Hey, you didn't think we'd ask you to go through all that trouble cooking a big meal for nothing, did you? Such a dinner is the ultimate setting for seduction. She's impressed by your culinary skills, taken with your confident and relaxed demeanor, and no doubt secretly yearning to touch your soft, mentholated face and exfoliated abdomen. You can turn up the heat by proposing an intimate bath for two.

Actually, bathing is a bona fide science. It's called balneology, and it represents the height of spa technology. According to Jonathan Paul De Vierville, Ph.D., owner and director of the Alamo Plaza Spa in San Antonio, Texas, the perfect bath has three components: time, temperature, and a therapeutic agent. To prepare yours, fill the tub with water slightly warmer than body temperature (about 100°F). Anything above this will promote perspiration rather than romance and relaxation. Fill the tub enough to put the water at neck level when you're both comfortably reclined.

It's best to think of drawing a bath as if you were making a cup of tea. De Vierville says that adding different herbs and oils can subtly alter your mood. Rosemary, for instance, is a stimulant, while lavender may have a tranquilizing effect.

According to Lana Holstein, M.D., a consultant at Canyon Ranch Health and Fitness Resort in Tucson, Arizona, such playful relaxation will lead to "exceptional sex." "It's an especially exhilarating way to finish the day," she says. "Exceptional sex happens when you combine the energy of the body-lust, if you will, with an intimate, heart-to-heart connection with your partner. You make this connection by taking your time and allowing yourself to feel the nuances of pleasure and sensuality—just as you've been doing all day."

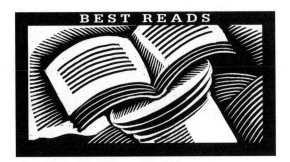

Don't Be an Old Fogey

Want a thousand laughs? Pick up A Man's Life: The Complete Instructions *(HarperCollins, 1996) by Denis Boyles. This pithy, wild collection of advice gets to the core of guydom in all its glory and misery. In this brief excerpt, Boyles provides the anti-aging advice we men really need: how to stave off fogeydom.*

Everybody's cultural life petrifies the minute they leave school. If you left college in 1977 or 1978, Bruce Springsteen's *Born to Run* is what pop music sounds like, *Star Wars* is what great movies look like, and Sol Lewitt is your idea of a crazy modern artist. Your wardrobe is likely to have frozen in time, too— not that you're still wearing bell-bottoms, but you don't dress the way this year's crop of grads dresses, either. And that, at least, is good.

But nothing tattoos your inability to adapt and learn as much as a time capsule mentality toward American culture, which, after all, just keeps right on truckin'—as somebody used to say. Here's how to go with the flow.

• Music. Give music videos or the local college FM station an hour a week. If you really don't understand what you're looking at or listening to, take along a guide: Go out to a newsstand and buy a rock mag—not *Rolling Stone*, which is, after all, for guys your age. But something you think a reasonably bright 20-year-old might read. If you've not been paying attention to pop music for the last decade or two, you'll be amused to see that what used to be bad protest poetry is now rap, what used to be bad club punk is now rock, what used to be rock is now country-and-western, and what used to be country is now folk music.

• Film. The introduction of cheap video cameras pretty much put an end to what used to be called "experimental" cinema. Once, a 16-millimeter camera was almost beyond all but the most ambitious film students. Now any kid with a job at Burger King can afford to moonlight as a "video artist." Pile an NEA windfall on top of that, and you have a video professional. So the real creative action has shifted to areas such as computer-assisted animation, where genuine skill is still required before anything intelligible may be displayed.

• Clothes. This is where guys over the age of, say, 30 get in hot water, since clothing is the one aspect of popular culture that is readily available and fairly easy to identify: Just dress like the boy next door. But that's exactly how dumb guys go wrong: They don't understand the difference between understanding youth culture and actually wearing it. Remember in the 1960s, how squirrely 50-year-old guys in love beads and tie-dyes looked? Well, those guys are all goners now. Don't let it happen to you.

Maximizing Mind and Memory

Nothing marks a man as an old man like that blank stare he adopts as he tries to remember something: his wedding anniversary, the name of that old college pal he went to Mexico with, the thing his wife asked him to do an hour ago. Sure, a little convenient amnesia is one of the perks of growing older, but when you need to re-member something, man, you want to be able to recall it with the speed of a super-computer. In her memorable book 12 Steps to a Better Memory *(Macmillan, 1996), author Carol A. Turkington outlines some simple strategies for keeping your mind sharpened to razorlike keenness—even as you age.*

While it's true that a person's memory can become less effective with age, memory loss is generally the result of disuse rather than disease. The important thing is to determine what is causing the memory problem and then deal with it. To counteract a problem in paying attention, you could develop what is called selective attention through observation. Identify situations in which you have memory problems, and then define what you want to remember, why, and for how long.

If your mental organization is decaying, you can learn specific recall strate-gies. And just as it's possible to strengthen a muscle by lifting weights, it's also possible to challenge the brain to become more efficient.

"The use-it-or-lose-it principle applies not only to maintaining muscular flexibility but to memory as well," says psychologist K. Warner Schaie, Ph.D., di-rector of the Gerontology Center at Pennsylvania State University in University Park. By running through some daily mental drills—sort of like practicing scales on a piano—a person can prevent intellectual breakdown. In fact, Dr. Schaie has discovered that you can reverse a downward mental slide through a combination of mental gymnastics and problem-solving skills. Physical exer-cise, too, when combined with mental stimulation, can play a role in improving memory function.

Stimulate Your Memory

Stimulating the brain can stop brain cells from shrinking with age; it can even lead to an increase in brain size, resulting in memory improvements. Animal studies in California have shown that rats living stimulating lives, with plenty of toys in their cages, have larger outer brain layers with larger, healthier cells. Rats kept in barren cages with nothing to play with were listless and had smaller brains.

Some scientists now believe that humans can achieve the same result, improving their memory function (and even reversing a decline) by challenging themselves with active learning or by living in an "enriched" environment, alive with colors, sounds, sights, smells.

Not only that: Research found that exercised brain cells have more dendrites (the branchlike projections that allow the cells to communicate with each other). With age, a stimulating environment encourages the growth of these dendrites, and a dull environment lowers their number. Researchers conclude that fewer, smaller brain cells are the price a person pays for failing to stimulate the brain.

That's why scientists believe that a person's socioeconomic status often predicts memory problems and mental decline, since people who don't have a lot of disposable income often can't afford very stimulating environments.

Liven Up Your Surroundings

The first step in bolstering your memory is to improve the health of your brain cells by making your surroundings stimulating—and the more stimulating the better. Here's how.

- The easiest way to liven up a room is through the use of color: Paint the walls a bright shade; add colorful curtains and pictures.
- A fish tank can provide soothing noise and a relaxing, constantly changing area of interest. Research has shown that simply sitting in a chair and watching fish can lower blood pressure.
- Fill your house with books, make sure there is music playing, and have videotapes available.
- Set up a chessboard—and play an occasional game.
- Put out lots of family keepsakes, heirlooms, and photos—even souvenirs from past vacations—and change them every week.
- Erect a bird feeder or birdhouses outside your window. Keep a pair of binoculars and a paperback bird identification book handy, and keep a "bird diary" to log each species sighted.

- Try jigsaw puzzles (the more complicated, the better) and three-dimensional interlocking puzzles.
- Equip yourself with a shortwave radio that can pick up international broadcasts, opening a window on the world.

Develop a Positive Attitude

Stimulation is not just about your physical environment, however. It's also about *attitude*.

- Work on maintaining a positive attitude, and try to stay flexible—don't get locked into a routine, refusing to deviate. Develop a willingness to explore new areas; get out and about and involved with life.
- Any kind of educational or recreational activity that requires problem solving is useful. What's not useful are passive or mindless activities. TV is okay if it is a program where you can guess what the contestants will do. *Jeopardy* scores a hit in the brain-building department. *The Flintstones* doesn't.
- Take a course. Not so hot at math or science? Try art history, photography, or cooking.
- Teach a skill. If you have some type of specialized skill (business, painting, writing, nutrition), try teaching a course at a YMCA or YWCA, senior center, community college, or an "open" or "free" college connected with a large university.
- Take an adventurous vacation. It doesn't have to be white-water rafting or mountain climbing. If you're not quite that adventurous, try an archeological expedition not too far from home. For an exotic change, how about a dolphin communication experiment in Hawaii? Seek information at travel agencies specializing in adventure tours.
- If you have extra time, volunteer. Check out the local volunteer service bureau, hospitals, nursing homes, service organizations, elementary or high schools, and day care centers.
- For the ultimate mind challenge, get a home computer. At the flip of a switch, there is an almost limitless number of games, programs, and types of information available. Go to the local computer store for a tryout—computers are much more user-friendly than they used to be—or visit a younger relative and ask for a demonstration. By their very nature, computer games improve eye-hand coordination, attention skills, and memory in such fun ways that it's not like learning at all. For a small extra fee, you can buy a modem to hook up to various computer networks that communicate over the telephone line. This is a great idea for those who are not so mobile, but whose minds are sharp. For the cost of a telephone call and a small monthly membership fee, a network provides instant

access to a host of information: financial tips, consumer reports, libraries, encyclopedias, banks, universities, news, cooking columns, free coupon offers, shopping networks, sports scores, and more. Special-interest "bulletin boards" (often free) allow members to receive and send messages to other members and can build up strong networks of friends among people of all ages around the country. If you can't afford a computer, see if the local library or school has one for use by the community. Explore renting and leasing options, or buy a used machine. Often, computer buffs who outgrow a perfectly good machine and move on to a more sophisticated model are willing to let their old unit go for a song.

• Join a group. Get involved with the community. Try politics, social clubs, service organizations, church or meditation groups, or animal protection leagues.

• Find a new talent. Work on carving, piano lessons, or soapmaking. What about a ham radio license—you'll profit from learning the Morse code necessary for the license, and a license will open up communication with other radio operators around the world.

• Learn American Sign Language (ASL). The visual language of the deaf community is great for developing eye-hand coordination, and the rigors of becoming fluent in ASL will quicken your mental reflexes. You can parlay this new skill into volunteering in the deaf community. (Don't expect to be able to learn enough ASL to function as a translator in a few months, however. ASL is a complex language and takes years to master. Still, many people find it fun to learn and a beautiful alternative means of expression.)

• Take a basic automotive-care course, offered at community colleges or technical schools (and sometimes dealerships).

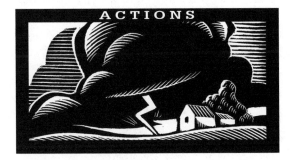

This Month

Day-to-day strategies can certainly make the difference in keeping you young in mind and body. But you can rejuvenate yourself on a monthly schedule, too. Over the next several weeks, make a point to try one of the seven suggestions below. Some you may have to plan in advance, so make an appointment or mark it down in your day log. Then, when the time comes, do it. You'll feel better. You'll feel younger. You'll live longer.

1. Get older, not wider. Why is it that when you were young, you could consume all the beer, pizza, and cream pies you wanted without gaining weight—but now every spoonful of chocolate-chip-cookie-dough ice cream seems to permanently park itself under your belt? A man's metabolism idles at a slower speed as he gets older. So fat gradually begins to accumulate and his gut gradually expands, even though he eats the same foods. The good news? Speeding up your resting metabolism to keep that weight off isn't that hard. Starting this month, gradually increase the time you spend exercising moderately, and slightly reduce your daily calorie intake, says Paul Fuss, co-author of a study, conducted by the Human Nutrition Research Center on Aging at Tufts University in Boston, on the relationship between aging and weight gain. Currently, no studies have been done to determine exactly how much you should increase your exercise amount or decrease your food intake, but the Tufts study showed that men age 60 and older retained an average of 87 calories more a day than men in their twenties who had eaten a similar diet. You can save 87 calories a day simply by switching from butter to fruit preserves on your toast and using skim milk instead of whole.

2. Stay short. Pick up the phone and make an appointment at your barber's this month. The older you become, the more important it is to keep yourself in order. Older men who become unkempt can look haggard, says Damien Miano of Miano-Viel Salon and Spa in New York City. Seeing a stylist or barber every month or so can go a long way to keeping you looking younger. You may also want to consider cutting your hair shorter and closer to your head, says Christina Griffasi, style director of New York's Minardi Salon. The shorter cut looks dramatic and has a much younger effect than trying to comb long strands of hair over a balding head, Griffasi says. Also, think about growing a closely cropped beard and mustache to balance the short hair on top.

3. Go with the gray. Here's another big fat hairy tip for you: When it comes to hair, remember that gray is a color, too, and not a bad one. When you think about it, gray goes with anything. But, if you choose to color your hair, invest in professional coloring. Over-the-counter products can give hair that's still naturally dark a blue-green or purplish tint. The idea isn't to get rid of all the gray, anyway, but to tone it down a bit. For instance, if you're 60 percent gray, you might want to think about reducing it to 30 percent gray, says Miano. Talk it over with your barber when you go for that haircut (have you made the appointment yet?).

4. **Go shopping.** To look younger, don't resort to the fashions of your youth. Instead, make a run to the mall and stock up on high-quality sweaters and turtlenecks, wool trousers, and a modest collection of sport coats, says *Men's Health* magazine's clothing and grooming editor, Warren Christopher. Muted, solid colors are best because they're more authoritative and can hide the little extra baggage we tend to put on as we age. Also, retire the shiny silk ties and opt for softer woven or knit ties, Christopher says. Dressing down smartly projects an image of being open to new things while retaining a casual elegance.

5. **Keep going and going and going...** As you look to the weeks ahead, make sure that you're leaving plenty of time in your busy schedule for amorous interludes with your honey. Those who regularly exercise their sexual systems while they're younger maintain much higher rates of sexual activity when they get older, writes Al Cooper, Ph.D., clinical director of the San Jose Marital and Sexuality Centre in California. The concern that too much sex at a younger age can result in a loss of penile sensitivity as a man ages is a widespread fallacy. Frequent sexual activity will not use up, damage, or in any way diminish your sexual potential or enjoyment, according to Dr. Cooper.

6. **Go to the opera.** If the thought of attending a performance of *The Marriage of Figaro* is only slightly more appealing than having a digital rectal exam, maybe you should reconsider—your life could depend on it. Research conducted by the department of social medicine at the University of Umeå in Sweden showed that attendance at cultural events may be the reason that some people outlive those who go rarely. They suspect that attending cultural events widens your social network and gives you the warm, fuzzy feeling of belonging to a group, which in itself could make you live longer. By the way, we don't think that poker night or an afternoon at the ballpark qualifies as a cultural event.

7. **Satisfy your curiosity.** They say that curiosity kills the cat, but new research suggests that it may actually help men live longer. Researchers compared curiosity levels in more than 1,000 men, averaging 70 years old, against their mortality rates after five years. They found that curiosity levels were higher in men who had survived than in those who had subsequently died. This suggests that curiosity helps maintain the aging central nervous system's health. So next time you're curious about the salary of the guy in the cubicle next to yours, give yourself a point for helping to ensure the health of your nervous system.

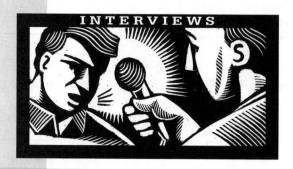

Michael Merzenich on
Thinking Yourself Younger

Many people complain that, as they get older, they gradually become more forgetful, less sharp, and less inclined to do new things and think new thoughts. We blame this phenomenon on aging, on the belief that our brain cells are either dying or moving away in droves. But it doesn't work that way, says neuroscientist Michael Merzenich, Ph.D. The brain, like a muscle, needs exercise. If you don't use it, you will lose it. But if you do use it, you can literally be as young as you think you are. In his work at the Keck Center for Integrated Neuroscience at the Medical Center of the University of California, San Francisco, Dr. Merzenich studies how one's individual skills evolve over a lifetime and how the brain learns new skills and abilities. According to him, old dogs can *learn new tricks.*

How does the brain change as a person ages?

You may worry about the physical changes going on inside your head, but the brain retains its fundamental capacity on a relatively high level. It is continually in play. The secret to maintaining that capacity is that you have to practice neurologically—exercise your brain—just as much as you have to exercise your physical body. You have to practice making decisions or else you lose the ability to make decisions. You have to practice finding your way around the world or else you lose your ability to find your way around the world. All of these skills require maintenance. They require exercise.

An aging person commonly limits his level of interaction with the world. This is most dramatic when a man's life revolves around his career. When retirement rolls around and a new life of relaxation replaces work, all of his highly developed cognitive abilities go unpracticed. The natural inclination is to get away from them. But if you want to be the same person 10 years from now, you have to practice the same kind of activities you admire in yourself today.

So people really do get "set in their ways" as they get older?

Yes. This happens when someone begins to limit the sort of activities he engages in, more and more. You become more and more conservative, more and more fixed in the range of things that you deal with. Consequently, you lose your capacity to deal with a wider range of things. Mental fitness is a critical part of maintaining a vigorous brain late into life. You have to practice operating at the same complex levels with the same ability that you operated on in real life earlier. You have to use it or lose it in the broader sense.

What kind of person is most likely to maintain his acute mental abilities as he ages?

Someone who stays active late in life, who maintains that vigor, makes decisions, and continues to do important things despite getting older. By doing so, he maintains a higher mental and cognitive ability, as contrasted with the person who's withdrawn from those things. Studies show that college professors who continue to work are less likely to become senile than others in the same age group who stopped working. Basically, the rate of occurrence of senility is less.

Can we give our readers any specific actions to take—perhaps go out and volunteer for something?

Yes. Find a niche and discover ways to use the skills and abilities that you applied in your career as much as possible. For example, if you're a bank director, don't volunteer to cook the soup in a soup kitchen. It is more appropriate to spend your time doing things on a more complex cognitive level, in line with what you used to do.

Any wisdom for those people stuck in a late-life rut? Is it too late for them?

It doesn't have to be. But if you limit yourself to watching television and taking a walk, pretty soon everything is diminished. Not just your capacity to make complex decisions or logical judgments but also your energy. You need to get active. Game playing is great to combat this.

What kind of games?

Games that really make your brain work. These include interactive computer games, card games (like bridge and pinochle), and strategic board games like chess. Find the kind of game, or a repertoire of games, where your weakness can be addressed. For people who worry that they have difficulties making decisions, choose a game that forces you to make decisions from among the kinds I just mentioned.

What are you doing yourself to age-proof your brain?

I'm in my fifties. I enjoy exercising my brain by playing computer games and card games and war games. You name it and I'll play it. I come from a family that likes games. I also try to read and think as much as possible.

Any parting wisdom?

Never stop learning. If you want to maintain the skills you're proudest of, keep practicing them and find ways to keep them in your life even as your life changes. Don't count on Mother Nature or God to keep you sharp.

Seth Matarasso on
Saving Your Skin

Life on planet Earth does its damnedest to age you faster than you ought to. Gravity, sunlight, pollution, daily stress, and numerous other forces conspire to make you look older than you really are. You can hold your own against the ravages of life, but it means paying attention to a part of your body you've always taken for granted. Unless you want to look and feel like a craggy old man, you're going to have to start taking care of the largest organ of your body. No, not that one. We're talking about your skin.

According to Seth Matarasso, M.D., dermatologist and assistant professor with the University of California, San Francisco, School of Medicine, you can treat your skin right in less time than it takes you to slap on aftershave. In fact, skip the aftershave, he says. Here are recommendations he gives his patients—and that he follows himself.

First, what are some of the things guys do to damage their skin?

Exposure to sunlight is the biggest contributor to aging. Smoking, pollutants, and stress also damage our skin. Some guys work out—they're in great shape—and after their workout they'll go to a tanning booth, which is just as bad as the sun.

What about skin conditions like acne? A lot of men get it even as adults. We can take care of that ourselves, right?

Do not manipulate your pimples. Do not do bathroom surgery. The normal life cycle of an acne lesion is 3 to 7 days. You mash on it, it's now going to last 7 to 10 days. You can initially try an over-the-counter product. Any benzoyl peroxide product, like Oxy-5 or Oxy-10. Leave your pimples alone. If it's painful, you can go to your dermatologist and have it drained.

Don't astringents help acne or oily skin?

I'm not a believer in witch hazel, alcohol, or astringents. A lot of men will put witch hazel or alcohol on their face. That tends to be very irritating and can lead to scarring and color alteration and even infection. I don't think they combat acne.

What if we have large pores? Can we shrink them to minimize adult acne?

No. You cannot shrink pore size. The pore is the opening to the sebaceous gland. This is genetically predetermined. It cannot be altered. No cream, no lotion, no potion, no peel or laser will alter the size.

So you can't shrink pore size. What are some other fallacies of skin care?

Here are the three big lies in my field of medicine. The first is that you can shrink pore size. Second, a diet with greasy foods and chocolate will give you acne. Third, if you drink a lot of water, it will clear out your skin and you won't get acne. Diet has no effect on skin.

Is there a way men should shave in order to protect their skin?

The two most important things about shaving: hydrating skin and shaving down with the grain of the beard. Do not shave up. Use tepid water for shaving. Mild soap without a detergent, not an antibacterial soap, not a deodorant soap. A glycerin soap is best. Wash your face and rinse off the soap. Then use a thick shaving cream. Let it sit a few minutes to hydrate. Shave down and wash off all residual shaving cream. You do not need to do all sorts of facial exercises to get every last nub and stub. I see guys in the gym shaving within an inch of their lives. You want a very nonabrasive shave. If you shave up, against the grain of the beard, often you will get an ingrown hair, which looks like an acne breakout.

Without making a big production about it, are there any quick and easy things that we can do to save our skin, to keep it from looking all wrinkled and shriveled up?

If you want to maintain your skin, put on an alpha hydroxy cream or lotion, low concentration, 8 percent to 12 percent, which is available over-the-counter. (For example, Neutrogena Healthy Skin Face Lotion with SPF, or sun protection factor, 15). Or use a topical vitamin C (Cellex-C or SkinCeuticals, for example, available through your dermatologist). The most important part of any man's regimen, though, is a sunscreen on top of alpha hydroxy acid or vitamin C.

How long is all this going to take?

Shaving takes me 4 minutes. Then putting on a vitamin C cream takes literally 30 seconds. Then putting on a sunscreen on top of that takes another 5 seconds.

If we're really strapped for time, what's the most effective low-maintenance option?

To keep the regimen simple, the most important thing is a sunscreen—that's prevention. The sunscreen I like men to use should be an SPF of 15 or greater. Then if you really want to fine-tune, pick a sunscreen according to your skin type. Are you oily? Then you need a gel. Are you dry? Then you need a cream.

The most we put on our skin is aftershave. What's wrong with that?

Aftershaves are nonsense. Their primary ingredient most of the time is alcohol or propylene glycol, and it braces your skin. But it's not closing your pores; it's not really cleansing your skin per se. You like the scent, you like the stinging sensation. That's just fine, but it's not really doing a heck of a lot for your skin.

Are there other ingredients we should steer clear of?

Lanolin. People with very dry skin should avoid products that contain lanolin because it can sting or burn their skin. People should stay away from products that contain formaldehyde or its derivative formalin, which are very common ingredients. These are the big offending agents—they make the skin drier.

Now at night, you can just wash your face, right?

Wash your face with a very mild glycerin soap and tepid water. Don't use an antibacterial soap. The antibacterial soaps tend to be abrasive. Wash your face, blot it dry.

Is there more we should do to our faces?

I have the vast number of my patients using a pea-size amount of prescription Retin-A (tretinoin). It's effective for acne, fine lines, and some of the mild pigment or color changes. Apply it to the whole face, including the forehead. This small amount is enough because Retin-A products tend to be a bit abrasive. First and foremost, apply it to dry skin. If you apply it to moist skin, your skin can get a little bit red and irritated. Start every other night and gradually build up to nightly.

What will happen to our skin over the years, and what can we do about it?

Skin tags, which are nothing more than excess skin. They're usually in the folds of the skin around the neck, armpits, and groin. They're pretty much genetic and can be removed readily by your dermatologist. Then there are keratoses—horny, callus-like growths—which can also be removed. These appear in sun-exposed areas such as the back of your hands, the rims of your ears, and your face.

What are those brown spots we're starting to see?

They are commonly referred to as liver spots. They're flat, brown spots that you see on your hands, chest, or neck. They are very similar in appearance to freckles. They are your body's response to chronic sun damage. Your body is trying to produce pigment to act as a protective mechanism. They are a sure sign of aging. Your dermatologist can use a chemical peel, freeze them off with liquid nitrogen, laser them off, or bleach them out with hydroquinone. A 2 percent hydroquinone cream called Porcelana is available over-the-counter. A higher concentration is available with a prescription.

How can we keep our hands from looking all gnarly as we age?

One of the biggest areas that will give away a person's age is his hands. Most men aren't going to get manicures, but just putting some petroleum jelly on the nails will prevent nicking and chapping and breaking of nails and cuticles. Keep the hands moist with a sunscreen. If you want to maintain your hands, wear gloves when you play sports like golf and also when you do something like yard work.

You keep saying use a sunscreen, but what about a moisturizer?

I tell people they don't really need a moisturizer. Another fallacy is that moisturizers prevent wrinkles. They mask wrinkles by filling in the crevices. You just get a sunscreen that has a moisturizer as its base, that is a cream or a lotion.

Anything else we can do to save our skins?

Get undressed, stand in front of a mirror, and begin systematically. Start at your face, work down to your chest and abdomen, look at one arm, flip the arm over, then look at the other arm, then look down one leg, then the other. If you are darker-skinned—Hispanic or African-American, for example—make sure to look at the soles of your feet for moles. Then take a mirror and look at your back. Start at the back of your neck, down your shoulders and back, and then thighs.

What are we looking for?

A mole that has become asymmetric, the border has changed, the color has changed, or the diameter has changed. Any one of these four changes warrants a visit to the dermatologist.

Let's say we take a spill or get in a fight or something. What can we do for bruises?

Ice packs. Keep an ice pack on for 10 minutes. Do this at least four times a day.

Why do we seem to look worse the next day?

You've traumatized the skin. You get breakage of blood vessels and leaking of blood. Initially, you don't see the leaking because it's under the skin. On day two, the blood comes to the surface and it becomes purple; that's when it becomes more apparent. The purple fades to brown, then to yellow, and then it disappears. But stay out of the sun because that can prolong healing.

You're kind of a stickler about staying out of the sun. We still want suntans. Isn't there anything we can do?

Do yourself a favor and get one of the fake tans in a bottle. They are basically a dye. There are some good products out there. Under no circumstances would I allow a patient of mine to get a real tan. No tan is good tan. Period. End of story.

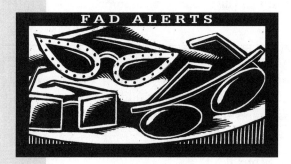

DHEA

 Men have been searching for the secret to staying young for ages. Legend has it that Spanish explorer Ponce de León was looking for the fountain of youth when he discovered Florida in the early 1500s. And no one has been able to beat the secret out of Dick Clark yet. Meanwhile, the modern-day hope for that elusive elixir of youth is DHEA (short for dehydroepiandrosterone). But its age-reversing powers may be as mythical as any fountain Ponce de León discovered.

Mail-order companies as well as some doctors who broadcast over the radio have touted this stuff as a wonder hormone. They claim that it can reverse aging, sharpen the brain, and boost sex drive. And after all, what guy wouldn't want to have the body of a twenty-something, along with the wisdom of increased age?

But don't believe a word of it. "There's no legitimate evidence that DHEA affects aging," says Arthur G. Schwartz, Ph.D., a DHEA researcher and microbiologist at Temple University in Philadelphia. Even worse, the body converts DHEA into testosterone, which could create serious problems. Dr. Schwartz thinks that long-term supplementation of higher than 25 grams per day (some believers take twice that amount) could eventually cause heart disease and prostate cancer.

"DHEA is snake oil at this point," says Elizabeth Barrett-Connor, M.D., professor and chief of the division of epidemiology at the University of California, San Diego, and a long-standing authority on the hormone. "There have been no long-term clinical tests in people, and the animal studies are meaningless—animals don't even have DHEA." However, proponents of the hormone are not swayed, so you can expect even more hoopla about DHEA for a while.

Facial Exercisers

 As you age, your facial skin tends to sag and wrinkle. Blame it on the sun, or blame Sir Isaac Newton if you want to. It's partly gravity at work. And there's not a heck of a lot you can do about it. But some gadget hucksters want you to believe that exercising your face will produce the same smooth muscles that exercising your quads does. Think again.

These gadgets resemble tiny exercise machines, and you're supposed to use them to flex your facial muscles or lift weights with your chin. But this won't work for your face the way that a full-size exercise machine might work on your body. The muscles in the face are very small, so even if you were able to pump them up using these types of devices, no one would notice. Instead, the repetitive movement of facial exercises takes its toll on the very thin layer of skin that covers the face and ends up promoting lines, creases, and wrinkles. Just think about how continual squinting contributes to the lines around the eyes, or how laughing helps to develop those lines that run from the nose to the lips. Facial exercisers have the same effect.

Sagging skin is caused not by sagging muscles but by genetics, aging, and sun damage. So while facial exercises may strengthen the muscles in your face to some extent, they won't get rid of sagging skin. Instead, they probably will give you more wrinkles. The bottom line is that when it comes to exercise, leave your face out of it.

Vision Training

 In this information-driven era, the secret to success is to read—and read voraciously. The man who's still reading the Sunday *New York Times* on Thursday evening will be left in the dust. And reading efficiency often seems to get poorer for the man entering his senior years.

"Even when you're a pretty good reader, as you get older your ability to process information slows down a bit," explains Harold A. Solan, O.D., distinguished service professor at the College of Optometry at the State University of New York in Manhattan. The eyes can lose their ability to stop quickly and accurately when they need to. Visual distractions cause an extra glance around a page or a quick look back at a series of words, which adds to the time it takes to get to the bottom of a page. "It's not that the eye muscles are weak—they just need to be re-educated," he says. But if the idea of taking a speed-reading class doesn't seem appealing, then consider a visual-training program.

In a recent study reported in *Optometry and Vision Science*, 16 people over age 62 took such a training program. Within eight weeks, people who had been complaining that the years had slowed down their reading speed were reading more efficiently with no drop in comprehension. While earlier studies had shown that young people report an increase in efficiency, this was the first proof that visual training could work with older people as well.

There are three types of vision-training procedures, says Dr. Solan, who led the study. The first is called flash training or perceptual accuracy. Numbers flash on a screen at decreasing exposure times. With practice, he says, a viewer learns to "process information more rapidly." A second is called eye movement training or visual efficiency. A number appears on the left side of the screen, a second number appears in middle of the screen, and a third appears to the right. Among those numbers, the number 2, for example, will appear several times. The viewer is asked to recall how many times the number 2 appeared. This trains the viewer to move his eye from left to center to right with increasing speed and to learn to recognize information as he's increasing the speed of eye movement. The third one is called guided or controlled reading. Sentences appear on the screen but a sliding slot allows only three words to appear at a time as it moves from left to right. "People often make too many backward movements as they read," explains Dr. Solan. "This teaches their eyes to move efficiently from one end of a line to the other."

Such training improves reading efficiency, says Dr. Solan. People read more rapidly, with better comprehension and with less fatigue after they're finished. "And they enjoy it more," he adds. He stresses that vision efficiency training is different from speed-reading, which includes such techniques as moving your finger beneath the words on a page. That strategy may help you move through the material, but it creates a dependence on the technique. It doesn't actually re-train eye movements or improve visual processing, notes Dr. Solan. If you want to learn more about this technique, talk to your eye doctor.

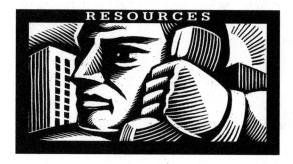

Worldwide Longevity

American Academy of Anti-Aging Medicine
World HealthNetwork Web Site
http://www.worldhealth.net

For a world of information on anti-aging and longevity research, call up this site, sponsored by the American Academy of Anti-Aging Medicine. Learn about the latest anti-aging drugs as well as upcoming research projects on extending life. This site is more than an information resource—it's fun, too. Take the test that tells you how long you're really going to live. Before you shell out big bucks for that self-help book that promises you a long, active life, read detailed book summaries (and even an occasional whole chapter) here and see if it's worth your time and money. And take a hop to other searchable health databases.

Natural Life Extension

Natural Health and Longevity Web Site
http://www.all-natural.com

For some unusual and alternative methods of turning back the hands of time, check this resource on natural life extension, run by the Natural Health and Longevity Resource Center. This resource has an index to articles on everything from holistic techniques for increasing longevity to the secrets of the world's oldest man.

Rejuvenating Data

The Rejuvenation and Longevity Foundation Web Site
http://www.anti-aging.org

This Web site provides a real public service: It synthesizes the latest anti-aging studies into articles that offer clear explanations on new age-reversal technologies in layperson's language. And if you join this nonprofit foundation for $17.50, you can get referrals to local doctors who are on the cutting edge of anti-aging technologies. This site also has a nice glossary of medical terms and an essay on the causes of aging.

Active Living

National Association for Human Development
Washington, DC 20036
(202) 328-2192

This nonprofit organization seeks to help people maintain physical and emotional health and vigor as they age, by conducting research and training programs. It also sponsors community awareness activities, such as "Active People over 60." They publish an assortment of booklets and manuals as well as a quarterly magazine.

Anti-aging

National Council on the Aging (NCOA)
Washington, DC 20024
(202) 479-1200

This is the granddaddy of anti-aging organizations, with scads of useful affiliations, such as the Health Promotion Institute and the National Interfaith Coalition on Aging. If you have a question about almost any aspect of growing old, the NCOA can either answer it or direct you to someone who can. For a $75 annual fee ($45 for retirees), you'll get access to a variety of council publications, such as their quarterly magazine, *Innovations on Aging*, which covers issues and developments in the field of aging.

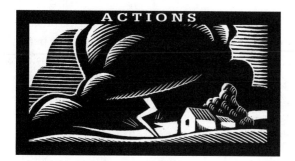

This Year

As time goes by, you'll want to work on long-term strategies to overcome old programming and ways of doing things that will make you look and feel older than you ought to be. Below we've suggested some mental and physical tweakings for you to work on this year. They won't all be easy to do, at least not at first. But stick with it. And don't think of these six actions as ways to waste time—but as ways to gain it instead.

1. **Stay open.** Passing stiff judgment on new trends and fashions is as good as getting on the expressway to Geezerville. Don't be a fuddy-duddy: Work on staying current, learning about what's new and hip, sampling some of the youth culture. "Being open-mined makes available a lot more energy and avoids the drain of negativity," says Ross Goldstein, Ph.D., a psychologist and the author of *Fortysomething: Claiming the Power and the Passion of Your Midlife Years.* That doesn't mean that you have to adopt MTV styles or take up bungee jumping, though. "It means adopting an attitude of curiosity, asking 'What's this all about?'" he adds.

2. **Examine your image of aging.** Do you equate getting older with becoming decrepit? "A lot of our thinking dates back to a time when 50 was considered old," says Dr. Goldstein. Mull that one over. Question the notion that chronological age determines vitality, he says. "There have been scientific, nutritional, and medical advances that allow us to remain quite energetic, productive, and enthusiastic throughout our life spans."

3. **Change your expectations.** Here's a sobering fact for you: People who thought they were destined to suffer from certain diseases died up to four years earlier than those who were more optimistic. A study of male Harvard graduates found that pessimistic participants developed diseases earlier and more severely than did more optimistic guys. That just goes to show you the power of your mind-set. Which one would you rather have?

4. **Look on the bright side.** Another argument for the power of positive thinking: Who cares that you don't wear size-32-waist pants anymore? It's better to think about what you have going for you now, says Dr. Goldstein. "Consider all the things that you do better now than when you were 20, how much more you know, and how much you have going for you as a result of maturity," he says. Focus on the benefits of aging—such as being 10 steps ahead of all those young bucks your company keeps hiring straight out of college.

5. **Don't get smoked.** Smoking may preserve meats, but it sure won't help you. Not only can smoking end your life prematurely, it can make you look older than you are while you're still alive. Preliminary results of one test conducted in Great Britain suggest a link between smoking and premature hair changes in people under the age of 50. Another study has shown that smoking may accelerate that process in men, causing their biological age to be older than their chronological age. And still another study followed 606 outpatients over the age of 30 for more than three months: Of the 152 men who smoked, 92 percent were either gray or bald, compared to 84 percent of the 112 nonsmoking men.

6. **Tackle the unknown.** If you want to live longer, keep the novelty factor in life high. Novelty is important, says Zaven Khachaturian, Ph.D., director of the Ronald and Nancy Reagan Institute for Research, part of the Alzheimer's Association, headquartered in Chicago. "Do things that are challenging, new, and different," he says. So, if you've wanted to learn fly-fishing ever since you saw *A River Runs through It*, now may be the time to cast your line.

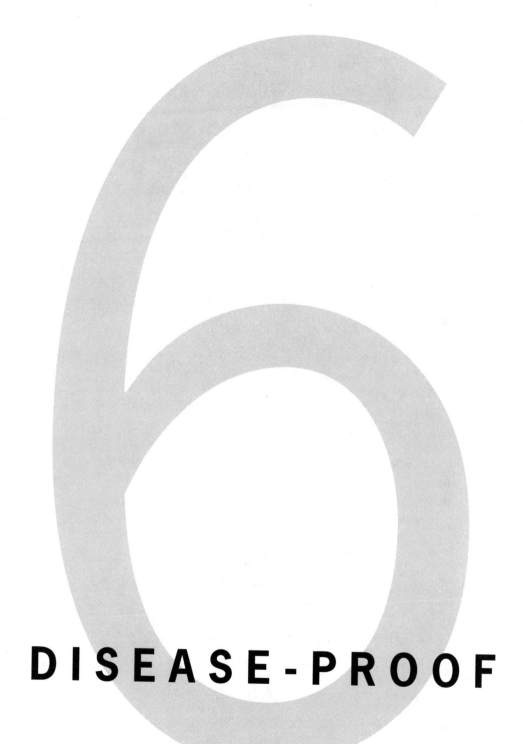

DISEASE-PROOF

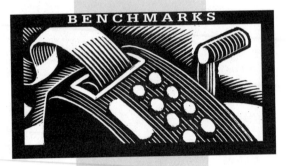

BENCHMARKS

AVERAGES

■ Average amount of time heart disease strikes earlier in people who are overweight: 1.9 years

■ ...in people who smoke: 3.1 years

■ ...in people with high blood pressure: 4.9 years

■ ...in people who don't exercise regularly: 5.7 years

■ Percentage of adults who smoked in 1964 when the first surgeon general's warning against smoking was issued: 40.3

■ Percentage of adults who smoke now: 25

■ Average number of young people who try cigarettes for the first time each day: 6,000

■ Number of the world's most polluted cities that are in Asia: 5

■ Percentage of overweight people in New Orleans: 38

■ Percentage of men who use multivitamins on a regular basis: 35

EXTREMES

■ Average number of neuro-active drugs that counterculture guru Timothy Leary ingested each day before he died of cancer: 8

■ The shortest life of a body cell: three days for cells found in the gut

■ The longest-living body cell: brain cells, which can last a lifetime

■ Most gallstones ever removed from a single gallbladder: 23,530

■ Cost of seven-year research conducted by R. J. Reynolds on the "smokeless" cigarette, Premier: $325 million

■ Amount of time Premier was on the market: four months

VITAL READING

Are Coronaries Contagious?

New research is finding that you might be able
to catch a heart attack just like a cold.

What if heart disease were not primarily caused by a lifestyle of excess? What if it had very little to do with cigarettes, alcohol, rich food, or laziness? What if the condition that provokes it (that is, the gradual blocking of arteries) were really the insidious work of a virus or bacterium that was passed from victim to victim—much like the common cold—by way of coughs, sneezes, and handshakes? And most important: What if the cure were as simple as getting an injection?

Such speculation may be closer to reality than you think, considering the mounting evidence from researchers around the world. "We're talking about the major killer in Western society and one that affects men in particular," says J. Thomas Grayston, M.D., professor of epidemiology at the University of Washington in Seattle, who has been involved in some of the most provocative studies to date. "If an organism could be found that was important in the cause of the disease, and if it was susceptible to known antibiotics, it could make a big difference."

The Pesky Pest

The chief suspect, so far, is a microorganism called *Chlamydia pneumoniae*. It's a different species of the same bug responsible for several sexually transmitted diseases. As its name suggests, this version is a common cause of pneumonia and other respiratory ailments, such as bronchitis and sinusitis. Everyone is probably infected by it at some point in his life, Dr. Grayston says. In fact, researchers speculate that each of us may be reinfected two or three times.

Scientists began to suspect a link between viruses or bacteria and arteriosclerosis (thickening and hardening of the arteries) in the late 1980s, when researchers in Finland detected *C. pneumoniae* while screening for infectious agents in heart patients. Then Dr. Grayston and his colleagues made their own remarkable discovery: When they looked at 56 samples of diseased coronary artery tissue, they succeeded in identifying the *C. pneumoniae* strain in 32 of them. But when they examined 31 healthy tissue samples, there was no sign of the bacterium. Other laboratories have since confirmed these findings.

The mystery (and the subject of much speculation and debate) is what role, if any, this microorganism plays in arteriosclerosis. There are three basic theories. Dr. Grayston surmises that white blood cells, the body's natural impurity police, ingest this bacteria/virus hybrid while it's in the respiratory system and innocently transfer it to other sites. (He has found evidence of it not only in diseased arteries but also in the livers, spleens, and lymphatic systems of men.) Since white blood cells are drawn to the body's trouble spots, any damage or problem in an artery wall would attract a legion of them. It's at this time, Dr. Grayston speculates, that the microorganism is somehow transferred, causing an infection that results in fat or cell buildup within the artery. This buildup may eventually lead to a blockage, which causes a heart attack.

A second theory suggests that this bug is not so much an underlying, stage-setting cause of artery disease as it is a trigger for a heart attack. In other words, its arrival in an already scarred and narrowed artery causes complications, such as additional inflammation, that prompt the blockage of that artery.

A final explanation, skeptics say, is that the presence of this microorganism is simply a coincidence. They argue that *C. pneumoniae* is nothing more than an innocent bystander that has been drawn to the site of an accident. And they point out that it's not unusual for diseased tissue to contain organisms that have no connection to the disease.

"The bottom line is that we just don't know for certain," admits Dr. Grayston, who is conducting animal studies and hoping to raise several million dollars for human clinical trials. "It's going to take more careful study before we can reach any conclusions."

An Idea That's Spreading

Even if *C. pneumoniae* turns out to be a false lead, the whole concept of infectious causes of certain chronic diseases remains an intriguing one. Stephen Epstein, M.D., chief of cardiology at the National Heart, Lung, and Blood Institute of the National Institutes of Health in Bethesda, Maryland, has been examining a member of the herpes family, called a cytomegalovirus (CMV), which may also play a role in arteriosclerosis. In fact, it has been suggested that immunization with a CMV vaccine could prevent artery disease altogether. Also being examined by experts for having possible infectious causes are arthritis, multiple sclerosis, irritable bowel syndrome, stroke, and even schizophrenia.

If all this seems out of the realm of reason, consider the fact that stomach ulcers, long thought to result from factors such as stress, spicy food, and too much smoking and drinking, are frequently caused by bacteria, specifically a spiral-shaped bug called *Helicobacter pylori*. This microorganism is transmitted via contaminated water, lives in the stomach for years, and, when given the opportunity, corkscrews itself into the intestinal lining, thus creating an inflammation. *H. pylori* is the cause of 80 percent of all gastric ulcers and 90 percent of all duodenal (upper intestinal) ones. Armed with such revolutionary knowledge, doctors can now detect its presence with a simple, 5-minute blood test and chase it from the body with common antibiotics.

"Who would have believed a few years ago that ulcers were an infectious disease?" asks David Spodick, M.D., professor of medicine at the University of Massachusetts Medical School and director of clinical cardiology at nearby St. Vincent Hospital, both in Worcester. "People laughed at those doctors in Australia who originally proposed it. But they were right."

Indeed, we may be on the verge of a revolutionary shift in medical thinking. Perhaps chronic diseases will increasingly be viewed as epidemics rather than persistent scourges. It might be more accurate, Dr. Grayston believes, to look upon coronary heart disease as an epidemic of the last 100 years. "It first became recognized in this country in the early part of this century, intensified through the 1940s and 1950s, peaked maybe 15 years ago, and has been on the wane ever since," he explains. But only about half of this decline, in his estimation, is attributable to lifestyle changes such as controlling dietary fat and cholesterol, getting more exercise, and cutting back on alcohol and tobacco. The other half is unexplained—except when you consider that it coincides with a widespread rise in the use of broad-spectrum antibiotics, which kill a variety of viruses and bacteria.

"It's intriguing speculation," Dr. Grayston says, "but I doubt whether avoiding heart disease and arteriosclerosis would ever be as simple as just getting a shot of tetracycline from your doctor. It would probably involve a combination of lifestyle changes and treatment."

"I don't think *C. pneumoniae* will turn out to underlie all or most of coronary artery disease," agrees Dr. Spodick. "Though it would be fortunate if it turned out to be a principle mechanism, it's probably one of a series. No doubt its investigation is just going to accelerate from here."

Defensive Measures

Rally your immunologic troops and stop cold,
flu, and major illness in their tracks.

As you read this, millions of tiny, vigilant warriors are marching through your bloodstream, tissues, and bodily fluids. There are generals, the T cells, who not only command their own forces but also issue orders to the body's brain and hormonal branches of service as well. There are intelligence officers, the B cells, who "fingerprint" invaders and devise targeted weaponry. There are look-outs, macrophages, who go around rooting out intruders and sounding the alarm. There are foot soldiers, the neutrophils, who come when summoned and kill as requested. And there are pockets of special forces, the natural killers, white blood cells who search and destroy viruses and tumors according to their own rules.

As diverse as these troops are, they have one common enemy: aging. After immunity peaks at about age 20, a gland in the neck called the thymus (a T cell academy of sorts) starts to shrink, graduating fewer and fewer future leaders. The older T cells count their stars and put their feet up. The B cells begin to lose their powers of perception, mistaking friend for foe and foe for friend. The rank and file thins out, and even the natural killers begin to lose their taste for adventure. The result is an increased susceptibility to infection, cancer, and autoimmune diseases such as rheumatoid arthritis.

Using simple measures, you can call your immune system back to arms. Research suggests that lifestyle changes, including exercising and eating less fat, can rejuvenate aging immune systems. And new fields of investigation into supplemental hormones such as DHEA (dehydroepiandrosterone) and herbal elixirs such as echinacea suggest additional means of refortification.

"It's how well we look after ourselves that decides how well our immune systems look after us," says Terry Phillips, D.Sc., Ph.D., director of the immuno-chemistry laboratories at the George Washington University Medical Center in Washington, D.C. So we asked experts in fields as diverse as psychology, nutrition, and exercise science to give you the latest advice on reviving your immunologic corps.

The Gatekeepers

Your first line of defense against contagious diseases, such as colds and flus, is a squadron of special proteins that are secreted by glands in the mouth and respiratory system. The higher your level of these proteins, called immunoglob-ulins (IgA), the better your chances of stopping viruses and bacteria before they cause a single symptom.

Take it easy. Anything that combats stress, whether that be meditation, reading a book, or getting a hug, increases IgA levels. Researchers have observed a spike in IgA levels in older people following a massage.

The Special Forces

Although most immune cells report back to and take orders from the T cells, one group, called natural killers, destroys according to its own rules. These cells circulate through the bloodstream and tissues hunting for viruses, foreign particles, and cancer cells, which they kill on contact. Many researchers believe that those with strong natural-killer forces can destroy small tumors. Try this to rally your renegades.

Fill up on garlic. Legend has it that in sixteenth-century Marseilles, during the peak years of the bubonic plague, four condemned criminals were forced to bury the infected dead. How did they keep themselves from catching the disease? By drinking a now infamous concoction of red wine and raw garlic.

Beyond recharging these killers, garlic provides natural antiviral, antibacter-ial, and antifungal compounds that researchers are just beginning to understand.

So how can you take advantage of garlic's full potential? Most experts agree that eating a recently chopped clove of raw garlic daily provides the cheapest, simplest immunity insurance. But if you can't stand the smell or balk at the taste, opt for an "aged garlic extract," such as Kyolic, advises Earl Mindell, Ph.D., professor of nutrition at Pacific Western University in Los Angeles and author of *Garlic: The Miracle Nutrient.* These formulations contain garlic that has been naturally cold-aged for up to 20 months to increase the potency of some benefi-cial chemicals.

Get plenty of sleep. When researchers cheated 23 men in a sleep laboratory out of 5 hours of sleep for four consecutive nights, they observed a 30 percent reduction in natural-killer-cell activity. Fortunately, it took just one good night's sleep (8 hours) to boost those cells back to fighting strength.

The Weapons Experts

Various types of T cells can mobilize a diverse array of forces when alerted to invading particles by large, jagged cells called macrophages. After you have reached adulthood and the thymus shrinks, there isn't much you can do to replace most T cells. You can intensify their power, however, by increasing the numbers of their right-hand men, the B cells. When alerted to trouble, these weapons' specialists manufacture made-to-order chemicals called antibodies that lock on to the invaders, making them easy targets for other immune forces. Here's how to give B cells a boost.

Pop a pill. Various studies have found that vitamins A, C, and E, plus zinc and copper, all supercharge B cells to make more antibodies. In one study, people over 60 who consumed a multivitamin daily for a year showed higher antibody responses to a flu vaccine than those who didn't take a pill. All had good, healthful "baseline" diets, leading researcher John Bogden, Ph.D., professor of preventive medicine at New Jersey Medical School in Newark, to speculate that older folks may need extra nutrients for optimal immune functioning.

Eat yogurt. Not all bacteria are bad; some, in fact, may help fortify your immune system. In one Italian study in which older adults downed capsules of *Lactobacillus acidophilus* and *Bifidobacterium bifidum* four times a day, researchers found a marked increase in the activity of B cells. And *L. acidophilus* redoubles its immune-boosting effects by producing four antibiotics of its own.

While supplementing with these helpful bugs is a good idea if you've just survived a bout of diarrhea or taken a course of antibiotics, a cup or two of yogurt daily is all it takes for most of us to keep our beneficial internal flora thriving.

The Grunts

Once an antibody has an invader bound and gagged, a cell called a neutrophil is summoned to polish it off. You can help your tiny terminators grow with the following tips.

Work out. Although heavy exertion can put a damper on the immune system, regular moderate exercise can be a real boon. "There's evidence that, in people who exercise moderately for up to 60 minutes a day, neutrophil function is elevated for as long as 9 hours," says David Nieman, Dr. P.H., director of health degree promotion in the department of health, leisure, and exercise science at Appalachian State University in Boone, North Carolina.

Stay away from sugar. Researchers have found that eating 100 grams of sugar (the amount in, say, a piece of cherry pie or two large sodas) on an empty stomach can dramatically suppress activity of neutrophils for up to 5 hours. "Sugar can act almost like a drug in our systems," says Ann Louise Gittleman, author of *Get the Sugar Out*. She suggests cutting back on sugar consumption and making sure that when you do indulge, it's at a meal that includes nonsugary foods and fiber.

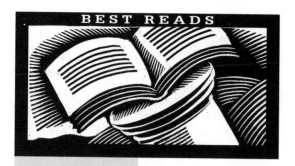

BEST READS

For Those at Risk
for Cardiovascular Disease

Andrew Weil, M.D., is at it again. Following on the heels of his 1995 bestseller, Spontaneous Healing, *comes his latest book,* Eight Weeks to Optimum Health *(Alfred A. Knopf, 1997). From being on the cover of* Time *magazine to appearing on talk shows, Dr. Weil is one of the most visible health professionals in the United States. In this excerpt from his new book, he tackles the problem of America's biggest killer.*

Cardiovascular disease is the number one killer in our society, producing a great deal of disability as well as premature death, and absorbing countless health care dollars. Its incidence rises sharply with age, affecting men earlier in life than women. Cardiovascular disease causes not only heart attacks and strokes (which might be better thought of as "brain attacks" because there are not emergency treatments for them that can be lifesaving if given with the same urgency as that with which we treat cardiac disasters) but also kidney failure, pain and gangrene in the lower extremities, and mental disability. The underlying disease process—arteriosclerosis (literally "hardening of the arteries")—damages arterial walls, making them inelastic, thick, and rough, eventually narrowing the channel within and decreasing blood flow. One component of this process is atherosclerosis, the deposition of fat and cholesterol in the walls of arteries, but the exact relationship between it and the larger disease is not clear. Arteriosclerosis is clearly a hazard of lifestyle, silent during its development, and of early onset in many people. Its prevention must be a high priority in any program designed to maintain optimum health.

It is clear that arteriosclerosis is multifactorial in origin. Among the contributing causes are heredity, diet, stress, lack of exercise, and toxins. The Eight-Week Program addresses all of these areas except heredity, of course, but in this customized plan I want to give you additional suggestions for prevention.

Projects

• Don't smoke, and don't inhale secondhand smoke. Nicotine directly affects arteries and is, in fact, one of the best-known toxins that accelerate arteriosclerosis; it is also a highly addictive drug. Besides nicotine, tobacco smoke contains other elements that undermine the health of arteries and many organs. If you smoke, set a date to quit, using any and all methods available to help you do so. If you live or work with smokers, do whatever you can to get them to quit or confine their smoking to the outside. If those strategies fail, protect yourself with an air filter.

• Never drink water that tastes of chlorine. Order bottled water if you are out, and protect yourself at home with a water-purifying system. As a powerful oxidizing agent, chlorine is another common toxin that promotes arteriosclerosis.

Diet

Very recently, the homocysteine theory of arteriosclerosis, first proposed decades ago, has begun to gain support from medical researchers. In brief, it states that homocysteine, an amino acid produced by the metabolic breakdown of methionine, an essential component of dietary protein, is an independent risk factor for cardiovascular disease, one that may turn out to be more important than serum cholesterol. Animal protein delivers significantly more methionine than plant protein, which may explain why vegetarians are less likely to suffer from arteriosclerosis even though they eat more fat than some doctors think they should. The production and disposition of homocysteine are controlled by three B vitamins: pyridoxine (B_6), cyanocobalamin (B_{12}), and folic acid. Mainstream Western diets, with their overloads of animal protein and deficiencies of fresh fruits and vegetables, may fail to provide enough of these vitamins to handle the amounts of homocysteine generated and clear them from the blood. I am much impressed by this theory and the history of rejection by the "cholesterol establishment"; I recommend watching for reports of experiments designed to confirm it.

• Tests for serum homocysteine are just becoming available. The normal value ranges around 10.0 micromoles per liter but must be adjusted for sex and age. If you have a family history of cardiovascular disease, ask your doctor to check your serum homocysteine.

• The dietary recommendations that follow from the homocysteine theory will be familiar to you from the Eight-Week Program. Note that they also may explain the effectiveness of the drastic diets that have been used to reverse atherosclerosis (fat reduction to 10 percent of calories or less, elimination of animal foods, and emphasis on fruits and vegetables). If homocysteine is really a major culprit, you may be able to relax about fat, enjoying the olive oil and salmon I recommend, and protecting yourself in other ways. Those ways are:

Reducing animal protein in the diet as much as you can. Moderate consumption of fish is okay. In fact, since vitamin B_{12} comes only in nonplant foods, some fish (or nonfat or low-fat dairy products) is desirable.

Eating plenty of fresh fruits and vegetables, including cooked greens, which are major sources of folic acid.

Increasing consumption of dietary fiber by replacing refined grains with whole grains as much as possible: less white bread, more whole-grain bread; less white rice, more brown rice.

Reducing consumption of white sugar and sweets in general. Diets high in sugar are most likely to be deficient in protective factors.

Reducing consumption of packaged and highly processed foods, which are similarly deficient. A heart- and artery-healthy diet must emphasize fresh foods, always your best sources of vitamins and minerals.

• Include in your diet as many protective factors as you can that reduce risk of cardiovascular disease by other mechanisms: garlic, onions, hot peppers, green tea, shiitake mushrooms, salmon, and sardines (or flax). All of them improve serum-lipid profiles and help keep serum cholesterol in safe ranges.

• If you drink coffee, try to switch to tea, especially green tea, which is much better for the cardiovascular system. At least substitute green tea for some of the coffee you drink.

• Remember to enjoy your food! A diet that is healthy for the heart and arteries can also be diverse and delicious. If you make yourself miserable through deprivation, your spirits will suffer, and you will not be experiencing optimum health.

Supplements

• For insurance against elevated serum homocysteine, take a B-complex vitamin supplement every day. I recommend a B-100 brand. Read the label to make sure it provides 100 milligrams of vitamin B_6 and 400 micrograms of folic acid. (Note that one of the components of this supplement, vitamin B_2, or riboflavin, will color your urine bright yellow for a few hours, a harmless change.)

• Be sure to take the recommended dosage of antioxidants. More studies support the role of vitamin E in preventing atherosclerosis, probably by protecting LDL (low-density lipoprotein, or "bad") cholesterol from oxidation. Vitamin C may protect the integrity of arterial walls, reducing their susceptibility to damage by whatever injurious factors may be circulating in the blood.

• Follow a low-dose aspirin regimen to reduce the chance of abnormal blood clotting. I recommend 162 milligrams a day—half of a standard tablet or two of the low-dose 81-milligram tablets.

• If you have any heart problems or a family history of them, take 100 milligrams a day of coenzyme Q_{10} (CoQ_{10}), a natural product that increases oxygen utilization by heart muscle cells. You will find this supplement in health food stores; shop around for the best value and the highest dosage form you can find so that you do not have to take more than one pill a day. (A side benefit of coenzyme Q_{10} is improved health of gums.)

• Do not take supplemental iron unless you have iron-deficiency anemia, diagnosed by blood tests. Iron is a risk factor for arteriosclerosis, by virtue of being an oxidizing agent that can increase oxidation of cholesterol into more harmful forms. Read labels of any multivitamin/mineral supplement you use to be sure it does not contain iron.

Exercise

• Do not neglect the exercise component of the Eight-Week Program. Regular aerobic exercise helps maintain normal weight pressure, increases the efficiency of the heart as a pump, and preserves normal elasticity of arteries. It is a key preventive strategy to reduce the risk of cardiovascular disease. Walk!

Mental/Spiritual

• Stress raises serum cholesterol and blood pressure and renders the arteries more susceptible to spasms that can initiate heart and brain attacks. Practice techniques of stress reduction and relaxation.

• Learn to control toxic emotions, especially rage when frustrated, which appears to pose a particular risk for the cardiovascular system. Psychotherapy, counseling, group work, and relaxation training can all be helpful.

• Practice loving yourself whenever you can; this is the basis for being able to have loving relationships with others. Consider that the heart first pumps oxygen-rich blood to itself through the coronary arteries, then sends it to the rest of the body. If it did not do so, it would be unable to supply all the needs beyond it. Self-love is not selfishness or self-centeredness but the basis for extending love beyond yourself. Here is a version of the Buddhist meditation on *metta* (loving-kindness), which you can memorize and recite silently if it appeals to you, envisioning your love extending to each widening circle in turn. Note how it begins.

My heart fills with loving-kindness. I love myself. May I be happy. May I be peaceful. May I be liberated.

May all beings in this vicinity be happy. May they be happy. May they be liberated.

May all beings in (name your place of residence) be happy. May they be peaceful. May they be liberated.

May all beings in (name your state or region) be happy. May they be peaceful. May they be liberated.

May all beings in (name your country) be happy. May they be peaceful. May they be liberated.

May all beings in (name your continent) be happy. May they be peaceful. May they be liberated.

May all beings on the planet be happy. May they be peaceful. May they be liberated.

May my parents be happy. May they be well. May they be peaceful. May they be liberated.

May my friends be happy. May they be well. May they be peaceful. May they be liberated.

May my enemies be happy. May they be well. May they be peaceful. May they be liberated.

If I have hurt anyone, knowingly or unknowingly, in thought or word or deed, I ask their forgiveness.

If anyone has hurt me, knowingly or unknowingly, in thought or word or deed, I extend my forgiveness.

May all beings everywhere, whether near or far, whether known to me or unknown to me, be happy.

May they be peaceful. May they be liberated.

Not a bad way to start the day. Give it a try.

Rx: Exercise

Feeling sick and tired too often?

Suffering chronic bouts with illness and infections? Have high blood pressure? Unhealthy cholesterol readings? Diabetes? Are you stressed out?

Ready to do something about it?

Take the exercise prescription.

As Richard Laliberte and Stephen C. George explain in this excerpt from The Men's Health Guide to Peak Conditioning *(Rodale Press, 1997), a regular workout routine can be a formidable shield against a host of afflictions.*

Okay, okay. It's true. Yes, even men who exercise religiously get sick at times. Some bully bacteria or virulent virus pounces when their guard is down.

But, you know what? Men who exercise get sick much less often than men who do not.

They have fewer sniffles, fewer aches, pains, fevers, colds, flus, infections, heart attacks, and so on.

They feel better, more vibrant. Their minds, muscles, and moods all function more effectively. Stressful situations don't faze them much. Their immune systems are stronger and more efficient.

And when they get sick, they bounce back fast.

We haven't created a special workout for disease prevention, since most any regular exercise routine will bolster your immune system. Instead, we'll explain how exercise affects your body's disease-fighting tools.

The Exercise Prescription

In 1995, two of the nation's preeminent health watchdog groups—the federal government's Centers for Disease Control and Prevention (CDC) in Atlanta and the American College of Sports Medicine in Indianapolis—issued a joint statement that gave formal endorsement to the exercise prescription. The statement formally marked a fundamental shift in the way the medical community views the role of exercise.

"They examined a persuasive body of scientific evidence and concluded that regular moderate physical activity is an important component of a healthy lifestyle—helping to prevent disease and enhance quality of life," says Jonathan Robison, Ph.D., an exercise physiologist, nutritionist, and executive co-director of the Michigan Center for Preventive Medicine in Lansing.

The exercise prescription is flexible, says Dr. Robison. You don't have to buy a stairclimber or take part in sports you don't like. All you have to do is accumulate a minimum of 30 minutes of moderate-intensity physical activity several days per week, he says.

"Let people know that they can garden, walk the dog, and so forth—they don't have to work out on stairclimbers and stationary bikes and treadmills to be healthy," says Dr. Robison.

The CDC and American College of Sports Medicine doctors determined that just 30 minutes of exercise—even if gathered in little snippets throughout the day—is enough to make us healthier and more disease resistant if done regularly.

"For the general population, we can probably be a little less obsessive about how high our heart rates are while we exercise or how long we're going for at a time, and focus more on just moving and having a good time and getting our breathing and heart rates up a bit," says Dr. Robison. "The recommendation for maintaining health is to accumulate 30 minutes of moderate physical activity most days of the week. All that really matters is that it's movement and that it is burning calories. You can walk for 30 minutes three times a week, or walk for 10 minutes nine times a week and probably get similar health benefits."

This is a recommendation for general health and, for instance, should not replace rehabilitative exercise routines prescribed for men following heart attacks or other specific conditions, notes Dr. Robison.

The best fitness routine mixes up lots of exercise types to make sure that you achieve all three tenets of fitness: strength, endurance, and flexibility. It turns out that that apparently is the best formula for disease resistance as well. "Mixing aerobic and resistance training may offer the greatest, long-term health benefits," says Dr. Robison.

But don't overdo it, cautions Charles Swencionis, Ph.D., head of the health psychology program at Yeshiva University in New York City and co-author of *The Lazy Person's Guide to Fitness*. "Exercise that is moderate will increase resistance to disease. But overdoing it to the point of exhaustion is not going to help the immune system," he says.

And, he cautions, don't overwork the heart when exercising. If your heart is pumping faster than usual—fast enough that you start to sweat in a few minutes—and yet not so hard that you can't breathe comfortably or carry on a conversation, you're in the right zone.

Why It Works

Here's why the exercise prescription works.

• Quite simply, "exercise is what the body is designed to do," says Dr. Swencionis. "It is not designed to sit at a desk, or use a computer, or ride in a bus, or drive a car. It's made for walking around, hunting game on the plains of Africa. That's really the kind of thing the body needs to do. When you deprive it of adequate physical activity, it develops all kinds of illnesses."

• The chemistry of the body is affected by exercise. The type and quantity of brain chemicals and hormones released changes—for the better—in a regularly exercised body. That, in turn, affects all sorts of systems. We produce more of a blood clot–dissolving substance. Our cholesterol balances change, making our blood thinner and easier for our hearts to pump. Our blood also is redder, more pumped up with fresh oxygen, bringing more life to each cell. We tax our immune systems less, thus they are more prepared for a major fight. And on and on and on.

• We make energy differently, more efficiently, when we're fit. We also tap into different fuel stores, particularly the fat stored around the belly.

• We lose weight, and that makes a difference in how our bodies work. "Aerobic exercise (combined with a low-fat diet) lowers high blood pressure and cholesterol and controls diabetes. Just a loss of 10 to 15 pounds can mean you can stop taking drugs for these conditions, or take much lower doses," says Dr. Swencionis.

• Aerobic exercise increases our sense of well-being, lessens tendencies toward depression and anxiety, and puts the brakes on immune-dampening reactions to stress.

Improve Cholesterol Levels

You probably know that HDL (high-density lipoprotein) cholesterol wears the white hat and LDL (low-density lipoprotein) wears the black one. But it's really not quite that simple, explains Covert Bailey, a popular fitness writer, in his book *Smart Exercise*.

Our bodies *need* cholesterol to digest fat and to manufacture male and female hormones, he says. But too high of an LDL cholesterol level is damaging. And too low of an HDL level is not good either. Physicians, says Bailey, recognize high levels of HDL cholesterol as a sign of good health.

So that's our goal with the exercise prescription—to raise the HDL and, maybe, to lower the LDL. If you have trouble keeping track of which is which, think of H as standing for healthy, and L as standing for lousy. It's a bit of an oversimplification, but a good memory trick.

The more unfit you are, the quicker and more dramatic improvement you will see in your cholesterol levels when you start exercising, Bailey says. That's encouraging. People who exercise all the time have to work hard to keep improving their cholesterol counts. Out-of-shape people will see improvement if they just start walking.

Low-intensity exercise won't produce great gains in HDL levels, Bailey says, but it will quickly lower LDL levels. And, by getting into the habit of shaking your booty, you may find it easier to make the transition to more vigorous exercise—which *will* raise your HDL, he says.

Lessen Stress Damage

Our bodies are equipped to snap into emergency supercharged mode in an instant in response to stressful situations. Glucose stores are released from the liver, the heart pumps faster, blood vessels to the muscles open wide, as do our pupils—so we can get a better look at what we're confronting or the path on which we're fleeing, notes Dr. Robison. Amino acids are sucked from tissues and burned for fuel.

All this is in response to hormones—like adrenaline—that spurt in response to stress, says Dr. Robison. In an emergency situation, the physical changes give us a tremendous edge. They're sometimes referred to as the fight-or-flight response.

The same physical changes occur, though, in response to emotional stress. Ideally, in an emergency, we use all that energy. We slay the dragon, save the maiden, outrun the attacker, whatever. But, with emotional stress, we just stew. If the stress is chronic, the physiologic changes can be debilitating and destructive to the immune system. Stressed-out people get sick more easily. Add unfit to the equation and you have a real whammy.

The good news, say the experts, is that regular exercise alters how our bodies respond to stressors. Studies show fit people are less flustered by emotional stressors and actually secrete fewer stress hormones in day-to-day stressful situations, says Bailey.

Even better, fit people produce an even more powerful response to unusual stressors, like real danger, than do nonexercisers.

And even better yet, says Dr. Robison, people who exercise regularly are more resistant to depression and anxiety.

Also important, Dr. Robison adds, are rest and relaxation. Exercise, rest, and relaxation all are crucial for optimal functioning of mind, body, and spirit—and optimal functioning is crucial for maximum immunity. The beauty is, it is within our control and reach.

Listening to the Heart

Exercisers have stronger, healthier hearts.

Regular aerobic workouts build powerful, resilient heart muscles. And regular exercise causes the body to create more of its blood-clot dissolving substance and slightly less of its clotting factor. Hearts celebrate both developments. Our hearts don't have to push so hard to pump thinner, cleaner blood.

Are we listening to our hearts? Our hearts want us to exercise.

A program of exercise is carefully designed and prescribed when a man is rebounding from a heart attack. Why wait? A little exercise now, and we may avoid heart trouble altogether.

Just remember Dr. Swencionis's caution not to overdo it—especially if you are not now in the exercise habit. Start slowly and carefully. "Enjoy yourself," says Dr. Robison.

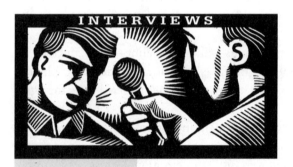

Karen Burke on
Beating Skin Cancer

Freckles on your shoulders that weren't there five years ago. A roughness to your facial skin that you've just started to notice. A mole that's been there since forever, but suddenly it looks larger. We don't want to scare you, but these might be early signals of skin cancer, and knowing about them and other signs of skin cancer can save your life. In fact, the overwhelming majority of deaths from skin cancers every year could be prevented if men took heed of their body's early warning system. Here, Karen Burke, M.D., Ph.D., a dermatological surgeon in private practice in New York City, discusses what you can do to protect yourself against skin cancer and what researchers are doing today to fight it in the future.

Who is more at risk for skin cancer: the man who works outside all day or the man who works at a desk but goes to the beach in the summer and gets burned?

That's a good question, because each person thinks it's the other one who's going to get cancer. The truth is that it's total exposure that, in the end, can do the most damage. Even though a suntan will actually provide you with some sun protection—comparable to wearing sunscreen with a sun protection factor (SPF) of 2 or 3—it's not enough to save you from the long-term damage from the sun.

Genetics play the biggest role in determining whether you're going to get skin cancer. Blacks and those with Mediterranean coloring (dark hair and olive complexions) aren't as susceptible, but anyone who gets a blistering sunburn will double his chance of getting skin cancer. The most important thing you can do is avoid the midday sun and always wear a sunscreen with an SPF of 25 to 30 that you reapply often.

The same thing is true of children, by the way. Since we can't keep our children indoors all the time, we should at least make sure that they don't get sun exposure without protection. While infants should never be exposed to the sun, you can start using sunscreen on your children at four months of age. Unfortunately, I think the rise we are now seeing in skin cancers is due to the early ages at which we're getting sunburns, especially because we travel more than previous generations and we take our children. For instance, in winter we take our children skiing, which involves reflected sun, or to hot, sunny climates to escape winter weather. Don't go outside in the midday and don't let your kids play outside in the midday. Instead, let them go out in the early morning and late afternoon. If you must go out, slip on a shirt, slap on a hat, and slop on some sunscreen to protect yourself.

A lot of men are scared of what might happen if they find something suspicious on their skin, especially if its on their faces. How does skin cancer advance from a spot on your skin to a deadly cancer?

We can never be certain about whether a small rough spot or darkening on the skin will become an actual cancer, nor do we know how long it will take to evolve from a precancer to a cancer. That's because we can't be sure of the time between when a person sees something and when he comes in to a doctor's office. Also, each individual and each lesion are different. Factors such as heredity, skin type, and degree of sun damage contribute to the many changes a lesion can go through. That's why, however, it's so important to see a dermatologist regularly. That means once a year from age 25 to 30 onward. It's also a good idea to have your children checked annually if they have a lot of moles. A dermatologist can take note of any areas of the body that should be watched. He'll ask you about past sun damage, because each blistering sunburn doubles your likelihood of developing a skin cancer.

If your doctor is concerned about a lesion on your skin, he'll do a biopsy. In other words, he'll remove some of the tissue and send it to a laboratory where a pathologist will examine the cells to determine whether they are healthy or cancerous. If the biopsy turns up cancer, the dermatologist determines the optimal method of treatment, depending upon the type of cancer, the size, the location (body part or face), and the depth of the lesion. Some cancers are best treated by freezing, while others need to be cut and stitched.

When a dermatologist can't determine where the edges of the cancer are, it's becoming more common to do what's called "Mohs," named for the doctor who developed the technique. We simply cut off the cancerous part sliver by sliver, continuing to check each layer for disease. In this way, we can stop cutting once we get to a healthy area.

All skin cancers start out small. If you have regular examinations, any suspicious lesions can be biopsied immediately and quickly removed, if necessary. You may not even have a scar afterward.

I realize that with the changes in our health care over the past few years, a lot of people rely on their primary care physician to check the spots and growths on their skin, but general practitioners aren't prepared, for the most part, to eyeball or remove things that are really small. Dermatologists, on the other hand, have the instruments to take care of the job more efficiently.

And, by the way, the many lesions that are on your skin that grow quickly and look ugly are not necessarily precancerous or cancerous, but you can only tell which ones are by having them checked and treated.

A big study came out in 1996 that looked at the relationship between selenium and skin cancer. Can you tell us about that?

Selenium is an essential mineral that I advise many people to take because it has a protective effect against sun damage and skin cancer. If you take about 50 to 100 micrograms of selenium every day, you give yourself extra protection against a blistering sunburn. Also, my research and that of other researchers have shown that topically applied L-selenomethionine is more effective than Retin-A (tretinoin) when fighting photoaging. However, this topical selenium preparation is not yet on the market.

The study released in 1996, which was conducted by the Nutritional Prevention of Cancer Study Group, showed that people who had skin cancer already didn't gain a protective effect against recurrences of skin cancer by taking selenium supplements. However, the researchers did show that the selenium provided a major protective effect against other forms of cancer—notably prostate, colorectal, and lung.

Most people don't get enough of this important trace mineral. In fact, many of the people who took part in this study had too little selenium in their diets and were, consequently, deficient in selenium to begin with. It's important to remember, however, that while many people in Florida, for example, don't get enough selenium, Midwesterners can actually get too much. That's because it's abundant in midwestern soil, but not in southeastern soil. So depending on where the majority of the food you eat is grown, you could end up with a selenium deficiency. Selenium is also found in lean beef, wheat germ, seafood, legumes, nuts, and milk products. So, before you start taking supplements, talk to your dermatologist about whether you need selenium.

Are there really skin cancer vaccines being developed?

Very active research is under way to develop a vaccine to treat metastatic melanoma. Early findings show that potentially 25 percent of melanoma patients might benefit and that these patients might be identified by testing each patient when their primary melanoma is surgically removed. In one study of 40 patients, 3 patients had complete responses and 4 patients had partial responses. About a three- or fourfold increase in survival time was found in 89 stage IV (terminal) melanoma patients treated with a vaccine. A variety of experimental vaccines have been tested with encouraging results thus far. One such study showed that vaccine-treated patients survived approximately 50 percent longer than those without it. Several large randomized studies are currently being conducted to establish the true effectiveness of some of these vaccines.

Although melanoma is at the forefront of cancer-vaccine research, there is also a great deal of interest in vaccines for more common tumors of the colon, stomach, pancreas, and prostate. Also, researchers are seeking vaccines to prevent cancers—particularly those caused by viruses (about 10 percent to 15 percent of all cancers). For example, a vaccine to prevent feline leukemia is being used by veterinarians today and a vaccine to prevent hepatitis C, a very carcinogenic virus, is being developed. Other cancers suspected to have viral etiology are masopharyngeal cancer, Burkitis lymphoma, and B-cell lymphoma.

Gerald Fletcher on
Outsmarting Heart Disease

Sobering fact of the century: Cardiovascular disease is the number one killer of men. According to recent statistics, more than 2,600 Americans die of cardiovascular disease every day—that's roughly a million deaths every year. In con-

trast, all forms of cancer combined kill only about half that number of people a year.

While the health you inherit plays a major role in your susceptibility to all diseases, in the end, having a strong, healthy heart is ultimately a result of how you respond to your genes. In other words, you have to think about what you eat, think about how to spend your leisure time, and use your mind to monitor your emotions and your response to stress.

To get perspective on some of the more recent news regarding heart disease, we turned to Gerald Fletcher, M.D., a cardiologist at the Mayo Clinic in Jacksonville, Florida. He also tells how, if worse comes to worst, you can boost your chances of survival during a heart attack.

We've heard a lot about the French Paradox—the fact that the French can eat such high-fat food, yet still be 2½ times less likely to develop heart disease than an American. Why do the French get all the luck?

No one answer has stood out, but we have some good ideas about the factors that seem to protect French men from heart disease. First, and I think most important, they lead less stressful and more laid-back lives than American men. They don't measure success in terms of moving at a fast pace and accomplishing so much. Research has definitely shown the link between stress and high blood pressure and heart disease. Now stress reduction is one of the key components of most heart disease–prevention programs.

Second, the French drink red wine, which contains flavonoids and other related substances. Flavonoids are found in foods and, like vitamin E, act as antioxidants. (Antioxidants are molecules that fight the effects of free radicals, which essentially "rust out" the inside of blood vessels and contribute to various diseases.) There are hundreds of flavonoids in plant foods, and each one seems to provide its own protective effect against various processes that contribute to disease, including hardening of the arteries and tumor growth.

Red wine has numerous flavonoids, but so do many other foods, including fruits and vegetables. Despite a love of cream sauces and beef, the French also manage to consume the recommended daily amounts of fruits and vegetables, something that Americans still don't do.

Finally, the French have a different style of drinking than Americans. It isn't as if red wine is a medicine to be used without limits. They drink a glass or two with dinner, rather than going out and drinking to excess on Saturday night. Moderation is the key to healthy drinking. In fact, drinking too much red wine won't help nearly as much as drinking one or two glasses a day.

Likewise, wine doesn't increase your weight the way beer does. Researchers at the University of North Carolina don't know why, but they have found that wine drinkers have the smallest waistlines when compared to men who don't drink and men who drink beer.

By the way, French people who live more like Americans have American rates of heart disease. The same is true for Japanese men who come to live in the United States. In other words, these nationalities may be genetically predisposed to less heart disease, but it's clear that the American way of life has a detrimental effect on any ethnic group.

We've heard that folic acid, a B vitamin, may help prevent heart disease. Why is this, and how much of it do we need?

Well, even though folic acid, also known as folate, has made a lot of headlines recently because it has been found to prevent some birth defects, the jury is still out on what it can do to prevent heart disease. However, to set the record as straight as possible: Recent studies have shown that people with low levels of folic acid have higher levels of the amino acid homocysteine in their blood. In turn, studies have shown that people with a high level of homocysteine have higher rates of heart disease.

According to the most recent data, when homocysteine levels are high, plaque buildup is more frequent along artery walls. So, to keep your homocysteine levels lower, be sure to eat at least five servings of fruits and vegetables a day. You can also take a multivitamin that has 100 percent of the Daily Value for the B vitamins. Roughly half of American adults get less than the recommended 400 micrograms of folate per day.

As of January 1998, folate will be a part of the national food-enrichment program. It will be added to many grain foods, which already have most of the other B vitamins along with some minerals. Even this addition to the food supply, say most nutritionists, won't guarantee that you'll get the Daily Value. If you want to eat more folate, you'll find it in lentils, oranges, leafy green vegetables, and wheat germ.

We've heard that vitamin E is helpful in preventing heart disease? Is vitamin C as effective?

As of yet, there isn't the same kind of compelling research showing that vitamin C can prevent heart disease. We do know that vitamin C works with the body to help absorb vitamin E—and both are antioxidants—so it's important to get at least the Daily Value of vitamin C, which is 60 milligrams.

If you feel symptoms of a heart attack coming on (chest pressure or full-ness, unusual shortness of breath, or new onset of extreme fatigue), we know that taking an aspirin can help you. Can you take other pain-relieving med-ications, too? Are some better than others?

Taking an aspirin within a few hours of the first chest pain has significantly reduced deaths in heart attack patients. But in fighting heart disease, or even a heart attack, aspirin isn't working as a pain reliever. It's working as a clotting control mechanism, which means that it prevents excessive clotting. So no, other painkillers won't replace aspirin. We recommend taking 325 milligrams of aspirin, which is one tablet, at the first sign of chest pain. Of course, you should also seek immediate medical attention.

The other drug that people often take at the sign of chest pain is nitroglyc-erin, which is a prescription drug that works differently than aspirin. Nitro-glycerin helps dilate or widen the arteries. If you've been prescribed nitroglycerin by your doctor, you should take that *and* an aspirin at the sign of chest pain. Fortunately, nitroglycerin and aspirin can work together to fight off the effects of a heart attack, although nitroglycerin works much more quickly than aspirin.

As of July 1997, American Airlines became the first airline in the United States to equip several of its planes with portable defibrillators. Only three other airlines in the world have them on their planes. If you suffer from heart disease, is it important to try to take planes that carry portable defibrillators?

A defibrillator is an electronic device that helps the heart start pumping in a normal rhythm when the heart has stopped or the heartbeat is rapid or ineffec-tive. Fortunately, the technology is so advanced now that anyone with minimal training can use it to help a person out. Once hooked up to the victim, the state-of-the-art machine knows whether a shock is needed and how powerful that shock needs to be. Some fire and ambulance crews are also being trained to use portable defibrillators, which can increase survival by almost 20 percent, ac-cording to a study done by the Mayo Clinic.

The thing is, if you're going on vacation and have heart disease or are at risk for having a heart attack, it's not a plane that you should worry about but the places where you're going. Suddenly being at a high altitude can cause more of a problem for people with heart disease than a plane, which is pressur-ized. That's because the low oxygen concentration at high altitudes can strain a person's heart. So if you're going to the mountains, for example, you should avoid physical exertion like skiing or hiking for a few days. That will give your heart time to adjust to the new amount of oxygen it's getting. And, of course, most cardiac patients are aware of the dangers of deep-sea diving and scuba diving. Again, the pressure difference and the lower oxygen concentration puts a real strain on your heart.

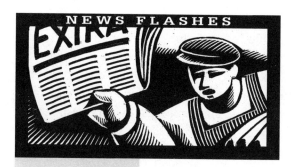

Dark Beer Keeps Arteries Clear

MADISON, Wis.—Here's a good reason to sidle up to the bar and order a Guinness. Dark beer seems to keep blood vessels clear of clots. Obviously, this is great news for beer-lovers who are at risk for coronary artery disease.

Researchers at the University of Wisconsin Medical School used machines and drugs to give anesthetized dogs narrowed, clogged arteries. Eleven of the canines then were given the dark Guinness Extra Stout, while five were given a lighter lager by Heineken. Clot formation was completely prevented in dogs given the dark beer, while the average number of clots in the dogs given the lighter colored beer was only reduced, from seven to four.

Organic compounds called flavonoids, more abundant in the darker beers than in their fairer cousins, may be responsible for the heart-healthy results. Research has shown that flavonoids are the mighty defenders of immunity, battling everything from inflammation to cancer to, yes, heart disease. Also, the alcohol in the beer may deserve some credit. Alcohol has been known to raise levels of good artery-cleansing cholesterol in the bloodstream.

While much research already shows that drinking moderate amounts of alcohol can reduce the risk of heart disease, the Wisconsin study is one of only a handful that looks at whether the color of beer is significant. Though dark beer definitely seems promising, researchers still recommend lowering your risk by reaching for spuds, not suds. Eat plenty of citrus fruits; dark green, leafy vegetables; and yellow and orange vegetables such as sweet potatoes, carrots, and squash.

Pet Iguanas Can Give You Salmonella

ATLANTA—If you keep suffering from bouts of the runs, your kid's pet iguana may be to blame, not the sour milk you put on your cereal this morning. Importation of iguanas climbed from 41,183 reptiles in 1982 to 569,774 in 1994. Alas, so too did the cases of salmonella. The Centers for Disease Control and Prevention (CDC) in Atlanta have now linked a certain type of salmonella infection with owners of iguanas, the most popular reptile pet.

The CDC studied 32 patients infected with this particular strain of salmonella, nearly all of whom suffered from diarrhea. Eighty-eight percent of them were exposed to an iguana the week before their illness. Direct contact was not necessary to contract the infection, nor was having the animal or its cage in an area where food was being prepared. And although most owners washed their hands before and after holding or feeding their reptilian pets, the infection was still transmitted. One patient contracted the infection after eating cake at the home of an iguana-owning family.

Reptile-associated salmonella poisoning affects more men than women, possibly because more men own reptiles and handle them differently than women. If you own a reptile, the CDC recommends the following precautions.

- Always wash your hands after handling your pet and its cage.
- Do not let iguanas roam freely around the house. Especially keep them out of kitchens or other places where food is eaten or prepared.
- Do not bathe your reptile or any of its personal effects in the kitchen sink. If your reptile prefers to bathe in the tub, make sure that you disinfect your tub thoroughly afterward.
- Think twice about owning a lizard if you live with a pregnant woman, young children, or someone with a compromised immune system.

Seeing Red Warrants Visit to Doctor, Survey Warns

PORTLAND, Oreg.—Have you noticed and ignored blood on the toilet paper within the past 6 months? If so, you are among the majority of men who keep themselves as well as their doctors in the dark about a symptom that points to gastrointestinal problems.

A 10-year study conducted at Portland's Veterans Affairs Medical Center and Oregon Health Sciences University looked at 200 men and one woman who had rectal bleeding but didn't seek medical attention. After thorough examination and a 6- to 12-month follow-up visit, the doctors discovered that 47 of the participants had serious gastrointestinal problems. Twenty-six had polyps, 9 had irritable bowel disease, and 13 had colon cancer.

We know you hate seeing the inside of a doctor's office. But if you see blood, you really also should see the doctor. Patients who have noticed blood should be thoroughly examined and then re-examined regularly.

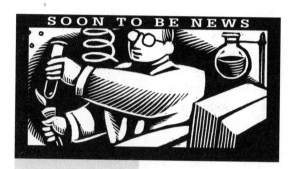

SOON TO BE NEWS

A Warming Trend?

With an overbearing boss, keeping your cool is a good survival tactic. But when you're undergoing the knife, you want to be warm. Research shows that keeping warm during surgery significantly reduces your risk of bleeding, infection, and other postsurgical complications.

Common hospital procedure is to allow a patient's body temperature to cool several degrees, which may promote wound infections, a common complication of anesthesia and surgery. A study conducted at the Thermoregulation Research Laboratory and the department of anesthesia at the University of California, San Francisco, found that warming the body to around its normal temperature decreased the number of infections in patients undergoing colon surgery. As a result, their hospital stays were shorter. Forty-two patients were kept cozy with forced-air covers and warm fluid. Of those 42, only 4 had complications. Of the 38 patients who were operated on with the normal hospital procedure, 9 had postsurgical infections.

The study found that patients with infections were hospitalized one week longer than other patients. The cost of prolonged hospital stays certainly exceeds that of this warming method, which costs about $30 in the United States.

In the future, more hospitals may adopt warming procedures to cut down on surgical complications and longer hospital stays.

Time to Face the Muzak?

Could elevators across America hold the sought-after cure for the common cold? Preliminary research shows an intriguing link between your immune system and Muzak, those airy musical renditions commonly heard on elevators and "on hold" calls.

Researchers at Wilkes University in Wilkes-Barre, Pennsylvania, found that students who listened to Muzak had an increase in immunoglobulins (IgA), antibodies that are major players in fighting off upper-respiratory infections. The students who listened to 30 minutes of the tape, described as "smooth jazz," had a 14.1 percent increase in IgA. Interestingly, students who listened to a radio station playing a similar type of music had an increase of only 7.2 percent. This could mean that some types of music will increase levels, while others will not. Students who were subjected to 30 minutes of silence had a decrease in IgA of 1 percent, and those listening to alternating tones and clicks had a decrease of 19.7 percent, implying a negative effect on the immune system.

The researchers say that their preliminary work could reveal an interesting new mode of defense against various diseases.

The results of this study are so compelling that more research investigating the responsiveness of the immune system to sounds in the environment is planned.

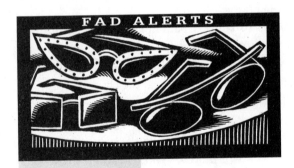

FAD ALERTS

Flu Vaccinations

 We don't know how it was where you live, but around here last winter, everyone was in bed with the flu. And that made many of us start to think: Do we all need vaccinations?

We think so. Each year about 40 million Americans get hit by some strain of influenza—chills, fever, nausea, and congestion—it isn't pretty. It's nothing to sneeze at either. The flu may seem like an everyday kind of illness, but it gives your immune system a real run for the money. The truth is that about 2,000 people each year—mostly the very old and the very young—actually die from the flu. Even a mild case can consign you to bed, with nothing to do but watch *Days of Our Lives* or Oprah—a cruel fate in itself.

Getting a flu vaccination, on the other hand, will likely shield you from these perils. At least one recent study found that when healthy, working adults got a flu shot, they missed almost half as many workdays due to upper-respiratory illness as those who didn't get the shot. The Centers for Disease Control and Prevention in Atlanta recommend the vaccination for people 65 and over, the chronically ill and their families, and all health care professionals. But millions of people actually get the shot each year.

But not everyone is a good flu shot candidate, so it's very important to talk to your doctor about whether it's right for you. For example, people allergic to eggs shouldn't take the vaccine because it's grown in egg-based cultures. There may be some discomfort afterward, too—some people get a fever and minor swelling at the site of the shot. And of course, a lot of people just hate needles. In which case, you'll be glad to know doctors are also developing a flu vaccine that can be administered by nasal spray, which may be even more effective than getting jabbed.

Blue-Green Algae

 Has someone recently tried to sell you pond scum? Did he tell you that it would give you more energy and help detoxify your body? Those are just a couple of the health claims made by the manufacturers of blue-green algae, a dietary supplement sold both in health food stores and by individual distributors. The problem is that there is no documented proof that blue-green algae has any health benefits.

The foul-tasting, expensive capsules (cost: $20 to $40 a month) contain a variety of algae, such as Spirulina, Anabena, and Aphanizomenon. While these are natural, microscopic plants, they are most closely linked, biologically, to bacteria. Sure, they're necessary to the good health of ponds and rivers, but do our bodies need algae? It's doubtful. One of their main ingredients, chlorophyll, isn't even a human nutrient.

"Blue-green algae contains minimal amounts of protein," says Varro E. Tyler, Ph.D., distinguished professor emeritus of pharmacognosy at Purdue University School of Pharmacy and Pharmacal Sciences in West Lafayette, Indiana, and author of *The Honest Herbal*. But that's about the only beneficial nutrient you'll get from it. Dr. Tyler says that most of the people who claim to have more energy as a result of taking blue-green algae are probably kidding themselves.

Saint-John's-Wort

 In Germany, pharmacists fill approximately 30,000 prescriptions each month for Prozac (fluoxetine), that well-known depression lifter. But that's a drop in the bucket compared to how many prescriptions they fill for Saint-John's-Wort, an herb that seems to be particularly useful in fighting mild depressive symptoms. Close to 200,000 prescriptions are filled each month for just *one* brand of the herb.

Saint-John's-Wort, which is also known as hypericum, functions partially as an MAO (monoamine oxidase) inhibitor, much like other antidepressive medications. MAO is an enzyme in the brain that destroys various "feel-good" compounds, such as serotonin, epinephrine, and dopamine. As with other MAO inhibitors, says Dr. Tyler, if you are taking Saint-John's-Wort, you should refrain from drinking red wine, eating strong cheeses and certain beans, or taking ephedra, another herb. There is a slight chance that using Saint-John's-Wort will also make users especially sensitive to sunlight, Dr. Tyler adds, so be sure to use sunscreen while taking it. Also, it's harmful to pregnant women.

You can buy Saint-John's-Wort as a tea, liquid, or in capsules without a prescription (look in health food stores). Look for the word *hypericin* on the label, because that's the active ingredient inside Saint-John's-Wort. Dosages will vary. Follow what's recommended on the label.

However, if you feel that you are suffering from depression, before using Saint-John's-Wort, you really should discuss your symptoms with a physician or psychiatrist. Severe depression warrants special care and medication, and you shouldn't try to deal with it on your own.

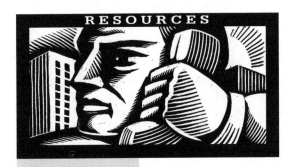

RESOURCES

Safe Water

U.S. Environmental Protection Agency (EPA)
Safe Drinking Water Hotline
(800) 426-4791

Don't drink the water without first checking this EPA hotline. They can answer your questions about federal drinking water laws and send you brochures about drinking water and groundwater issues. And if you're wondering how safe the drinking water in your area is, they'll provide a local contact to give you that information. Call Monday through Friday, 9:00 A.M. to 5:30 P.M. Eastern time.

Sexually Transmitted Diseases

American Social Health Association (ASHA) Web Site
http://sunsite.unc.edu/ASHA

Learn the ABCs of STDs. ASHA's Web site provides information on every sexually transmitted disease from antigens to urethritis. The site also provides a complete list of telephone hotlines nationwide for help with confidential and anonymous questions on sexual diseases. Read current news releases and the latest research on STDs, too.

Headache Relief

National Headache Foundation Web Site
http://www.headaches.org

Here's one example where time spent on the computer might prevent a headache, not cause one. The online Headache Information Center of Chicago's National Headache Foundation (NHF) offers free fact sheets on specific headache conditions, contact information for local support groups, lists of educational materials you can buy, sample articles from the Foundation's newsletter, and general information about the NHF and how it can help. Founded in 1970 by physicians, the NHF is devoted to helping headache sufferers, increasing public awareness of the debilitating effects of headaches, and promoting research into possible causes and treatments.

Lung Problems

National Jewish Medical and Research Center Lung Line
(800) 222-5864

Get the latest facts on asthma, emphysema, bronchitis, and other lung ailments. Operated by the highly respected National Jewish Medical and Research Center (formerly known as National Jewish Center for Immunology and Respiratory Medicine) in Denver, the Lung Line can send you free information on lung, allergic, and immune diseases. You can also get a nurse on line to answer your specific questions.

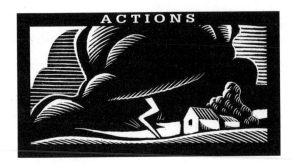

We know, we know, you've heard it all before: Eat lots of fruits and vegetables, be sure to exercise, blah, blah, blah. Underneath those tired old rules, though, is a mountain of other hints that can make a big difference in the quality of your health. Here are 13 of them right now.

1. Tap your feelings out. We're not going to tell you to hit a local Barnes and Noble to buy a journal with poetry quotes on each page. But the next time something frustrates you, sit down at your computer and tap your feelings out on that keyboard. Studies show that people who keep journals (or those who write about traumatic events) visit the doctor less. That's because keeping your feelings inside is a big emotional no-no that can wreak havoc on your immune system. "Disclosing your thoughts and feelings on paper or computer can be especially beneficial to men who otherwise have a tough time sharing their feelings," says James Pennebaker, Ph.D., professor of psychology at Southern Methodist University in Dallas and an expert on the mental and physical health benefits of journal keeping. So think of yourself as Jack Kerouac. Just start writing until you don't feel the need to write anymore. No one's going to read it, so your writing doesn't have to sound perfect or contain good spelling. In fact, you don't even have to save the file.

2. Wash your mouth out. Dental researchers have found that people who suffer from acid reflux (stomach acid coming up to the throat or mouth) have lots of erosion in their teeth. In fact, stomach acid can actually dissolve the mineral structure of teeth. So if you suffer from chronic heartburn or frequently have stomach acid come up to the back of your throat, make it a habit to rinse your mouth with a cup of water. Want to make that rinse even more beneficial? Adding a teaspoon or two of baking soda to 8 ounces of water will neutralize the acid in your mouth, says Esther Rubin, D.D.S., a dentist in private practice in New York City.

Unfortunately, acid reflux doesn't just hurt the stomach (or the teeth). About 50 percent of people who suffer from heartburn several times a week actually have burns on the lining of their esophagus. Of course, trying to fight the heartburn itself, rather than just the tooth decay, will help you solve both problems. So if you have chronic heartburn, talk to your doctor about possible causes and solutions.

3. **Pet a dog.** You talk, she listens. You want to relax, she lies down by your side. You want to go for a walk, she'd open the door for you if she could. Yup. That's what having a dog is like. What's more, if you have a heart attack, she helps you live longer.

It's true. When researchers at Brooklyn College in New York City looked at 369 people who had heart attacks during the previous year, they found that the people who owned dogs fared better than those who didn't. In fact, the death rates differed by 6 percent.

Furthermore, in a study done at the University at Buffalo, researchers found that dogs relaxed men more than the presence of their spouses did. It seems that we all fully understand that a dog won't judge us the way a person will—and that helps us relax.

4. **Drink tea, fight hot dogs.** Tea has strong antioxidant powers—that means it fights off carcinogens and free radicals that can cause cancer cells and other diseases to proliferate in your body. In fact, if a man drinks 3 or more cups of the low-caffeine beverage every day, he will completely block the carcinogenic action found in foods such as hot dogs, salami, and barbecued meat.

Two-and-one-half cups of tea—black, green, or herbal—actually have the same amount of antioxidants as one serving of fruits and vegetables. Tea also seems to help fight heart disease, esophageal cancer, senility, and some bacteria and viruses. Another reason that tea is especially helpful to men is that it fights the absorption of iron, a mineral many men eat too much of.

So why doesn't coffee, that other well-known caffeinated drink, work as well as tea? Because the antioxidants are roasted out of the beans.

Caution: Adding milk to your teacup might negate the potential benefits of the drink. Italian researchers found no discernible antioxidant benefits to tea with milk. They think that the protein in milk makes the antioxidants indigestible. Finally, chemicals specific to black tea seem to help form kidney stones. So if you're prone to them, switch to herbal or green, says John Weisburg, M.D., Ph.D., senior member of the American Health Foundation in New York City. And, drink lots of water.

5. **Sniff Play-Doh.** It will relax you—if you're between the ages of 18 and 68. It seems that smells from childhood help many people feel calm. It's called olfactory-induced nostalgia. So, if you grew up sniffing candy such as Pez and

Sweetarts, Alan R. Hirsch, M.D., neurological director of the Smell and Taste Treatment and Research Foundation in Chicago, says that you can bring it all back by taking a good whiff.

Okay, so Play-Doh's not your thing. Maybe these scents are: If you grew up on the East Coast, then the scent of fresh flowers will bring you back to those heady days of youth. Midwesterners adore the smell of farm animals. Kids from the West Coast favor the smell of meat barbecuing. In the South? Fresh air. Lavender, on the other hand, relaxes almost everyone.

6. **Gassy? Check your gum.** Although it's a great way to clean your teeth after a meal, chewing sugarless gum that contains the sweetener sorbitol can lead to problems with your colon. While our stomachs can't absorb sorbitol, the bacteria in our colons are able to break it down. But that causes the release of gas. Alas, these same bacteria can also cause diarrhea.

The solution: Eliminate anything you eat, chew, or drink that contains sorbitol. Check those labels.

7. **Watch your drugs.** While medicine may rid your body of infections, many prescription and over-the-counter medications can also deplete the body of important nutrients. For instance, laxatives contain mineral oil, and that impedes absorption of all fat soluble vitamins (A, D, E, and K). Some types can also deplete the body of potassium. Other medications can be problems: Diuretics, found in weight-loss and anti-allergy drugs, can rob the body of sodium, calcium, potassium, and magnesium; prescription anticonvulsants deplete vitamins D and K and folate. Lipid-lowerers (cholesterol-fighting drugs) deplete folate, beta-carotene, and vitamins A, B_{12}, D, and K.

While it's probably not a bad idea to supplement with a multivitamin and mineral tablet while you're on medication, be sure to ask your doctor about particular nutrients that you might especially need.

8. **Pull some strings.** We can't say it enough: Flossing is just as important as brushing your teeth when it comes to saving your gums. "Just do it," says Dr. Rubin. It should be a habit. It doesn't only remove food but it removes bacteria that collects daily. And it's bacteria that cause cavities and gum disease. Here's a flossing crash course: Bring the floss up into the gum and scrape down each side of the tooth, using a sawing motion as you go along. You're not trying to clean *the space* between the teeth, Dr. Rubin adds. "You're wiping down the side of the tooth and getting into the gum where the bacteria collect."

9. **Pay attention to your race.** It may not be politically correct to say so, but it so happens that we are somewhat different under the skin. The truth is that African-American men suffer from vitamin D deficiencies much more often than pale white guys, and that might lead to their having higher rates of prostate cancer.

Our bodies manufacture vitamin D from sunlight. One form of the compound, vitamin D_3, has been shown to retard the progression of prostate cancer cells. But men with darker complexions need a lot more sunlight to make enough of vitamin D_3. This is also true, actually, for fair-skinned men over 60. Their bodies don't efficiently absorb D_3.

To remedy this situation, all you need is a few minutes of sunshine (without sunscreen) every day. And don't forget to drink lots of milk; it's usually fortified with vitamin D.

10. **Be a switch-hitter.** Has your back become a pain in the neck? A lot of guys who are stuck at desks all day start to feel twinges in their lower backs over time, but there are a couple of ways to fix that. First, stop sitting so much. It may be difficult, but force yourself to take a walk around the floor every hour or so, says Dan Spengler, M.D., professor and chairman of the department of orthopedics and rehabilitation at Vanderbilt University Medical Center in Nashville. Park further away from the office so that you have to take a few extra steps to get to the building. Going straight from your car to a desk doesn't give your body a chance to loosen up.

Finally, when you get outside for a game of tennis or baseball, switch sides once in a while to prevent a strain. "And if you're a runner, try walking backward on a track for a lap or two," says Joseph Askinasi, a member of the American Academy of Sports Medicine and a chiropractic orthopedist in New York City. "I have recommended this to my back patients for years—and with great success."

11. **Stop licking your lips.** It's always the little things in life that drive you nuts. You have a great job, great woman, great kids, but man...your lips feel like sandpaper. Chapped lips are like an addiction: You lick them to keep them moist, but that just dries them out further. Instead of trying to lick the problem, try switching toothpastes. Some formulas, especially tartar-control pastes, can irritate your lips. Most important, drink lots of fluids. "Dry lips are the number one sign of dehydration," says Dr. Rubin. "It just means that you need to drink more water."

12. **Get a hobby.** Stress is the number two health concern, after prostate cancer, say readers of *Men's Health* magazine. Oddly, one of the best ways to control the stuff that's on your mind is to put your mind to use somewhere else.

In other words, find a hobby that absorbs you so completely that you forget to ruminate on what Smedley did at the office today, or how much it's going to cost to replace that window your kid broke. Make shelves. Build a shed. In fact, if you cultivate a hobby that's also a physical activity, such as gardening or walking, then exercise will become a pleasurable activity, and you won't have to make time in your life for both your hobby and exercise.

Whatever hobby you choose, whether it's stamp collecting or playing touch football on Saturdays, make sure that it isn't watching television. TV can actually make you feel more stressed out because it's so passive and boring. "If you really want to reduce stress in your life and make more leisure time, cut out TV," suggests Earl Mindell, Ph.D., professor of nutrition at Pacific Western University in Los Angeles.

13. **Submit to the scope.** Sorry, but it's true: After 50, you need a colonoscopy. It's only once every five years, and it's worth it. Colorectal cancer kills 27,400 men each year (it's the third-deadliest cancer in men), and those who survive do so with little bowel control. But if you get the test (a tube is inserted into your colon through the rectum), then you have half the chance of developing cancer that progresses to a fatal stage.

To check for colon cancer, a doctor will have you submit a stool sample brought from home, and a laboratory technician will check it for blood. Then, the doctor will insert a flexible sigmoidoscope (a thin tube) into your rectum (it just takes a few minutes) to see if he sees any polyps (there, it's over already).

7

MENTAL
TOUGHNESS

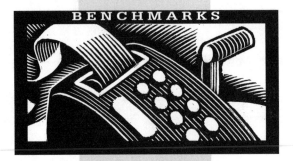

BENCHMARKS

AVERAGES

■ Percentage of Americans who say they are at their best in the morning: 56

■ Watts of power used by the human brain when it is engaged in deep thought: 14

■ Chances that an American "always feels rushed": 1 in 3

■ Percentage of Americans who say they want their boss's job: 29

■ Average number of books a man reads in a year: 12

■ Number of faces the average person learns and remembers throughout his lifetime: 10,000

■ Percentage of Americans who say they have a good sense of humor: 85

■ Percentage of Americans who often feel that they did something exactly right: 55

■ Number of nightmares the average adult has in a year: 1

■ Percentage of Americans who feel overloaded with work: 42

■ Americans who think that their presence at a sports event influences its outcome: 1 in 4

■ Percentage decrease in a household's television viewing after a personal computer is brought into the home: 40

EXTREMES

■ Longest time spent motionless: Radhey Shyam Prajapati stood motionless for 18 hours, 5 minutes, 50 seconds at Ghandi Bhawan, Bhopal, India.

■ Fastest talker: Stephen Woodmore of Orpington, England, spoke 595 words in 56.01 seconds on a 1990 British television program called *Motor Mouth*.

■ Most prolific author: Charles Harold St. John Hamilton, alias Frank Richards, wrote nearly 75 million words during his lifetime in Great Britain.

Handle Stress at Every Turn

Fast-action techniques to stay on top of your game, all day long.

In an age of uncertainty, trust one certainty: You can run but you can't hide from stress. Each day, in fact, is a sort of Darwinian stress test. And on any given day, stress can arrive on an almost hourly basis. Lynda H. Powell, Ph.D., associate professor of preventive medicine and director of the section of epidemiology at Rush–Presbyterian–St. Luke's Medical Center in Chicago, counts 30 "hooks" or "ephemeral events" throughout the day that can gnaw at our peace and equilibrium—niggling little annoyances and aggravations that trigger stress attacks. Dr. Powell breaks them down into the two I's: injustice and incompetence. Injustice: The Super Bowl is interrupted by a meaningless news flash. Incompetence: The IRS has misplaced your appeal for a three-month filing extension.

"Over time, little stressors can make you as ill as big ones—perhaps more," says C. David Jenkins, Ph.D., adjunct professor of psychiatry at the University of North Carolina at Chapel Hill.

A man's only defense against stress is learning to anticipate it and being prepared to manage it when it arrives. So before the cumulative effect of these "stressettes" makes you sick, let's take a look at a typical guy's stress-filled day and some solutions to deal with it.

6:00 A.M.: BBRROOINNGG!! Oh, no, the annual budget report is due at a lunch with Doolittle, your boss. And you have to make the Fairweather presentation to the board this afternoon. And you have to drop the check to your kid's private school in the mail by 5:00 P.M. or his chances at Stanford will look as good as yours for advancement. Worrying generates a steady hum of anxiety, says Daniel Goleman, Ph.D., author of *Emotional Intelligence*. Now, worry is not a bad thing in itself. As a constant vigilance against impending stressors, it's a basic survival instinct. But when it becomes an endless loop, it can trigger what Dr. Goleman calls a neural hijacking.

Studies conducted at Pennsylvania State University in Universtiy Park found that the best way to break the cycle is to catch the fret as near to its beginning as possible. The minute a vision of doom and gloom arises, stop and challenge your concerns. Question their plausibility. Is there really a chance in hell that the dreaded event will happen? What constructive steps can you take to make sure that it doesn't? By becoming aware of it when it starts and applying a dose of healthy skepticism, you can nip worry in the bud.

Right now, there's only one intelligent choice: the snooze button.

6:30 A.M.: Wake the kids. Wake the wife. Put the coffee on. Kiss peace and quiet goodbye. Hello, mayhem. Experts say that there's a key to managing the family rush hour: Expect your children to do the unexpected and you'll never cry bloody murder when they spill the milk—because they will spill the milk. Jon Kabat-Zinn, Ph.D., director of the Stress Reduction Clinic at the University of Massachusetts Medical Center in Worcester and author of books on stress coping and relaxation skills, suggests that you practice what he calls mindful parenting. Before you go to bed, think through the variety of tasks that you and the kids will need the next morning. "Plan what time they go to bed so that you can wake them up with enough time to do everything as unhurriedly as possible," Dr. Kabat-Zinn says. "Whenever you can, get things ready beforehand."

10:00 A.M.: You have 2 hours to finish the budget report for a noon lunch meeting with Doolittle. They don't call you the Joe Montana of the accounting department for nothing. But this is cutting it close. Performing under pressure requires a supreme belief in your ability to, well, perform under pressure. And therein lies the secret: knowing you've been here before and lived to face another pressure performance. Chicago Bulls coach Phil Jackson shares this tip he culled from Michael Jordan, perhaps the league's preeminent pressure player: "He often calls up images of past successes in his mind during high-pressure situations," says Jackson. "Rather than cloud his mind with negative thoughts, he says to himself, 'Okay, I've been here before,' then tries to relax enough to let something positive emerge."

12:05 P.M.: You put the finishing touches on the report and race downstairs to meet Doolittle for lunch. By the time you arrive at the restaurant, butterflies the size of pterodactyls are practicing maneuvers in your stomach. You can't afford to further upset your already-upset stomach. You're going to need the blood that would ordinarily flow to your digestive system to head to your brain, which will be working on overdrive. "I've seen a lot of potentially successful business luncheons destroyed by people eating the wrong food," says Linda Prout, nutrition consultant at the Claremont Resort and Spa in Berkeley, California. If you want to stay mentally sharp, eat protein—but avoid carbohydrate-rich foods such as pasta, rice, and potatoes. Protein, sans carbohydrates, has been shown to elevate levels of catecholamines, neurotransmitters that stimulate brainpower. So stick with the fish and broccoli, or the lean cut of beef and any other vegetable of your choosing. Also, politely refuse drinks with sugar, whether in iced tea or soda.

2:10 P.M.: The Fairweather presentation begins in 10 minutes. Nervous? You? Was Nixon nervous before debating Kennedy? You betcha. You have just enough time to either heave your lunch or calm down. Here's an easy way, although we realize it sounds crazy. "Our research shows that when athletes were happier, felt better about themselves, and were in good health, they went to the next level of performance," says sports psychologist James Loehr, Ed.D., president of LGE Sports Science in Orlando, Florida, and author of *Toughness Training for Life.* So go into the men's room, look in the mirror, and repeat, "I can do this. I want to do this. I love this." This is not a time for self-doubt, adds Dr. Loehr. "The fear of failure creates failure. Even if you're not, pretend you're confident. You may just fool yourself."

4:49 P.M.: You wrap up work with enough time to run to the post office and mail the check to your kid's school. But on your way out the door, you bump into Doolittle, who chided you last week for running personal errands on company time. By the time you lie your way out of a close call and reach the post office, the doors are locked, and no government employee—not even the one you can see walking away from the glass door—has ever cut a civilian a break. There's that ol' foxhole buddy again—anger. "Anger is the most seductive of the negative emotions," notes Dr. Goleman. "Anger is energizing, even exhilarating."

Energized or not, you're pissed. Your head is pounding, and you want to pound anybody. That postal worker will do.

Wrong thought, says Mark Epstein, M.D., a psychiatrist in Manhattan and author of *Thoughts without a Thinker.* "There is a widespread belief that the way to rid oneself of anger is to express it," explains Dr. Epstein. It's not. In fact, catharsis—the vent to rage—typically pumps up the brain's arousal, leaving people feeling more angry, not less. Dr. Epstein suggests neither venting nor suppressing anger. "People afraid of their anger act prematurely, trying to get rid of it," he says. "The point is to recognize the anger coming on. Take note of it. Then become aware of its effect on your body. Yup, same old signs. Heart and head are pounding, you're sweating and clenching your jaw, viselike. This will take you out of focusing on what's happening in your mind and get you into your body." Relax your jaw. Let your heart return to normal. Okay, what's next?

6:20 P.M.: You're on the highway, headed home from the park and ride, and there's a tortoise driving the car in front of you. To get him to speed up, you tailgate. Bad move: You have to be ever ready, muscles tensed for the possible meeting of metal against metal. Will you arrive at your destination any faster?

'Fraid not. Instead, take some advice from the researchers at the General Motors Research and Development Center in Warren, Michigan: Stay 2 seconds behind the car in front of you, and work off the tension by fidgeting. "Sitting in one position for too long can put a big strain on your muscles and skeleton," says David Viano, Ph.D., a research scientist at the center. Rock from buttock to buttock. Slide down in your seat and then back up. Take advantage of the cruise control to stretch first one leg, then the other. Do this seated macarena every 15 minutes to take stress off your body and keep your blood moving.

8:00 P.M.: The blur of helping with dinner and eating it is over. Now it's time to do some domestic chores. "Chores can be the bane of our existence," says Robert Bramson, Ph.D., an organizational behavior consultant and author of *The Stressless Home.* "They can tear a relationship apart, or they can provide a shared sense of completion." The problem is that what she expects from you and what you think is required are often two different things. For example, you finally take out the garbage, and she's still miffed. Why? Because to her, taking out the garbage also means replacing the plastic trash bag. You didn't replace the bag. To avoid conflicts, Dr. Bramson suggests that the entire cleanup committee answer three critical questions before slipping on rubber gloves.

1. Who's supposed to do what around here? Gather everyone into a room and make a list of all the chores. Pick your chores or draw lots to see who is responsible for what.
2. Who gives orders to whom? This is the power-and-control question, the one that especially trips up men, says Dr. Bramson. Optimally, no one tells anybody what to do. You discuss it. You negotiate. You compromise. Nobody is happy cleaning the cat's litter box. The key is to parcel out chores so that everyone thinks he or she is being treated fairly The least stressful way to do this is to make a chore list that matches everyone's preferences.
3. How will you know if a job has been done satisfactorily? When you all sit down to delegate responsibilities, outline exactly what each chore entails, even if it makes you appear a little compulsive. "Everyone has a different notion of a job well-done," Dr. Bramson observes. "It's a matter of perception."

Getting a Grip on Business Problems

The most common workplace dilemmas are often the easiest to solve.

Today's work environment is more stressful than at any other time in history, except for next year, when it will be worse. Your father wouldn't recognize the place. The career ladder has been replaced by a career trampoline. Under the new flat organizational hierarchy, you're one of 25 guys reporting to a man who mistook you for a waiter at last year's Christmas party, and it's slowly dawning on you that job security means that the guys from security will be happy to escort you from your job now that you've been replaced by an undergraduate with his own laptop.

But the modern workplace isn't a complete madhouse. It only seems that way because the first thing most of us do when job stress revs up is dumb down. We jettison common sense as if it were a crazy aunt, forget everything we've learned, and redouble our efforts at the very things we're doing wrong. If we took only a moment to catch our collective breath, we'd see that most common workplace problems have unexpectedly simple solutions. So listen up because, as Yogi Berra may once have said, sometimes you can see a lot just by observing.

Problem: I'm spending half my day on the damn phone.

Solution: Prepare an interruption.

I used to have a deal with Rich, a guy in my office. We'd walk by each other's door four or five times a day. If I found myself on the phone with somebody who wanted to lose weight by talking himself thin, I'd flash Rich the time-out sign. Whereupon he'd stick his head in and say in a loud voice, "Don wants that memo now, man. He's been trying to get you." I'd do the same for Rich. It got to be fun as we invented new scenarios. ("Don's screaming your name. He's armed.") It's easier with a straight man, of course, but you can do the same thing with an imaginary interruption. Or try one of these tactics.

Stand up. It has a magical way of shortening calls, according to Lyle Sussman, professor of management at the University of Louisville and co-author of *Smart Moves.* "You're less likely to shoot the breeze, and you get to the point faster," he says.

Set a time limit. Tell your caller that you have a meeting in 5 minutes, then remind him after 1 minute. This isn't rude; it's efficient.

Create a phone-free zone. If you have tasks that can't be postponed, have your secretary or voice mail announce that you will be returning calls after 11:00 A.M. today.

Problem: My brain is on siesta, but this project is still due at 5:00 P.M.

Solution: Adopt the three-week breakfast plan.

Many men report that they tend to pack their mental bags for catatonia around 3:00 P.M. no matter how light or healthy their lunch was. "Oh, I run into this one all the time," says Elizabeth Somer, R.D., author of *Food and Mood.* "The answer is not what you should eat now that you're in an energy slump, but what you didn't eat before. And that's breakfast."

Somer is a soft-spoken woman who turns tough when the subject is the first meal of the day. "Breakfast is paramount to energy levels all day long," she explains. Without it, you're begging for fatigue, junk-food cravings, and general irritability. "The only fuel the brain uses is glucose, and by the time you wake up, it has been 8 to 12 hours since you've provided it with any. So you're basically asking your body and brain to run on fumes. Even if you eat an excellent lunch, you'll never regain the energy you would have had by eating breakfast in the first place. By this time, the whole system is too stressed."

When you wake up, your brain automatically signals its desire to be fed. If you don't feel hungry in the morning, it's because you've simply overridden the message for so long that the brain, in a huff, has stopped sending it. She says it takes two to three weeks of eating a sensible breakfast to reprogram your body to be hungry. So what's a sensible breakfast? A bowl of cereal with low-fat milk and a banana. An English muffin with peanut butter and orange juice. Even a tortilla with some cheese and an apple. "Concentrate on eating complex carbohydrates and some protein," advises Somer. Carbohydrates energize your body but sedate your brain. A little skim milk or yogurt will counteract this effect and keep you energized all day. "And if it takes more than 5 minutes to prepare," Somer says, "you're spending too much time."

Problem: I have 18 things due by tomorrow, and I can't stop sucking my thumb.

Solution: Observe the 80/20 rule.

This problem is a natural outgrowth of downsizing, in which the work stays the same but there are fewer people to do it, says Peter Wylie, Ph.D., an organizational psychologist and management consultant. We're so overloaded with responsibilities that we're not sure where to start. The answer is to borrow an old adage from management textbooks known as the Pareto Principle. No one knows exactly why, but if you're like most people, 80 percent of your effectiveness will come from 20 percent of what you do.

The trick, then, is to concentrate on the 20 percent of the work that really matters. Dr. Wylie suggests that you take an hour to organize the Matterhorn of paper on your desk into three piles. The first is This-Will-Make-a-Big-Difference-Today. Pile two is Some-Fool-Wants-Me-to-Do-This-but-It-Won't-Help-Much. The third is I-Don't-Think-So. Congratulations. You've just figured out where your efforts should go.

Problem: I'm feeling overwhelmed, I'm not sure exactly what I'm doing, and my boss is a moron.

Solution: Redefine your job.

With the company changing directions weekly with all the poise of a drunk trying to parallel park a Cadillac on a cul-de-sac, small wonder you're not sure where you fit in. As for your boss, did you really think he took the job because of a lifelong dream to lead, nurture, and inspire? Of course not. He saw a chance for a Lexus and a corner office and jumped on it, same as you would.

What you have to do is make yourself fireproof. Your boss wants a low-maintenance employee who makes him look good. Your only salvation is to become this guy, says Stan Silverman, professor of social science at the University of Akron in Ohio and co-author of *Working Scared: Achieving Success in Trying Times.* Sit down with your manager and tell him three things:

1. What you see as your role in the company
2. Exactly what you should be doing to fulfill this role
3. The precise results by which you'd like to be judged

"This kind of initiative-taking will delight most bosses and considerably lessen your stress level because it puts you back in control," says Silverman. "You'll find out whether you're aligned with the organization and stop doing unproductive work. Better still, you'll stand out from the herd as somebody who wants to make a difference for the company. This is a nice place to be when it comes to handing out the raises." And after your discussion, remember to fire off a follow-up memo so that you have in writing exactly what you two agreed upon. In case your entire department goes up in smoke, you'll have clearly noted what you were—and weren't—responsible for.

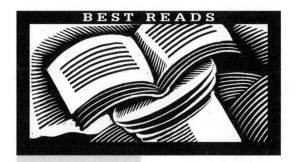

BEST READS

Cultivating Confidence

When looking for good "mental toughness" books to excerpt, we naturally turned to golf books. Why? First, golf is not a game of brute strength or skill; probably more than any other sport, it relies on mental toughness to do well. Second, and it sounds trite, but golf really is a good metaphor for life. Third, and perhaps most telling, there are a whole lot of great books out there on the "mind game" aspect of golf (when was the last time you saw a book on mental toughness for football?). Golf Is Not a Game of Perfect (Simon and Schuster, 1995) is one of those books. Written by Robert Rotella, Ph.D., director of sports psychology at the University of Virginia in Charlottesville, it offers some striking wisdom about attitude, confidence, and stress. While the following excerpt on cultivating confidence is couched in golf language, it clearly has universal applications.

I will be revealing no secrets by stating that good golf requires confidence.

Coaches and athletes in all sports have long recognized that teams don't win and athletes don't perform well without confidence.

All of the ideas and techniques I teach to golfers, from free will to the preshot routine, are intended to produce confidence. Without confidence you can't trust your physical ability. You can't perform at your best.

But a lot of golfers that I speak to about confidence have misconceptions that hold them back.

They think that confidence is an attribute that they cannot choose to seek and acquire. They think it's something that descends on an athlete like a revelation from above after he's performed perfectly for a long time.

Sometimes, a player struggling with this kind of misconception will ask me which comes first, confidence or success. They understand that a player cannot win tournaments without confidence. But they think that you have to win tournaments before you can get confidence.

If that were true, no one would ever win a tournament for the first time.

In fact, anyone can develop confidence if he or she goes about it properly. Confidence isn't something you're born with or something you're given. You control it. Confidence is what you think about yourself and your golf game.

Confidence at the level of any single shot is nothing more than thinking about your ball going to the target. If you're thinking about the ball going to the target, you're confident.

A lot of golfers find this too simple. They have good educations. They've learned how to analyze and question. They want to apply what they know about probability and statistics.

This kind of person might engage me in the following argument.

"Doc, are you confident when you stand over a 40-foot putt that you're going to make it?"

"Yes," I reply.

"Well, then, would you bet me your house that you'll make it?"

"No."

"Then how can you say you're confident?"

The answer is that while I wouldn't bet my house, that doesn't mean I'm not confident.

Being confident doesn't mean that I don't know that 2 percent is a good average on 40-foot putts. It means that when I'm standing over a 40-foot putt, no one is asking me to bet my house, and I'm not thinking about averages. I'm thinking about putting the ball in the hole. And that's all I'm thinking about.

Great athletes think this way. It would never occur to one of them to ask me whether I would bet my house on a 40-foot putt.

People would understand this better, I think, if confidence guaranteed success. It doesn't. Standing on the tee and thinking about your drive going to the target doesn't guarantee that it will go there. It only enhances the chances. If it guaranteed success, people would more readily get the idea. But they try thinking confidently, and as soon as a shot doesn't succeed, they think, "Well, that doesn't work."

But look at it another way. If you're not thinking about your drive going to the target, what are you thinking about? Obviously, you're thinking about it going somewhere else—into a lake, maybe.

And that kind of thinking definitely works, assuming you want to hit the ball in the lake. Negative thinking is almost 100 percent effective.

In a larger sense, your confidence is the sum of all the thoughts you have about yourself as a golfer. You have to think about what you want your golf game to be. You have to think about driving it well, wedging it well, being a great bunker player, being a superb putter.

If you are a competitive player, you have to think about winning tournaments, about shooting low scores, about being able to stay cool if you get off to a rocky start and still come in with a good number.

I frequently tell touring players that when they're off the course, if they can't think about playing great golf, they shouldn't think about golf at all.

By its nature, golf will try to sap your confidence. On every round, even the best golfer will mishit some shots. Over the course of a year, even the best golfer will lose more tournaments than he wins. So, maintaining confidence in golf is like swimming against a current. You have to work hard to stay where you are.

I tell players to try to feel that their confidence is increasing over the course of every round, every tournament, and every season. I want them to feel that they are looser and more decisive on the 18th tee than they were on the first. I want them to feel more capable of going low on Sunday than they did on Thursday. I want them to feel more likely to win the last tournament of the season than they did in the first. As golfers grow in skills and experience, they must make certain that their confidence grows along with them.

They can do this if they learn to be selective about their thoughts and their memories. They have to learn to monitor their thinking and ask themselves whether an idea that springs to mind is likely to help them or hurt them in the effort to grow more confident.

If it won't help them, they have to make a conscious choice to put that thought out of their mind and turn to one that will enhance their confidence. They have to focus on what they want to happen, be it a particular shot or an entire career. Everyone thinks this way some of the time. Doing it consistently is a habit that requires disciplined effort.

This is what Nick Price has learned to do over the past few years. Nowadays, he tells me, the only thoughts that enter his mind on a golf course are thoughts about what he wants to do—where he wants to place his tee shot, where he wants his approach to land, and how he wants his putt to fall. The prospect of hitting a drive into the woods or running a putt way past the hole simply does not occur to him.

It can sound a little bit like self-deception. But it isn't. It is simply the way that great athletes, or successful people in any field, have trained themselves to think.

Expecting the Unexpected

If there's one thing you can count on in this life—besides death and taxes—it's the fact that nothing ever goes as planned. When your schemes and dreams go awry, you want to be prepared with a back-up plan that covers every contingency. In this chapter from Stress Blasters *(Rodale Press, 1997), Brian Chichester and Perry Garfinkel tell you how to be ready for anything.*

There is something manly about being prepared. British war hero Robert S. S. Baden-Powell knew it. That's why he made "Be Prepared" the motto of the group he founded, the Boy Scouts. He wanted boys to be ready "to take on any kind of duty at any time...and help other people at all times."

We all admire a man with a plan. But we hold a man with a Plan B in the highest esteem. The guy who appears to be cool, calm, and collected while everyone around him is running about madly either doesn't fathom the severity of the situation or knows something that everyone else doesn't. He remains unscathed by stress because he has thought about what could go wrong and has a backup plan. He knows where the escape hatch is.

He is James Bond toting every techno-gadget known to man, Bill Gates with a computer system that the competition hadn't anticipated, or a Boy Scout who wrapped his matches in a plastic bag in case of rain.

"Having an alternative backup solution is always a good idea," says Stephan Rechtschaffen, M.D., president of the Omega Institute in Rhinebeck, New York, which teaches healthy relaxation techniques, and author of *Time Shifting: Creating More Time to Enjoy Your Life*. "We spend so much time stressing out about things that may go wrong, things that we had not expected. We would spend that time more wisely coming up with a detailed contingency plan."

But being prepared—poised like a cat ready to pounce, thinking several steps ahead—requires all senses to be alert, present and accounted for, ready to rock and roll. And that can take a toll on your body and mind.

Surprise! Surprises Are Stressful

Why are unexpected events and surprises stressful? "Because they throw your body out of homeostatic balance," explains Robert Sapolsky, Ph.D., professor of biological sciences and neuroscience at Stanford University and author of *Why Zebras Don't Get Ulcers: A Guide to Stress, Stress-Related Diseases, and Coping*. Homeostasis, for those who claim that biology wasn't offered at their high schools, is the ideal level of oxygen, acidity, temperature, and other physiological factors that our bodies maintain under normal circumstances. Surprise—by definition a deviation from the norm—triggers our bodies into the classic fight-or-flight stress response. We're ready to run either from it or after it, whatever "it" is. This stressful response, when confronted with unexpected situations, is true of zebras, lions, and humans.

But humans, says Dr. Sapolsky, add a stressor that zebras and other animals don't deal with. "We have this great propensity to worry ourselves sick," he says. "So we have to include as a stressor the anticipation of bad things happening. When we see things coming, we can turn on just as robust a stress response based merely on anticipation."

Butterflies in the stomach before a speech, clammy palms before a job interview, and accelerated heartbeat as you knock on the door of a blind date illustrate the point in the short term. Looking ahead also can trigger stress: Will you get the raise at the end of the quarter? Will the IRS audit you...again? How long will your parents be around? The same goes for looking far ahead: Will it be any better in your next incarnation?

Men specifically deal with yet another mental stressor, says Samuel Osherson, Ph.D., honorary research psychologist at Harvard University Health Services and author of *Wrestling with Love*. "Men translate unexpected events to mean a loss of control, and that's a significant stressor for us," he notes. "We have a choice: to let go of trying to control everything, or do all that we can to prepare."

Be Prepared

When life's vagaries cause us to lose hair—or turn what's left of it gray—we are called anxious, neurotic, paranoid, worrywarts, or worse. When we plan for the unexpected and it happens, we are called forward-thinking visionaries. Since there are about 1 million young men enrolled in the Boy Scouts and more than 92 million alumni, you'd think that more of us would have what George Bush used to call that vision thing. Here are some key tips to keep in mind as you work toward your stress-reduction merit badge.

Be street smart. In police lingo, it's called coming up, explains Detective J. J. Bittenbinder, formerly with the Chicago Police Department, now an inspector and lecturer assigned to the Cook County Sheriff's Department in Illinois. "On the streets, police are more focused," he says. "You become more aware. You pay attention to your surroundings. If something seems unusual or out of the ordinary, you should wake up, come up a notch with all your senses. When you recognize something as a potential threat, it's not as big a threat because it can't take you by surprise," adds Bittenbinder. The same holds true in life. Practice such preventive behavior and you minimize surprises.

Turn to family planning. Contingency plans are critical if you're a parent, as anyone who has had the pleasure of trying to get children off to school morning after morning can attest. "Take into account things that might go wrong," says Jon Kabat-Zinn, Ph.D., director of the Stress Reduction Clinic at the University of Massachusetts Medical Center in Worcester who is also an associate professor of medicine, lecturer, and author of *Full Castastrophe Living: Using the Wisdom of Your Body and Mind to Face Stress, Pain, and Illness* and *Wherever You Go, There You Are.* "Get up earlier, and get everything ready beforehand. Plan what time they go to bed so that you can get them up with enough time to do everything as unrushed as possible."

Practice visualization. That's the advice of 1996 NBA Coach of the Year Phil Jackson of the Chicago Bulls. "If you visualize what's going to happen, you can react to it quickly without thinking, because you've seen it in your mind," he says. "If you think of enough variables, you've covered every possibility so that nothing will be unexpected."

To increase the number of possibilities, he suggests following Japanese Zen master Suzuki Roshi's wisdom to empty your mind and think like a beginner. As Roshi said, "If your mind is empty, it is always ready for anything; it is open to everything. In the beginner's mind, there are many possibilities; in the expert's mind, there are few."

Take the time to make a Plan B. People have anxiety about making plans "because plans govern the future and most of us look to the future with fear," says Dr. Rechtschaffen. "What if our plans don't work out? What if something unexpected comes along to stop us? What if...?"

He suggests coming up with plans that aren't so specific that they "become a weight that keeps you from seeing alternatives."

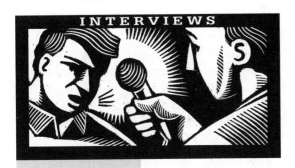

Daniel Goleman on
Getting Smart, Emotionally Speaking

Ever since he earned his Ph.D. in psychology from Harvard University in 1975, Daniel Goleman wondered why some people with high intelligence quotients (IQs) attain both emotional satisfaction and financial success while others founder.

During the years since then, Dr. Goleman, who covers behavioral sciences for the New York Times, *became intrigued with how exciting new research in brain physiology could inform his inquiry. His own answers are contained in his book* Emotional Intelligence, *which was on the* Times *bestseller list for more than a year.*

Dr. Goleman's point is that society has placed too high a value on intelligence as measured by IQ tests, Scholastic Aptitude Tests, and Graduate Record Examinations, and not enough on the emotional skills that can spell success in our interpersonal relationships at work and at home. With some mindful attention, he says, we can raise our EQs—our so-called emotional quotients.

Why do otherwise intelligent people sometimes "lose it," as the saying goes?

Emotional explosions are basically the result of neural hijackings. That is, before you have a chance to think something through rationally, a wave of body chemicals floods the limbic center in the brain, called the amygdala, which is the seat of all passion. In those moments, even smart people do things that they admit later were very stupid.

What is the effect of negative emotions on mental clarity?

When unsettling emotions overwhelm concentration, what is being swamped is "working memory," which is the ability of the mind to hold all information relevant to the task at hand. The prefrontal cortex of the brain executes working memory. It's also where feelings and emotions meet. So when you're in emotional distress, it's natural that one cost is in the effectiveness of working memory. Literally, we can't think straight. At its worst, like when terror overtakes you, your mind can go into a sort of a paralysis. That happened to me once when I walked into a calculus test completely unprepared. A tape loop of fear and doom left me motionless, like a frozen animal.

This makes it sound as though we are prisoners of our own hormones. How can we prevent these hijackings from happening?

There are several things we can do to gain some modicum of control over such emotions. The first step is to recognize that an emotion is being triggered, instead of being caught in a state in which all you are thinking is, "I hate you, you S.O.B." If you can stop yourself and simply say, "Oh, I'm angry," you are beginning to practice a kind of self-reflection called mindfulness. Just by activating this self-reflexive awareness, you're triggering areas of the brain that actually short-circuit the reactive emotional centers. This mindful awareness opens the door to the other ways to prevent emotional hijacking: managing anger and handling anxiety, the ability to motivate yourself through hopefulness, empathy, and developing the kinds of social skills that enable people to feel good about your interactions with them. These are the components of what we're calling emotional intelligence.

You're talking fantasy scenario for men, right? Ask most men in the midst of an intense emotional encounter to respond this rationally and they'd say to you, "Easier said than done."

It's true that men may find this difficult. In emotionally charged situations, many men are more likely to shut down—to stonewall it, as the expression goes. Men may be justified in responding this way. Once flooded with emotion, men secrete more adrenaline into their bloodstreams, their heart rates jump more quickly, and their physiological recoveries take longer than those of women. I suggest that men in that state just take time out from the troubling situation, at least long enough to let their heart rates slow down. It's literally a cooling-off period. Ten to 20 minutes later you can come back and deal with your boss, your lover, your own anger at yourself more calmly, with more emotional intelligence.

What emotion separates some people from others when it comes to achievement?

In studies of Olympic athletes, world-class musicians, and chess grand masters, their unifying trait was the ability to motivate themselves to pursue relentless training routines. The earlier they started in their lives on rigorous programs, the better they became. What seems to set those at the very top of competitive pursuits from others of roughly equal ability is the degree to which they can stick with an arduous routine for years and years. The emotional trait that distinguishes them is enthusiasm and persistence in the face of setbacks.

There's another factor: optimism. It means having strong expectation that things will turn out all right in life, despite setbacks and frustrations. It's a buffer against apathy, hopelessness, and depression. Optimistic people see failure as a result of something that can be changed. Pessimists, on the other hand, take the blame for the failure, pointing the finger at some fatal character flaw of theirs that they cannot change. These opposing viewpoints can make a world of difference in the outcomes of things, as it turns out. People's beliefs about their abilities have a profound effect on those abilities.

What's a good emotional indicator of whether a child will grow up to succeed in life?

There is perhaps no psychological skill more fundamental than resisting impulse. It is the root of all emotional self-control since all emotions by their very nature lead to one or another impulse to act. I reported on a remarkable study in which four-year-olds were challenged to resist a marshmallow for the 15 minutes that it took an experimenter to leave the room and run an errand. They were told they could eat the marshmallow if they couldn't wait. But if they waited, they could have two. Twelve to 14 years later these same children were tracked down and interviewed. The results: Those who resisted temptation were found to be more socially competent—that is, better able to cope with life's frustrations than their marshmallow-grabbing schoolmates. This can translate in adult life to staying on a diet, pursuing a medical degree, or any number of other scenarios that require us to delay gratification in return for bigger rewards.

Can you teach emotional intelligence?

Absolutely. There is already a strong emotional-literacy movement. For example, at the Nueva Learning Center, a private school in San Francisco, fifth graders take a class called Self Science. They report on and talk about the emotional fabric of their lives: being left out, envy, disagreement. The lessons are small but, like good child-rearing techniques, when repeated over a number of years, they become ingrained. The lessons become neural habits that their brains apply at critical times throughout their lives.

You can also teach optimism and hope, which we talked about earlier. Granted, some of it may be inborn temperament. But the belief that we have mastery over the events of our lives and can meet challenges as they come up—psychologists call it self-efficacy—begins early in life. Parents play a significant role in assuring their children that they can develop competencies that strengthen their sense of self-efficacy and make a person more willing to take risks and seek out challenges, knowing he can do well in them. Surmounting those challenges, again, increases that sense.

We've all had domineering or abusive bosses who we wish had learned emotional intelligence in school before they joined the workforce. What are the chances of offering such courses as part of management training?

Better now than 20 years ago. I recall a study of 250 executives in the 1970s that showed that most felt that their work demanded their "heads but not their hearts." I think that attitude is outmoded. There's a new competitiveness in the workplace that doesn't just encourage emotional competence; it demands it. When they're emotionally upset, people cannot remember, learn, or make decisions clearly. This certainly can destroy careers, if not corporations. For starters, it behooves managers to master the art of constructive criticism. If their criticism sounds like a character attack, employees lose hope and stop trying. But an artful critique can motivate someone.

To that end, here are some suggestions. Be specific; pick an incident that illustrates a key problem that needs changing rather than deal in vague generalities. Offer a solution that makes everyone happy. Be present when offering a critique; tell the person face-to-face rather than in an e-mail or memo. Be sensitive; think about the impact of what you're saying as though it was being told to you. In other words, have some empathy.

Steven Ungerleider on
Playing the Mental Game

Steven Ungerleider, Ph.D., is a thinking man's jock. Since his days as a college athlete, he's always been fascinated with why some men and women who are gifted physically may not excel as well as others of the same ability. The difference, he decided, was how they play the game in their heads. He has spent the better part of his professional career as a research psychologist studying and analyzing the phenomenon—and using what he has learned to help train elite athletes.

Since 1984, he has served on the U.S. Olympic Committee Sports Psychology Registry and is currently director of Integrated Research Services in Eugene, Oregon. His research into the winning strategies of Olympians, conducted with Jacqueline Golding, Ph.D., of the University of California in San Francisco, was published as Beyond Strength: Psychological Profiles of Olympic Athletes. *He is also the author of* Mental Training for Peak Performance, *in which he shares mental exercises that top athletes use to excel at their sports. In this conversation, he gives us a glimpse into the psyche of some of the world's greatest athletes—and how we can apply their lessons to our lives.*

You talk about how successful athletes prepare mentally for a game. How would that work in the lives of most of us who don't compete in athletics?

Doing mental homework helps me in almost everything I do. Even for this conversation, I prepared by asking myself questions that you might ask me and thinking of various answers that I might offer. At work, you can plot what you need to get done in a day, allot certain amounts of time to each task, figure out how you're going to get from point A to point B. Whether it's routine daily tasks or major projects, you have to play it through step by step in your head first. What we learned from studying athletes was that those who actually made the U.S. team and competed in the Olympics were doing more mental practice as part of the final stage of preparation than those who didn't make the team.

Can you explain what you mean by mental practice?

The basic principles, which can apply to almost any sport or any other endeavor, are simple. They involve a cognitive step-by-step dress rehearsal of the physical actions you plan to take to complete a move or task. I encourage drawing on all of your sensory modes—the smell of flowers, the feel of wind in your face, the feel of your feet on the ground, the sound of lovely classical music—to really put yourself in the moment. I rely strongly on the visual sense: I ask you to use visual imagery to "see" yourself running or giving a speech in your dress rehearsal. I ask you to focus on perfect performance—not tripping over words—so that the image of the well-executed activity is what your brain remembers.

If you were going to give a talk to your board of directors, for example, I'd have you first picture a comfortable, nonthreatening setting. Then imagine different people in the boardroom. Identify how much intimidation or threat you'd feel. Now recall that comfortable relaxed feeling. Move back and forth between these two feelings. With people or situations that cause you stress and tension, simply let the feeling of relaxation wash over you until those hot spots cool down, until you feel self-confident.

Why or how does this kind of mental practice work?

There are two theories. One is called symbolic learning theory. It states that every move we make is coded—like a blueprint—in our minds and nervous systems. When we rehearse the symbolic gestures, we are making them familiar to our body chemistries. Repeating the gesture mentally encodes it in us, making it almost automatic. The other is called psychoneuromuscular theory. Even sitting still, when we mentally go through the moves, we produce small muscle contractions just like those we would produce if we actually ran or swam or gave a talk. These mental faxes, if you will, travel at lightning speed and command the muscles to perform in the appropriate sequence. This has been shown to be true for athletes who've had their electrical activity recorded with an electromyograph, an EMG, while they are doing these mental rehearsals.

Can you talk yourself into success?

Yes, absolutely. You can give yourself a personal pep talk that, in effect, affirms your ability to do well. We call these little self-talks affirmations, and many of us already do them and we don't even know it. On the tennis court, when you miss a shot and say out loud, "Come on, I can hit that cross-court shot," you are affirming your ability. But it depends on your intention. If you're beating yourself up, punishing and scolding yourself, you're not helping yourself. But if you are really reminding yourself of the level of play you are truly capable of, then you can do it. The trick is to reprogram your inner dialogue to positive statements and self-affirmations.

Some of us think that our minds get in the way of our success. We want so much to win at sports, at life, that we think our way into a tangle of nerves. How do we get out of that trap?

Good question. Yes, a lot of us let stress—not our opponent or a colleague—defeat us. There are a number of techniques for relaxing your mind. Breathing is a simple one. Meditation is another form of relaxation. Repeating a certain word, or just focusing on your breath, helps you shut out the external world, allowing you to reduce distractions. Once you assume a quiet calmness, there is a feeling of letting things just happen, of letting go of things that are not in your control. A simple phrase like "Easy does it" or "I'm doing fine" may be enough to remind you to find that inner calm. By doing all this, you relax your muscles. Tension starts in your head and moves down to your muscles, making them constrict, thereby impeding your ability to move freely in response to what comes at you. So, ironically, the more you worry about performing well, the more difficult you make it for yourself to perform well.

One of the best techniques is called progressive relaxation. Here's how it works: Sit in a chair or lie on the ground. Tighten your right hand and fist for 10 seconds. Then release it completely and let it go limp. Now do the same for your left hand, tightening it and letting it go limp. Notice the before-and-after difference. Notice a relaxed flow of energy through your hand. Do the same thing, starting at one end of your body and moving to the other—from feet, to calves, to thighs, to buttocks, to stomach, to lower and upper back, the arms, shoulders, neck, head, and facial muscles. It's like a self-massage. This is terrific for circulation and for helping focus your mind on your body—and not on all your worries.

Why do some guys "choke"?

We're just scratching the surface on that phenomenon. In our research with athletes, we're finding that some of it has to do with their relationships with their mentors or coaches. When they get to a certain critical moment, if they sense that their mentors will be angry at them if they fail, they will fail. Excelling to make someone else happy or proud of you may not be beneficial after all. On the other hand, people who feel that their mentors or coaches support them, win or lose, may do much better. I've heard athletes say, "I knew my coach was there for me, regardless of the outcome. He or she knew exactly what I needed to hear to pick me up." It's a delicate balance. Sadly, in our society today, we are mentor-starved. We need more role models who encourage young men and women to strive for their personal best.

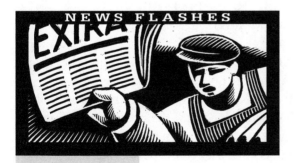

Coping Strategies Can Cure or Kill

PERTH, Australia—In the movie *Falling Down*, Michael Douglas plays a regular guy with a regular job who is particularly stressed out. He yells. He smashes groceries with a baseball bat. He kills people, but that's another story. Which is going to kill him faster, you wonder, the stress or the self-destructive things it causes him to do?

Researchers at the University of Western Australia and West Australian Heart and Research Institute in Perth had the same question. They studied the most stressed-out 337 men and 317 women they could find—people working in a tax office—to see whether work stress or their coping methods caused their blood pressure to skyrocket.

The conclusion: The coping methods appeared to be the culprit.

The tax workers filled out questionnaires telling how stressed they were and how they dealt with it. Researchers arranged the coping strategies into five groups: solution-oriented (reorganizing work), social (having stable relationships), attitude (taking positive time out), consumption (using drugs, alcohol, caffeine, or food), and denial (suppressing emotions).

Although the men and women had similar job-stress levels, after 10 weeks the men had higher average blood pressures than the women. The main difference between the men and the women, researchers found, was the way the men coped with their work-related stress. They drank more. They smoked more. They ate worse. They denied the fact that they were stressed out.

Women, on the other hand, used more positive coping strategies, and their blood pressures went down.

So if your job bears a striking similarity to the set of *Falling Down*, try more positive solution-oriented or social approaches to stress—practice effective time management, take up a new hobby, or seek social support. And lock that gun cabinet.

Too Much Self-Esteem Can Be Bad for You

BOSTON—Men who look in the mirror and see the fairest one of all—and the funniest, smartest, sexiest—may be in for a shock. Researchers at Northeastern University and the University of California at Berkeley found that people who view themselves the highest often are only fooling themselves.

Researchers studied more than 100 people for five years, interviewing them each at age 18 and 23. First, they determined how the people saw themselves: negatively, positively, or somewhere in between. Then they called in the experts. Four to six trained clinical examiners interviewed the people and assessed their personalities. When they compared the two, if the person saw himself better than the trained examiner saw him, that showed that he was self-enhancing, said C. Randall Colvin, Ph.D., co-author of the study and assistant professor of psychology at Northeastern University.

Then they called in the real experts—they asked the people's friends what they thought of them. It turned out that the individuals who saw themselves in the most positive light were described by their friends in negative ways, and those who saw themselves most accurately were described in positive ways.

"If you self-enhance, it may bolster your self-esteem and make you feel good temporarily. But it will push away those who are close to you," Dr. Colvin says. "Sometimes self-enhancing is useful. If you suffer a blow—your boss puts you down, for example—it's okay to think, 'That's not true. I am a good guy.' So in a short time span, self-enhancing is fine. But over the long term, if you continue to self-enhance, that means you'll never see any flaws in yourself and, therefore, you'll never be able to improve yourself.

"It's good to have a positive view of yourself, but it's also important to acknowledge your strengths and weaknesses and to view yourself as a 'work in progress,'" Dr. Colvin says.

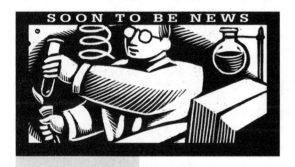

Internet Addiction: A Genuine Affliction?

You probably know at least one Internet junkie. He's glued to his screen for hours at a time, fixating on one Web site after another—from Virtual Lego to Psychotronic Cinema to tales of the latest Elvis sightings.

But is he truly addicted? Mental health professionals and Internet devotees are beginning to raise concerns about the growing trend of computer users who seem caught by the druglike lure of the World Wide Web. The issue has spawned numerous Internet sites—some serious, some tongue-in-cheek. Ironic as it seems, there is a growing trend for "Netaholics" to reach out for help using the very medium that they feel may be impairing them.

Reports that heavy online users were behaving something like drug addicts prompted Kimberly S. Young, Ph.D., assistant professor of psychology at the University of Pittsburgh at Bradford and founder of the Center for Online Addiction, to study the trend. By adapting a questionnaire based upon American

Psychiatric Association criteria for determining substance dependence, Dr. Young surveyed Internet users to judge whether they were nondependent or dependent. She found that dependent users reported an inability to control their computer usage and felt impaired by their computer use in five lifestyle areas: school, relationships, finances, work, and physical health. Dr. Young concluded that while the Internet itself is not addictive, its use can result in behavior common to recognized addictions like pathological gambling.

Other professionals doubt that Internet Addiction Disorder (IAD), as it has been dubbed, warrants all of the concern that has been raised. "What we are seeing is merely the continuation of a decades-long trend of people spending increasingly more time with technology than with other humans, " says A'isha Ajayi, professor of information technology at the Rochester Institute of Technology in New York. "This shift away from the family and peers to mass media technology as the primary socialization agent can be traced to the radio in the 1930s, followed by television in the 1950s, and the computer networks today." Nevertheless, Ajayi, who teaches a human-computer interaction course, acknowledges the seductive nature of the Internet. She notes that it provides an outlet for people to experience life from a different perspective or with a different persona. "It's almost like having an electronic alter ego," she says.

"I believe the problem will only grow as more individuals gain access to 'the Net,'" *predicts Dr. Young. "As more people learn about the technology, more problems will* *emerge in households trying to deal with new electronic relationships and their impact* *on the family system." And just as it took over a decade for pathological gambling to be* *viewed as a bona fide disorder, says Dr. Young, it will take more time, more research,* *and a larger number of affected people for Internet addiction to gain credibility.*

A New Definition of Depression?

Psychiatrists are studying just how low you have to go before you suffer the disabling affects of depression. And there's increasing evidence that it doesn't take much. Mild or minor depressive symptoms, sometimes known as subsyndromal symptomatic depression (SSD), may be taking more of a toll on public health than previously thought.

Researchers, who interpreted nearly 2,400 interviews gathered by a National Institute of Mental Health program in Los Angeles, found very little difference between the problems of depressed men and women and those with just a few depressive symptoms. Both groups of people experienced more irritability, poorer health, lower productivity, and greater home and financial stress than study participants without any of the commonly recognized symptoms of depression.

During an episode of SSD, a person's relationships, job, and other priorities can become distressing and difficult. Some people expend great amounts of energy just to keep up the appearance of being effective. The most common SSD symptoms reported are insomnia, fatigue, and trouble concentrating. Some studies have found that the incidence increases among people in their thirties before dropping off and recurring later in life. The prevalence of the problem is unknown but has been found to be more common than major depression in some settings.

The American Psychiatric Association's most recent edition of the Diagnostic and Statistical Manual of Mental Disorders *includes research criteria for a proposed minor depression–disorder category, challenging experts to study the condition and determine whether it should become an official mental health category.*

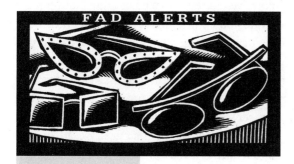

Promise Keepers

What's wrong with this picture: Some 50,000 men and *only* men filling to the brim RFK Stadium in Washington, D.C.—but there's no sports event? What's wrong may be what's right. Or it may just be the latest spin in the ongoing social trend known as the men's movement. That's the loose amalgam of groups of men throughout the country that get together to figure out what it means to be a man today, whether through academic conferences exploring masculinity issues, or through banging conga drums in the woods and getting in touch with what poet Robert Bly, author of *Iron John*, calls our "wild man."

These latest men's gatherings are called Promise Keepers, a Christian-based outreach organization. Through stadium conferences, educational seminars, local church meetings, and the dissemination of other materials, the organization espouses seven principles focused on commitment to family, ethical values, racial and denominational respect, other men—but first and foremost to Jesus Christ. While non-Christians are welcome to attend stadium events and other meetings, full participation is limited to only those who are willing to honor that last commitment.

Promise Keepers started in 1990 in Boulder, Colorado, when then University of Colorado head football coach Bill McCartney brought together 72 men to develop a plan for hosting giant gatherings of men—not to play or watch violent sports or bang drums but to seriously examine deeper spiritual issues that affect men. In 1991, some 4,200 men attended the first conference in the University of Colorado event center. Since then, the movement has grown exponentially. More than 2 million men have attended Promise Keepers stadium conferences. In 1997, 18 stadium events were scheduled. The organization's professional staff has grown from 22 in 1993 to 452 four years later. Its budget has skyrocketed from $4 million to an estimated $117 million. Headquartered in Denver, it has 36 regional offices throughout the United States, with independent Promise Keepers groups in Australia, New Zealand, and Canada.

So what's the big draw? "I think we've tapped into a basic issue that men are grappling with," says Rod Cooper, Ph.D., a counseling psychologist who is the organization's national director of educational ministries. "That is: How do you be a man of integrity in these complicated times? The problem is that many men have isolated themselves. They feel like islands unto themselves. When they become part of these large events they can say, 'Gee, I'm not the only one struggling with these concerns.' There's a sense of permission—permission to connect, permission to drop that typical male competitive stance. We encourage men to develop buddyships that go to a deeper level."

That Promise Keepers promotes what it calls accountability—taking responsibility for one's own actions and inviting other men to do the same—is a message that all men can stand to hear. But it has taken flak for narrowing its appeal only to men who are of strong Christian faith.

That doesn't phase Promise Keepers, and it apparently hasn't slowed its growth. Dr. Cooper says that, by the year 2000, they "hope to have impacted every church in America." The direction will be away from large stadium gatherings and more toward small group meetings in local churches. Those interested in attending should leave their conga drums at home.

Subliminal Tapes

 They don't work. Period. That is the conclusion of Clifton Mitchell, Ph.D., counseling psychologist at East Tennessee State University in Johnson City. He studied literature on the effectiveness of audiotapes claiming to contain life-improving subliminal messages and published his findings in *Perceptual and Motor Skills*, a professional journal.

These audiotapes typically claim to carry inaudible messages that somehow penetrate to the listener's subconscious, where they help motivate people to lose weight, quit smoking, start exercising, or simply relax.

The problem, Dr. Mitchell emphatically states, is that "there is no scientific evidence to support the efficacy of auditory subliminal tapes as they're marketed."

To illustrate why, he first explains how they are made. Manufacturers tape-record a suggestive voice message containing a phrase such as "I will stop smoking." That message will be repeated many times. Over that recording, they will then record the sounds of ocean waves, mountain streams, or mellow New Age music—so loud that they will drown out the voiced message.

"The theory is that you'll unconsciously hear the first message, that it will bypass your conscious awareness," he says. But it doesn't, Dr. Mitchell contends, and here's why. The human eardrum works mechanically. It vibrates when air waves hit it. Those waves then get converted to neurological electrical impulses that then tell the brain something is banging on that drum. If the waves don't hit the drum, the brain never gets the message. Dr. Mitchell makes this analogy: If he and you were talking next to railroad tracks when a loud train went by, drowning out your conversation, you wouldn't be able to hear what each other said. "Those louder train vibrations would eat up the softer ones of our voices," he says. "You'd never physically hear my words, so they'd never get to your brain." It's the same with so-called subliminal messages.

In the study he devised, he used the highly suggestible message of itching. One group heard a tape that contained only music. Another heard a tape with music and a so-called subliminal message (but they weren't told it contained a message). The third heard the tape with background music and a clearly audible message and were told what the message was. The groups were observed listening to the tapes. There was no difference in the amount of scratching observed among all three groups.

Nonetheless, people buy these tapes. Why? "The advertising of subliminal tapes works because people are susceptible to magical remedies," says Dr. Mitchell. "They're offering you the ability to break habits without making you exert any willpower and with no suffering."

But really (*buy another copy of this book*), wouldn't they be great (*buy two more copies of this book*) if they did work (*buy a whole stack of this book*)?

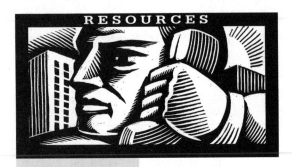

Mental Health

National Institute of Mental Health
(800) 421-4211

For free literature about depression and where to get effective treatments, call this hotline anytime. The Information Request Line will help you with panic disorders, anxiety, obsessive-compulsiveness, post-traumatic stress disorder, and phobias.

Grief Relief

Grief Recovery Institute
(800) 445-4808

This toll-free number will put you in touch with counseling services to help you cope with your loss. Call Monday through Friday, 9:00 A.M. to 5:00 P.M. Pacific time.

Help for Dad

Parents Place Web Site
http://www.parentsplace.com/readroom

Here is a forum for all parents. Parenting professionals answer your questions. Read advice from lawyers, gender experts, doctors, preschool teachers, and others. Reading rooms cover needs such as stepparenting, parenting teens, single parenting, and raising adopted children. There are more than 20 reading rooms for information and guidance. You can find science and nature activities to do with the kids.

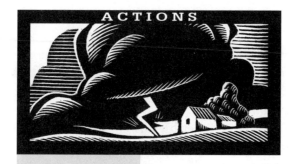

ACTIONS

If the 1980s were known as the Greed Decade, the 1990s may well be remembered as the Mental Toughness Decade. As the world—and our lives—move faster and faster toward the millennium, "The guy who maintains sharp focus, strong discipline, and passionate commitment will not just survive but thrive in these times," says Steven Ungerleider, Ph.D., a research psychologist based in Eugene, Oregon, and author of *Mental Training for Peak Performance*. That means making sure that your mental muscles are as well-toned as your arm, leg, and back muscles. Here are 14 suggestions for winning life's mental Olympics.

1. **Count on mental warmups.** If you wake up feeling as though your thought processes are moving at glacial speed—and they need to be moving at the speed of light—try some mental warmups "to get the fuzzies out," says B. Alexis Castorri, a mental health counselor in Fort Lauderdale, Florida, and author with Jane Heller of *Exercise Your Mind: 36 Mental Workouts for Peak Performance*. (Among her trainees: tennis great Ivan Lendl.) "Warming up your mind will allow you to perform more effectively when it really counts," she says. She calls the following warmup "Getting Your Mind in Gear." Take about 5 to 10 minutes when you first wake up for this (do each as quickly as you can).
- Count out loud backward from 100 to 1.
- Recite the alphabet out loud, accompany each letter with a word that starts with that letter.
- Name out loud 20 men's first names, numbering each as you go.
- Do the same as above with women's names.
- Do the same for types of food.
- Choose one letter of the alphabet and name 20 words that begin with that same letter.
- Shut your eyes and count to 20. Open your eyes. Take on the day.

2. **Break negative thought cycles.** Negative thinking saps your energy and draws your attention to exactly the opposite of what you should be focusing on. Castorri says that the next time someone or something ticks you off and gets you thinking in a dark downward spiral, follow this five-step process. Command your mind to:

- *Stop* letting this unpleasant thought affect your behavior.
- *Cancel* any negative feelings you have toward this person, experience, place, or thing.
- *Release* any residual feelings from your body and mind.
- *Relax* your whole body by taking several deep breaths.
- *Refocus* on what is important here—namely, the positive movement of your life toward the goals you want to achieve, whether they be rich and fulfilling personal relationships or satisfying work experiences.

3. **Keep the faith.** Researchers at Dartmouth Medical School in Hanover, New Hampshire, found that older folks who derive at least some strength and comfort from religion are three times more likely to survive longer after cardiac surgery than those who do not. The study also found that those involved in social and community groups—whether government or church groups, historical societies, or senior centers—had three times the survival rate of nonjoiners. Those with both faith and friends enjoyed a 10-fold increase in survival. Researchers on the project concluded that these social and religious factors could be as important as the risks of cigarette smoking and high blood pressure. The take-home message is clear: A social network and religion may not yet be the kind of medicine your HMO will prescribe, but they may help you live a little longer just the same.

4. **Learn to breathe.** You thought it came naturally. You've been breathing since the doctor spanked your butt. But did you know that breathing exercises can help reduce a slew of ailments—like generalized anxiety disorders, panic attacks, agoraphobia, depression, irritability, muscle tension, headaches, and fatigue? To review, there are two types of breathing. Chest, or thoracic, breathing is associated with anxiety or other emotional distress. It's shallow, irregular, and rapid and causes the shoulders to rise. Newborn babies and sleeping adults do the other type of breathing—abdominal, or diaphragmatic, breathing—naturally. They draw air deep into their lungs as their diaphragm contracts and expands. This is the breath of fresh air your life needs: It's the way to go. You can tell which way you're breathing by bringing your right hand to your abdomen and your left to the middle of your chest. If your right hand rises and falls, you're breathing in a relaxed style. Continue with slow deep breaths; if your left hand is rising, that's chest breathing. Not good. Do two full exhalations to push out the air from the bottom of your lungs. The vacuum created by that shift will force you to breath in deeply through your belly. Stay with that.

5. **Change for good.** Approximately 50 percent of Americans make New Year resolutions every January 1, according to John Norcross, Ph.D., professor of psychology at the University of Scranton in Pennsylvania and co-author of *Changing for Good.* His studies show that after the first week about 25 percent of them give up. From then to the six-month mark, it's a slippery slide into sloth-dom. By July 1, only about 40 percent will have kept their resolve to quit smoking, shed some pounds, undertake exercise regimes, or drop bad habits. "Willpower does not come in a bottle," says Dr. Norcross. "We see discipline as a series of behaviors that can be taught and learned." Here are some specific stick-to-it tips.

- Face the facts. "The first step is to be aware that you have a problem," says Dr. Norcross. Gather information that convinces you, for instance, that smoking is bad for your health or that those extra pounds are taking a toll on your heart. "Everyone is great at denial and rationalization," he adds, "but the facts are more difficult to refute."
- Look both backward and forward. You have to be repulsed by the bad habit you want to stop and "drawn to the light of change," says Dr. Norcross. That's why Janus, the ancient Roman god after whom January was named and resolutions were inspired, is two-faced. "We've found that relying on either alone is not as effective," he adds.
- Avoid negative influences. Keep away from people participating in the behavior you'd like to quit and situations that trigger your urge to renew those behaviors. Keep "tight environmental control," said Dr. Norcross. "Avoid tempting people, places, and things that try to seduce you back into what you're trying to give up.
On the flip side, he adds, buddy up. Exercise with a regular partner or abstain from smoking or eating in conjunction with a friend. Social support provides reinforcement, concrete advice, and a sense of togetherness and mutual struggle.

6. **Cut yourself some slack.** When you're committing to change, don't try to force absolutes on yourself, says G. Alan Marlatt, Ph.D., professor of psychology and director of the Addictive Behaviors Research Center at the University of Washington in Seattle. "Be gentle on yourself," he says. Some people punish themselves for missing a workout or sneaking a Twinkie by quitting the regime, the ultimate cutting-off-your-nose-to-spite-your-face gesture. Self-blame is demoralizing and works against you, says Dr. Marlatt. You have a better chance of keeping your resolve if you view a relapse as a slip from which you can recover. In fact, he has observed, an occasional slip may enhance the ability to be successful in the long run, provided that it's rectified as quickly as possible. He adds that wanting something to come true is not enough; you need a game plan: "It's not enough to say, 'Where there's a will, there's a way.' There has to be a will *and* a way."

7. **Add these motivational weapons to your artillery.** Steve Edwards, Ph.D., professor of sport psychology at Oklahoma State University in Stillwater, adds still more factors that spur the motivation to exercise.

- Catharsis. Vigorous exercise helps you work off steam. You can vent feelings of frustration at work or home by sweating out a few more reps with weights or extra minutes on the treadmill.
- The aesthetic attraction. "There's a beauty to the body in motion," says Dr. Edwards. That doesn't only apply to NFL films of football players moving in slow motion to a ballet soundtrack. It also includes the close-up view of bulging biceps—yours!—curling 25-pound weights. Why do you think they put mirrors on all the gym walls?
- The ascetic attraction. Discipline is a reward in itself. Getting off your butt, sticking to the regimen, facing down the demons of sloth and torpor "is where the strokes come in," Dr. Edwards says. "There's a big perk in just being able to say, 'I did it!'"
- Pursuit of vertigo. There's a rush, a thrill, to taking on a new challenge. Each time you lift a heavier weight or add resistance to your stationary bike, "you are creating a risk-taking situation," explains Dr. Edwards. "It's more psychological than physical risk. It's also the risk of failure or embarrassment or giving up."

8. **Remember this tip.** Forgetfulness is a fact of life. As we age, we start to lose neurons, brain cells that send signals to each other. Vitamins, mnemonics (tricks for remembering things), tying a string around your finger—these little strategies help. But when it comes to a critical wedding anniversary or birthday, sometimes you need a friend to tap you on the shoulder. Better yet if it's a techie friend. Enter Blake David Mills IV, who created "Remind U-Mail," a World Wide Web address that—for free!—sends you an e-mail reminder of important events such as anniversaries or your sister's piano recital. Once you sign up—and did we mention it's free?—you enter the date that you want to be reminded of and a brief description of it. Once a year up to 2001, you'll get an e-mail message shortly before the date. Mills started the service while at the University of Pennsylvania. The Web site is http://calendar.stwing.upenn.edu. You can contact the service by e-mail at blakem@calendar.stwing.upenn.edu. It's free.

9. **Command respect.** Marines call good posture command presence, and "it leaves no question about who's in total charge," says Gunnery Sergeant David

Camacho, who trains drill instructors at the Marine Corps Recruit Depot on Parris Island, South Carolina. This ramrod-straight position—the basic military stance from which all other positions are taught—may not guarantee respect, but we guarantee that you will look taller. These, says Sgt. Camacho, are the official directions to attain command presence.

- Bring left heel to right heel.
- Turn feet out equally to 45 degrees. Keep heels on same line and touching.
- Legs should be straight but not stiff at the knees.
- Keep hips and shoulders level and chest lifted.
- Arms should hang naturally, thumbs along trousers seams, palms facing inward toward legs, and fingers joined in a natural curl.
- Keep head and body erect. Look straight ahead. Keep mouth closed and chin pulled in slightly.
- Stand still and do not talk.

10. **Drive smart, not fast.** When you get cut off in traffic, do you try to catch up to the other guy, cut ahead, honk your horn, or salute him with a digit other than your ring finger? You're not alone, but neither are you helping your own case, says Raymond Novaco, Ph.D., a psychology professor at the University of California at Irvine. He found that about 40 percent of the men he surveyed did the same thing at some time. That kind of behavior makes commuting feel like a Darwinian survival test. Here are some of Dr. Novaco's tips for how to make it less so.

- Avoid peak driving time whenever possible.
- Set your expectations for traffic and calmly adjust to the unexpected. Most anger comes from the way we perceive things.
- Make the condition in your car as comfortable as possible with music you enjoy, a good backrest, a seat cushion, and other ergonomic adjustments.
- Work out stress before you get in the car by working out at the gym. (And you'll avoid those traffic jams after work, too.)
- Use a car phone in cases when you're going to be late, to forewarn others of your delay.

11. **Leave the driving to someone else.** If the above tips don't apply to you because you take public transportation, you may still be under stress when you miss the train or get crammed in between two people who apparently don't own soap. "Mass transit stress is a control issue," says Richard Wener, Ph.D., professor of environmental psychology at Polytechnic University in Brooklyn, New York, who has surveyed train commuters. He suggests taking control to the degree that you can.

- If the train stops between stations and there's no explanation, find a conductor and ask why there's a delay and when it will be resolved. You may not get an answer but, Dr. Wener says, you'll feel better for having asked.
- Make as few transfers as possible. Every time you switch from one train to another, or from bus to train to bus, you relinquish control and increase the possibility of delay.
- Try to get on the bus or train at a station where your chances of getting a seat are improved. Standing the whole trip will stress you out all the more.

12. **Practice "office aikido."** If that dweeb in accounting is trying to sabotage your career, don't wait in hiding in the parking lot and attack him. (After all, he *is* the boss's nephew.) Better to practice "office aikido," according to James Campbell Quick, Ph.D., professor of organizational behavior at the University of Texas at Arlington. Aikido is a martial art in which you use the force of your opponent's attack to let him overthrow himself. Use it when someone at work—or anywhere—is trying to get the best of you. Rather than counterpunch, let him make the mistake. In other words, explains Dr. Quick, instead of being defensive or aggressive, let him destroy himself. So when he comes up with a memo that tries to undercut you, ask him or his boss if he has considered the implication of his memo on the new marketing plan (which your friend in marketing has slipped you and which buries his memo).

13. **Play music that moves you.** Louder and faster or slower and quieter do not necessarily make a difference in the power of music to pump you up or settle you down. So says Suzanne Hanser, Ed.D., chair of the music therapy department at the Berklee College of Music in Boston. In a study she conducted, she found that progressively louder, faster, more complex music causes people to have heart rate and respiration responses that are remarkably similar to those they experience when they listen to progressively softer, more mellow music. What made the difference was people's history with the music. "It's the associations we make with music that influence its physiological and psychological effect on us," she explains. So it's your pick: Brahms's lullabies or the Beastie Boys. Whichever moves you emotionally.

14. **Play with your houseplants.** According to Bill Wolverton, Ph.D., retired senior research scientist for NASA and now head of Wolverton Environmental Services in Picayune, Mississippi, houseplants "give off substances that we haven't identified yet" that he believes contribute "to euphoric feelings." So water them; hang out with them. But when you find yourself asking them for advice, it may be time to hose yourself down.

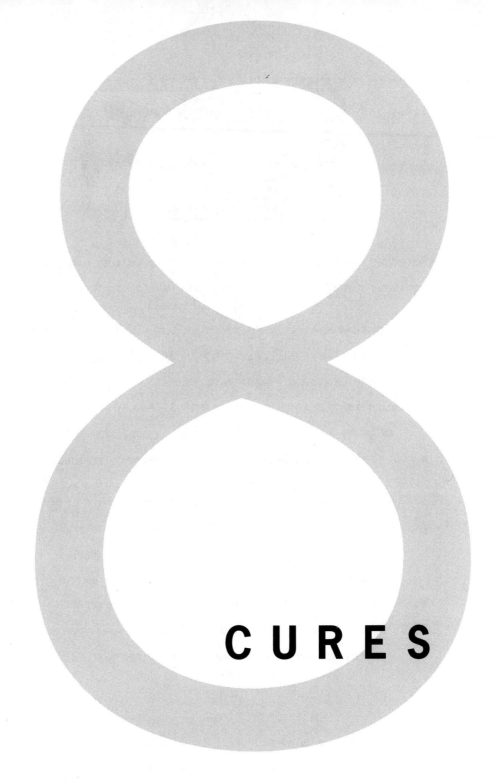

CURES

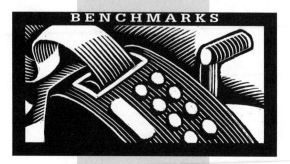

BENCHMARKS

AVERAGES

■ Percentage of Americans who would like to have more time for stress-reducing activities: 25

■ Number of users worldwide of the popular antidepression drug fluoxetine (Prozac): 24 million in 107 nations

■ Cost of depression-caused absenteeism and productivity losses: $23.8 billion

■ Number of men having hair transplants or restorations in a year: 197,276

■ Average cost for a hair implant or restoration: $2,150 to $8,000

■ Number of surgical procedures in the United States annually: more than 25 million

■ Chances that an American will undergo invasive surgery this year: 1 in 8

■ Maximum amount of sulfur in one human exhalation before it is considered bad breath: 130 parts per billion

■ Number of Breath Savers mints Americans consume annually: 2.9 billion

■ Percentage of Americans who believe they will get cancer: 59

■ Percentage of American men who actually do get cancer: 48.2

■ Death rate drop for testicular cancer since 1973: 66 percent

■ Percentage of Americans who believe they are likely to get AIDS: 4

■ The lifetime chance of dying from heart disease for the average American: 1 in 3

■ The ratio of chronic constipation between men and women: 2 to 1

EXTREMES

■ The most likely month for dying: January

■ The least likely month for dying: September

■ Amount by which one standard chest x-ray increases your risk of cancer: approximately 1 in 1,000,000

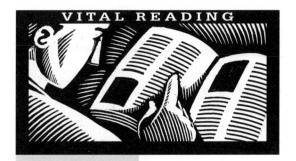

VITAL READING

Surprising Side Effects

Look to your diet for answers to what's causing unusual symptoms.

Sometimes the male body is a mystery, even to those of us who live in one. We think we have a pretty good handle on how our bodies function, but occasionally a symptom shows up and we can't figure out what's causing it. Unexplained pains. Slow-healing sores. Foul odors adrift at inopportune moments. Nothing bad enough for us to rush to the doctor about, but then again, not the kind of thing a guy wants to live with for too long.

That's when you have to slip on a trench coat, muss up your hair, and play a little Columbo. And often, the first place to look for evidence is your diet. What you eat, and the quantities you eat it in, can not only have a long-term impact on your body but also cause or cure numerous niggling short-term health problems. Eradicating these symptoms can be as simple as chowing down on more or less of what's good for you.

The symptom: Leg cramps

What could cause it: A lack of calcium, magnesium, sodium, or potassium in your diet. These minerals are the electrolytes that your body needs to spur normal muscle contractions. As you drip your daily sweat, your body doles out these minerals like campaign funds. Simple dehydration can also add to the misery.

What could cure it: First, drink plenty of water before, during, and after exercise. Second, eat a banana or some low-fat yogurt during your postexercise ritual. Both pack the necessary minerals to keep your muscles functioning properly. Other good choices include sports drinks, baked potatoes, and whole-grain foods.

The symptoms: Diarrhea, gas, and bloating

What could cause them: Lactose intolerance. Your body may not produce enough lactase, the enzyme necessary for digesting dairy products. It's especially likely if you're of Native American, African, or Asian descent.

What could cure them: If you suspect that you can't handle dairy foods, try not eating any for a day or two, then slowly add them to gauge your body's reaction, advises Franca Alphin, R.D., director of nutrition at the Duke University Diet and Fitness Center in Durham, North Carolina. If the problems return with gut-wrenching certainty, then reduce or eliminate dairy products, switch to lactose-free milk products, or try one of the over-the-counter lactase preparations that make up for the missing enzyme in your digestive process. In any case, make sure to find alternative sources of calcium in your diet. Some top dairy-free alternatives include calcium-fortified orange juice, canned salmon, and broccoli.

The symptom: Stinky feet and pits

What could cause it: Too many visits to that trendy Thai restaurant. Peppers, onions, and garlic can cause some funky odors to emanate from your pores, often up to 24 hours after a meal. Spicy foods that make you sweat can kick-start the pungent bacteria that occur naturally on your skin.

What could cure it: Either stick to mildly seasoned versions of your favorite dishes or stock up on antiperspirant—and keep your boots on.

The symptom: Cavities

What could cause it: Not your sweet tooth but your carbo-loading fetish may be the culprit. Any sticky, carbohydrate-packed food, such as dried fruits, fig cookies, and the like, can leave a wealth of debris clinging to your teeth long after your snack. While these naughty, nougaty things linger, your body will swamp your mouth with acid. This acid can damage your tooth enamel, and eventually bacteria will find the time and place to invade the soft dentin in your teeth and set up light housekeeping.

What could cure it: Well, brushing and flossing will help, as will cutting down on snacks. But when you're someplace where this isn't possible, choose your carbohydrate sources more wisely. Go for fresh, crunchy fruits and vegetables, such as apples, which help scrape debris off your teeth.

The symptom: Poor morning performance

What could cause it: If you've had a good 8 hours of rest and still find your head on your keyboard all morning long, either you're skipping the most important meal of the day or you are Keith Richards.

What could cure it: Don't eat one breakfast, eat two. Breaking your fast when you first get up will help make you less hungry the rest of the day and give you long-burning energy. But to keep yourself extra sharp during that morning meeting, grab a second light meal—a bagel and juice, maybe—a half-hour before your big presentation. A study of school students showed that those who ate breakfast a half-hour before a test performed better than students who ate 2 hours beforehand, thanks to the quick boost in their blood sugar.

The symptom: Blushing

What could cause it: Too much niacin. Niacin is used to treat high cholesterol because of its ability to reduce low-density lipoprotein (LDL, the artery-clogging kind) cholesterol and boost high-density lipoprotein (HDL, the artery-clearing kind) cholesterol. But in high doses, niacin can cause you to blush like a priest at a panty raid. How much is too much? "It's individual," says Janice Joneja, Ph.D., director of the allergy nutrition research program at Vancouver Hospital and Health Sciences Center. "A few people respond even at the multivitamin level."

What could cure it: Lay off the niacin-enriched multivitamins and keep track of how much tofu, beans, cottage cheese, fish, and chicken you're eating. Niacin is necessary for good nerve function and metabolism, but you need only about 19 milligrams to fill your daily quota (about what you'd receive in just 5 ounces of chicken). More than 100 milligrams a day can be toxic. If you're taking prescription niacin for cholesterol control, consult your doctor.

The symptoms: Fatigue and pallid skin

What could cause them: Anemia, an exhaustion of red blood cells. Iron-deficiency anemia is one of the most common dietary pitfalls in the world. Though it's rare among men in the United States, it's found occasionally in endurance athletes and men on strict vegetarian diets. A simple blood test can tell you if you are anemic.

What could cure them: If you're a vegetarian, you can either start eating filet mignon or try drinking more orange juice. Meat contains a kind of iron readily taken into the bloodstream; the iron in beans and plant sources is more difficult to absorb. The vitamin C in orange juice makes it easier for your body to extract the iron and put it to use.

The symptom: Slow-healing cuts and scrapes

What could cause it: Your body could be crying out for zinc, which is believed to promote rapid healing. Rigorous athletic training, especially in conjunction with a vegetarian diet, can deplete your body of the zinc it needs to repair cells and grow new ones. Zinc deficiency is also linked to infertility and low testosterone levels.

What could cure it: If you're on an intense body-reshaping program, review your diet and build up your zinc levels by consuming more oysters, wheat germ, and fortified breakfast cereals.

The symptom: Dull, dry hair

What could cause it: A lack of protein in your diet. Without enough protein, your hair may turn dull and dry-looking and could begin to fall out. The protein-heavy diets of North Americans have pretty much sent this malady packing, but protein deficiency has been noted in anorexics and crash dieters.

What could cure it: Start ingesting more lean meats and beans for protein. A 3-ounce serving of sliced turkey breast has 1.5 grams of fat and 19 grams of protein. Likewise, a cup of cooked black beans provides only about a gram of fat and 15 grams of protein. But remember, vegetable proteins aren't the same as animal ones. You'll need to couple the beans with rice and a veggie to create a complete protein.

The symptom: Yellowing teeth

What could cause it: The high-powered company that your teeth keep: coffee, tea, and sodas. Sodas contain acids that can weaken the surface of teeth, making them susceptible to contamination. Tea and coffee contain tannins, long famed for staining teeth mildly brown.

What could cure it: Drink water instead. If the only alternative to caffeine is decking a co-worker, however, chase your high-test beverage of choice with a swig of water. Water dilutes the acids left in your mouth, preserving the enamel and the pearly whiteness. Fluoride can also cause mottling of the teeth in children and endurance swimmers, but contrary to urban legend, the fluoride in tap water isn't nearly strong enough to cause this problem.

The symptom: Strange odors or colors when you pee

What could cause it: Your kids put Kool-Aid in the toilet again, or you've been eating asparagus or beets. Asparagus can be smelled in urine 30 seconds after it's ingested (in a study that thrilled the pathologist, no doubt). And beets can tinge the urine red, which some people mistake for blood. Deep yellow, brownish urine can also indicate dehydration, so make sure to gulp down plenty of fluids during the day.

What could cure it: Leave the asparagus spears and borscht to those who enjoy being surprised.

Headache Relief

Instead of running for the pill bottle, try these pain relievers.

Right this minute, 1 in 15 men has a headache. If you're one of them, you don't want to hear about how you should have slept more, had less to drink, or left your computer screen a few hours ago. You want to know how to stop the pain. Here's your checklist.

Change your lighting. The constant, barely perceptible flickering of fluorescent light tubes can bring on a blinding headache. Kill the overhead light and bring in a few lamps with regular incandescent bulbs, suggests Lawrence Robbins, M.D., author of *Headache Help*.

Muster some hot thoughts. Visualizing yourself on a hot beach can actually raise your body temperature, which might take the edge off a headache. Or just fantasize about the rhythmic gymnast in accounting.

Apply ice. Wrap a bag of crushed ice in a towel and hold it to the area of your head that hurts. Works best for dull throbs. The cold reduces the inflammation of the blood vessels that causes pain.

Drink some joe. Caffeine has a slight constricting effect on the arteries in your head, which can relieve headaches, says Dr. Robbins. In fact, caffeine is an ingredient in some pain relievers, including Excedrin and Anacin.

Turn to peppers. Rubbing capsaicin (the stuff that makes ground red pepper hot) on your nose can relieve cluster headaches. Just be careful not to get it in your eyes, as it will burn. Ask your doctor for a capsaicin preparation. It helped 75 percent of patients in one study.

Focus on your breathing. Breathe deeply six times, silently counting to four as you inhale and again as you exhale. "Concentrating on your breathing is an old trick to relieve tension, which is responsible for most men's headaches," says Dr. Robbins.

If your headache persists, go ahead and pop that pill. But new remedies are on the way.

Seek out magnesium. See your doctor about this one. A study at the New York Headache Center found that a shot of magnesium can relieve severe migraine or cluster headaches within 15 minutes. The shots worked only for people with low magnesium levels, but there's a 50/50 chance that you're one of them, says Alexander Mauskop, M.D., who directed the study. Oral supplements don't have the same effect, but daily doses may prevent migraines. Dr. Mauskop recommends 500 milligrams of chelated (check the label) magnesium, divided into two or three doses through the day.

Keep an eye on lidocaine. Researchers at Kaiser Permanente Medical Center in Woodland Hills, California, gave migraine sufferers nasal drops with 4 percent lidocaine, an anesthetic for skin conditions. About half of the headaches vanished, though many of them resurfaced within an hour. "We believe that the anesthetic dulls a large nerve in the nasal passageways," says Morris Maizels, M.D., lead physician in the study. Lidocaine is available, but you'll have to wait until the Food and Drug Administration approves it for headache treatment.

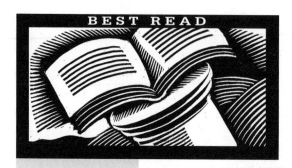

BEST READ

Self-Care Massage of the Head and Face

There are few things more aggravating than a stiff neck from staring at a computer screen all day. Instead of popping a painkiller, try something a little different—like massaging that tension away. In this excerpt from Massage for Pain Relief *(Random House, 1996), Chinese massage master Peijian Shen relates these techniques to relieve stiff necks, headaches, and other ailments through self-massage. Here's how to give pain the rubout.*

Kneading the head. Place the heel of your right hand on the top of your head, midway between your ears. This covers the acupoint known as Du20 (*Baihui*). Apply moderate pressure and knead the area slowly with 10 circular clockwise strokes, and then 10 counterclockwise strokes.

In Chinese medicine, the brain is called "Reservoir of Marrow." Du20 is the key acupoint that controls the flow of Qi passing through the reservoir. This massage therefore has a beneficial effect on the brain. It also enhances the memory and prevents high blood pressure.

Kneading the temples. Put your thumbs on either side of your face on the temples, one thumb-width away from the outside edge of the eye and level with the top of the ear. This is the position of the extra acupoints known as *Taiyang*. Knead both points slowly in a clockwise direction and with moderate pressure. Repeat 30 times.

Taiyang is very effective in treating a variety of disorders in the head region. This massage helps to prevent headaches, insomnia, and eye problems such as shortsightedness. It also relaxes the brain.

Combing the head. Let your fingers curl naturally. Then, using your fingertips, apply moderate pressure and comb your head from the forehead hairline to the back of the neck. Repeat 20 times.

All the Yang Channels meet in the head, which in Chinese medicine is called the "Converging Place of All Yang." This massage relaxes the brain, improves the memory, and prevents neurosis.

Pushing the eyebrows. Place the tips of your middle fingers on the inner ends of your eyebrows. Then, with gentle pressure, push along your eyebrows to their outer ends. Repeat 10 times.

This simple massage stimulates three acupoints along the eyebrow. It relaxes the eyes and prevents eye diseases and headaches.

Rotating the eyes. Close your eyes and slowly rotate your eyeballs clockwise three times and then counterclockwise three times. Repeat three times and then open your eyes and look ahead to finish the sequence. Repeat the whole sequence three times.

In Chinese medicine, the eyes are called the "Doors of Life." This exercise relaxes the eyes and keeps them in good condition.

Wiping the face. Rub your hands together until they are warm. Then place your palms on either side of your nose and slide them across your cheeks toward the ears with a smooth, wiping action. Massage your face 10 times.

This gentle massage increases the circulation of blood to the face. It also improves the elasticity of the skin and helps to prevent wrinkles. (*Caution:* Do not perform this massage if you suffer from acne or pimples.)

Pushing the nose. Place your index fingers on either side of the bridge of your nose. Push down the sides of your nose toward the nostrils. Apply moderate pressure and speed, and repeat the stroke 20 times.

This massage, which in Chinese is called "Pushing the Life Longer," stimulates several acupoints including LI20 (*Yingxiang*). Use this massage to prevent respiratory disorders.

Pinching the ears. With your thumbs and index fingers, pinch your ears with moderate pressure. Start at the top of your ear and work down to the lobes. Repeat 10 times.

The ears are home to numerous acupoints, which relate to all the other organs and parts of the body. This massage, by stimulating your whole ear, benefits your overall health. More specifically, it also prevents high blood pressure.

Pressing the ears. Place your palms over your ears with your fingers pointing toward the back of your head. Press your palms down tightly and then remove them quickly. When you remove your palms, you may hear a sound like a drumbeat. Repeat 10 times.

This exercise improves your hearing and prevents various ear diseases, particularly tinnitus.

Rubbing the neck. Place your palms behind your ears on the back of your neck. This covers both GB20 (*Fengchi*) acupoints, on either side of the head. With your palms, rub back and forth over the acupoints 30 times. The rubbing action may make your neck feel warm.

This massage helps to prevent the onset of the common cold.

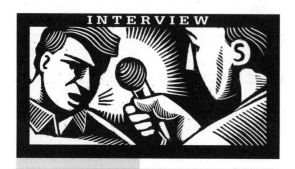

Steve J. Vodanovich on
Banishing Boredom

If ever there was a scourge upon mankind, it's that most debilitating of diseases—boredom. Forget curing the common cold: If someone could bottle a medicine to make the dull parts of life seem keen and interesting, we know we'd buy out the store. But tedium doesn't just strike like a cold or virus; it's part of you and your perception of life and its daily tasks. Even so, you can fight it. To make your life a little more interesting, we talked with Steve J. Vodanovich, Ph.D., associate professor of psychology at the University of West Florida in Pensacola and author of more studies on the topic of boredom than anyone else we know.

Why do we get bored with stuff? Is it mental? Is it physiological? Is there a step-by-step progression of events that take place in the brain and body when we get bored? What's going on inside us?

We don't really know. Friends in my department have done some studies to look at what happens physiologically in the brain when you have to do rote stuff, routine tasks—but that isn't quite the same as being bored. There is a lack of research on boredom in general, and particularly on the physiological aspects.

Okay, but tell us this: Do men get bored differently than women?

Research does indicate that men report feeling boredom more often than women. For example, there is some evidence that male infants adapt more quickly to complex and novel stimuli. When infants get exposed to something new, male babies seem to habituate more quickly. It may mean that males have a predisposition to get used to things quicker. Or maybe they just get bored faster. Of course, this is speculative.

So if we extend that speculation forward 20 years from the cradle, does it still hold true? Do men grasp things more quickly and consequently get bored more quickly?

I have found in the research I've done that males report being more bored with a lack of variety, a lack of stimulation. We feel more bored when things are mundane and monotonous than females do.

So, put the same task in front of a man and a woman, and the woman is going to get into it a little deeper; whereas the man will tend to dismiss it and get bored pretty quickly?

It depends on the task. But generally, some research has shown that men score lower on tests that measure how much they engage in and enjoy thinking. These test scores are linked to higher boredom. But it's still wide open to interpretation. However, one gender difference we do find consistently is that men report a greater need to seek out sensations. They are more inclined to be thrill and adventure seekers. Let's say that you're experiencing boredom. You say, "Gee, I feel bored. What do I do?" Men tend to seek out sensations: They'll go see a movie or turn on the TV and flick a station or two.

Or drive too fast.

Yeah, or jump out of an airplane, bungee jump—but they're all things that you can associate with stimulation and sensation seeking.

Numerous studies seem to suggest that boredom can have negative effects on our health and well-being. Can you give us more information about that?

It's not a pretty picture. The person who's more often bored than not bored doesn't do well in school, is more impulsive, experiences more states of negative affect—depression, hostility, anger, things like that. Even substance abuse has been associated with boredom. Overeating and eating disorders, in general, have been associated, too. Obviously, if these things are indeed true, we should be looking at efforts to help people identify when they're bored in the first place. I think that there is a tendency to minimize the importance of this issue. You can tell by the lack of research out there.

Certainly, there are specific types of things that universally cause boredom. Can you tell us about the most common events or scenarios that are likely to bore us?

People usually consider boredom to be temporary and something that they can escape from. It may be a class at school. It may be a task at a job. I did a study asking people to describe the time when they were most bored. Inevitably, it was either job- or school-related, and it was either a repetitive, monotonous task or just not much of a challenge.

Is boredom stressful? Or does boredom result from stress?

It can be thought of as a type of stress. Some people describe it as absence of feeling. It's a dissatisfying state. I wrote an article with a colleague that defined boredom, and one of our criteria was that it has to be dissatisfying, unpleasant.

Is feeling lethargic part of the definition?

Well, you could be not very aroused mentally or physically, but that may be a pleasing state—as in meditation. You wouldn't label that as boredom. Boredom must have the components of being unpleasant and dissatisfying. I actually think that boredom may be somewhat adaptable and may have a positive side.

How's that?

If viewed properly, boredom is a motivator. It encourages us to do different things. If you don't do things in vain—don't drink excessively, use drugs, or jump out of planes carelessly—but instead use boredom to drive you toward positive achievement, then it is useful. It can be used as an impetus, a sign that says, "Hey, you have to do something different."

Rattle your cage a little, shake you out of your misery.

Yes. Unfortunately, it is true of most people that you have to be in an unpleasant and dissatisfying state first in order to be motivated enough to do something daring and different. But if you observe boredom in people who respond positively, you'll see them go read a different book, see a different film. Or they'll make new friends, seek out new sensations, learn new things, new skills. That's the positive side of it.

Studies seem to indicate that people who get involved in educational activities—learning new things—seem to be less bored, better adjusted, happier. What else can we do to turn off boredom once it rears its ugly head?

Good question. In some situations, the easiest option is to just get up, move, escape. One other thing to do is work on concentration skills. Learn ways to absorb oneself in a task, to become interested in a task. Raise the level of challenge internally, if nothing else, to make it less boring. The internal, creative way of dealing with stimuli is probably the ultimate way of alleviating or avoiding boredom. Whether it be daydreaming or finding a different way of looking at something. There is some evidence out there that talks about how people perceive their environments. Some people perceive their environments as very black and white. Very one-dimensional. Other people have the tendency to see the world in all kinds of shades and colors. They see the complexity of a tree or of a book. People who perceive and process information in a multifaceted way—who see textures and colors and who purposely, actively try to see the world this way—are much less likely to be bored.

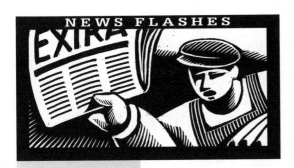

Antibiotics May Cure Periodontal Disease

DETROIT—It starts with swollen gums. Then plaque hardens into tartar, damaging those gums. Then infection causes full-blown periodontal disease, and you have to have surgery. Talk about pain and misery—and that's before you get the bill. But research conducted at the University of Michigan School of Dentistry and University of Detroit/Mercy School of Dentistry indicates that sufferers of periodontal disease may be able to avoid the scalpel with something far less invasive—antibiotics.

In a study sponsored by the National Institutes of Health, researchers had patients with periodontal disease take antibiotics orally and topically, applied directly to infected areas around the tooth. Those on antibiotics showed a 93 percent reduction in the need for surgery. Meanwhile, the number of teeth that had to be pulled was lowered by 81 percent. The results of this study open up new treatment options for people with gum disease. If you're suffering from periodontal disease, talk with your periodontist about the possibilities of antibiotic treatment—it may well be a viable option for the health of your gums.

Rubber Band Treatment Removes Hemorrhoids

PETAH-TIQWA, Israel—Hemorrhoids, the ultimate pain in the butt, will affect more than 50 percent of Americans at some point in their lives. Though they are most common in people over the age of 40, they can strike anyone who sits or stands for long periods of time, is overweight, or is frequently constipated. Researchers in Israel have found what may be the safest and most convenient way to get rid of the little tormentors.

Doctors at Rabin Medical Center treated 2,934 people with hemorrhoids, ages 12 to 86, with rubber band ligation, which involves placing a rubber band around the base of the hemorrhoid, cutting off blood supply. Without the nourishment of a fresh blood supply, the tissue forming the hemorrhoid falls off within several days. When researchers followed up a year later, 79 percent of the patients were completely cured of their hemorrhoids. Only 18 percent of the patients needed one or more additional sessions.

The researchers noted that if this method were used more frequently, it would save hundreds of hospitalization days and many thousands of sick leave days per year. Moreover, the procedure could help hemorrhoid sufferers avoid more serious and costly options, such as surgery.

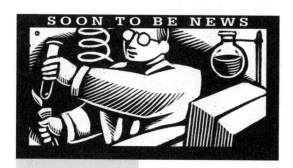

Can Heart Attacks Be Prevented?

A study that could become a landmark in high blood pressure research is entering its second phase. The Antihypertensive and Lipid-Lowering Treatment to Prevent Heart Attack Trial (ALLHAT) involves an estimated 400 doctors and 40,000 patients. The outcomes of this study could affect the millions of Americans being treated for high blood pressure and high cholesterol.

ALLHAT intends to answer several questions, including whether the newer antihypertensive drugs are as good as or better than traditional diuretics in controlling or halting coronary heart disease. Another main question that ALLHAT hopes to address is whether lowering low-density lipoprotein (LDL, the "bad") cholesterol in people who have moderately high cholesterol levels will reduce their risks of heart disease and death.

The 40,000 patients making up this trial all have high blood pressure. Fifty-five percent of the patients are African-Americans, who have a particular susceptibility to high blood pressure. Researchers will compare traditional diuretic treatment with three alternative treatments to determine if the alternative treatments are as effective or better in treating high blood pressure. A subgroup of

20,000 patients who suffer from moderately high cholesterol levels will take part in an additional study to determine if a cholesterol-lowering substance, prava-statin (Pravachol), can reduce death rates.

This study could change the way hypertension, especially among African-Americans and those with high cholesterol, is treated in the future. The ALLHAT study treatment and follow-up is scheduled to last for the next six years.

An End to Open-Heart Surgery?

Typical open-chest heart surgery involves making a foot-long incision in the chest. Then surgeons saw through the breastbone and pry open the rib cage. God forbid that you ever have to go through that. Soon, though, you may never have to, even if you ever do need heart surgery.

A research firm called Heartport, of Redwood City, California, has devel-oped a new method for performing several heart surgeries that usually involve cracking the chest wide open. But the new procedure, called Port-Access heart surgery, involves making only two to four small incisions between a patient's ribs to gain access to the heart. Tiny instruments—including a flexible scope to let surgeons see what they're doing—are then inserted into the incisions.

The benefits of Port-Access heart surgery include minimal pain, much less scarring, and easier movement after the surgery. The procedure also reduces hospital stays from 7 to 10 days to only 3 to 5. Port-Access also cuts down recov-ery time from months to only a couple of weeks.

Though Port-Access methods may not be available at your local hospital yet, doctors are being trained in the technique at Brigham and Women's Hospital in Boston, the Cleveland Clinic Foundation in Ohio, and Johns Hopkins Hospital in Baltimore.

Can Cancer Be Starved to Death?

Just the word *cancer* strikes fear into the hearts of most people. No wonder—according to the National Cancer Institute, almost half of all American men will develop cancer of some kind over the course of their lifetimes. But a new set of cancer-starving drugs may soon give tumors something to worry about.

These new drugs are called angiogenesis inhibitors. They work on the theory that tumors need a blood supply, usually from the body's capillaries, in order to grow. Not only does that blood supply provide the nourishment that tumor cells need to live; it also offers a route that cancerous cells can use to spread to other parts of the body. But if you can cut off that blood supply, or keep the tumor from sending out signals to make new blood vessels to feed itself, you can starve the cancer out. That's exactly what angiogenesis inhibitors are designed to do.

Already, several substances have been found that act as inhibitors, but one of the most powerful is called angiostatin. In laboratory animals, this substance stops almost all blood vessel growth in tumors and in the locations where the tumor has spread, essentially starving a tumor to death.

More research needs to be done on angiogenesis inhibitors, but right now scientists are studying the effects of these drugs on prostate, colon, and breast cancers that have been implanted in mice and allowed to grow. Angiostatin has been shown to reduce the tumors to microscopic size, and keep them from growing, for as long as the drug is administered. When these substances are approved and more widely available, they would be used in conjunction with more traditional cancer therapies, such as chemotherapy and radiation treatments.

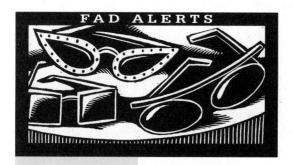

FAD ALERTS

Anti-Arthritis Supplements

Science calls them glucosamine and chondroitin sulfates. Millions of people with arthritis would like to call them cure-alls, and they've been buying these two expensive supplements in droves ever since a book by Jason Theodosakis, M.D., and others, called *The Arthritis Cure*, hit the bestseller list. In that book, Dr. Theodosakis, a sports medicine specialist and director of the Preventive Medicine Residency Training Program at the University of Arizona College of Medicine in Tucson, contends that these supplements are building blocks for cartilage—the tough, flexible tissue in your joints that keeps bones from grinding against one another and causing arthritis pain.

European studies have shown that glucosamine and chondroitin sulfate supplements are effective in reducing osteoarthritis pain for most sufferers, notes holistic physician Andrew Weil, M.D., director of the Program in Integrative Medicine of the University of Arizona College of Medicine and editor of the newsletter *Dr. Andrew Weil's Self-Healing*. Both substances have long been used by veterinarians to treat arthritis in dogs and cats, notes Dr. Weil.

While "cure" may overstate the case, Dr. Theodosakis contends in his book that the supplements can relieve arthritis symptoms. "Some patients who have suffered from arthritis for years have been able to use the supplements for a few months, go off them, and remain pain-free more than two years later," he says. Also, there is evidence of reversal of the cartilage damage that occurs from osteoarthritis. This is the basis for the bold title of Dr. Theodosakis's book. Obviously, he adds, no medical treatment, including this one, works on everyone.

Dr. Weil says that he recommends glucosamine and chondroitin sulfates to his osteoarthritis patients and has seen good results in his practice. A month's supply can be quite expensive (from $39 to $87), though, and not all brands contain adequate levels of the effective ingredients. To ensure its purity, make sure that the chondroitin label says that it's pharmaceutical grade.

In his book, Dr. Theodosakis offers a dosage chart based on weight. Some people may need more and some need less, but generally if you weigh between 120 and 200 pounds, he recommends 1,500 milligrams of glucosamine plus 1,200 milligrams of chondroitin sulfates. Dr. Theodosakis says that these supplements have no known adverse side effects.

Echinacea

This may be the best-selling herb in America and for good reason. It builds the immune system and fights both bacterial and viral infections. "A general immune system stimulant like echinacea is something that we don't have in conventional medicine," says Adriane Fugh-Berman, M.D., author of *Alternative Medicine: What Works.*

Early American doctors learned about echinacea (pronounced *eh-kin-AY-sha*) from Native Americans. Made from the roots of the purple coneflower, it was widely prescribed until penicillin was discovered and came into vogue in the 1930s and 1940s, along with other modern antibiotics. Now it's back, and it has science to back it up. More than 25 scientific trials have established the herb's immune-boosting ability. You can find echinacea in health food stores and drugstores in teas, capsules, tinctures, and combination remedies. And it's probably showing up on more and more of your co-workers' desks when they have colds.

Go ahead and use it for minor infections like colds and flu, says Dr. Fugh-Berman. Take it at the first sign of sniffles or scratchy throat, but never depend on it solely to fight a major infection like pneumonia, she warns. And when you do use it, follow these guidelines.

- Only use the herb for brief periods during infections, a week at a time. Used daily, it loses its effectiveness.
- Skip it if you have an autoimmune disorder such as lupus or rheumatoid arthritis—you don't need to hype up an immune system that already is overreacting.

• No one is sure how much you should use and various formulations have varying potency. The best recommendation for now, according to Dr. Fugh-Berman, is to follow the instructions on the package of commercial preparations.

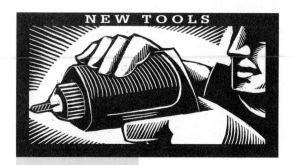

Saving Seeds

Ground Flaxseed

What tastes pleasantly nutty, is easy to sprinkle on cereals and other foods, cuts bad cholesterol significantly, wards off heart disease and autoimmune diseases like rheumatoid arthritis, is full of fiber, and has even been shown to shrink colon cancer tumors in animal and test tube studies? Ground flaxseed. You can order it at health food stores. Try to get between one level tablespoon and ¼ cup of the ground seed daily for maximum health benefits, researchers say. If you buy the seed pre-ground, make sure that it has vitamins C and E added to protect against oxidation, in which it mixes with oxygen, loses its nutritional benefits, and could even become harmful. Keep it refrigerated after opening and use it within six months. Sprinkle a tablespoon or more on cereals, soups, and yogurts and in fruit juices. Or buy the whole seeds and grind just what you're going to use each time in a coffee grinder. Price: $1.19 a pound for seeds in bulk at our favorite local health food store.

Ending Phone Pain

Wireless Headsets

If you spend the day on the phone, holding it on your shoulder by cocking your head against it to keep your hands free, we don't need to tell you about grumpy, crampy necks. Tilting the head in that awkward position actually causes the neck and shoulder muscles to get shorter and tighter, says Joel Press,

M.D., medical director of the Center for Spine, Sports, and Occupational Rehabilitation at the Rehabilitation Institute of Chicago. Telephone headsets have been available for years to help mitigate this problem, but many older styles have proved as clunky and awkward as the handsets they were meant to replace. Enter the lightweight, wireless, hands-free headset. These newer, nicer models are so light and liberating, you'll think someone implanted a phone in your head. One of our favorites, made by Plantronics, has a wallet-sized dialing unit that clips onto a waistband. Dr. Press even uses his while working out on a cross-country ski machine. If they're not readily in stock, you can special order them at most office supply stores. Price: $200 to $300. Or call the company at (800) 544-4660 to locate a distributor near you.

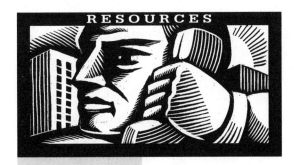

RESOURCES

AIDS Alert

HIV/AIDS Treatment Information Service (ATIS)
(800) 448-0440
http://www.hivatis.org

The HIV/AIDS Treatment Information Service provides health information specialists who answer questions on federally approved treatment options for AIDS. The staff is bilingual (English and Spanish) and uses the National Library of Medicine database and other federal resources to answer questions. The specialists can refer you to an extensive network of federal services, national organizations, and community-based groups for more treatment-related information.

Both the hotline and the Web site are part of a project sponsored by seven public-health agencies, including the Centers for Disease Control and Prevention in Atlanta. The Web site can link you to AIDS Clinical Trials Information Service for clinical trial studies and treatment options being researched. You can also access fact sheets on understanding viral load, protease inhibitors, and caring for an AIDS patient at home.

Cancer Treatments

CancerNet Web Site
http://cancernet.nci.nih.gov

The official Web site of the National Cancer Institute provides up-to-date information on cancer treatment and research for patients and professionals. Post questions to cancer specialists. Locate worldwide clinical trials or use a directory to find doctors and organizations providing care. The site even gives you access to PDQ, the Institute's comprehensive cancer database on treatment, supportive care, screening, and prevention. This information has been reviewed by oncology experts and is based on current research.

Diabetes Control

National Institute of Diabetes and Digestive and Kidney Diseases
National Institutes of Health Web Site
http://www.niddk.nih.gov

More than 3.5 million men in the United States have diabetes and don't know it. Explore this site and you'll find a wide array of information on types I and II diabetes, including news releases, upcoming meetings and conferences, and diabetes statistics. You can also find information on diabetic eye disease, renal disease, hypoglycemia, insulin-dependent and non-insulin-dependent diabetes, blood sugar control, and nerve damage due to diabetes.

Rosacea Resource

National Rosacea Society
(888) 662-5874

This common skin disorder causes visible blood vessels and pimples on the face. Symptoms usually begin in your thirties and worsen with age. Rosacea is especially severe in men because they delay treatment and end up looking like W. C. Fields, who had the disorder. Call the hotline and you can get a free newsletter, checklists of information, and a list of dermatologists in your area. You'll also learn about treatment options and risk factors. We learned, for example, that rosacea can be aggravated by stress, spicy foods, and alcohol but is highly treatable with topical antibiotics.

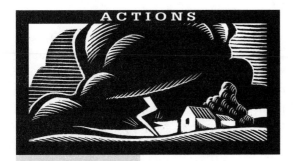

ACTIONS

Cures don't have to be miraculous acts of God or science. Sometimes they're as simple as changing what you eat for breakfast, drinking a cup of coffee, or even writing something down on a piece of paper. From the common cold to the recurring nightmare, here are 10 simple cures that are good for what ails you.

1. "C" your way clear of osteoarthritis. People with osteoarthritis probably know that the agony that condition causes is from disappearing cartilage, the padding on the ends of bones where they meet at joints. It wears away for some reason—no one knows exactly why—and the ends of the bones grind together painfully. Now researchers have discovered that you can drastically slow down the loss of cartilage simply by watching what you eat. For 10 years, researchers followed 640 participants in the Framingham Osteoarthritis Cohort Study. They found that those getting the least vitamin C in their diets had three times the risk of their arthritis getting worse and losing cartilage than people who had more vitamin C in their diets. In fact, according to Boston University's Tim McAlindon, M.D., lead researcher of the study, a diet containing 150 to 175 milligrams of vitamin C daily reduced the progression of osteoarthritis significantly.

It may not be the vitamin C itself that is responsible for the turnaround but other healing compounds in the vitamin C–rich fruits and vegetables. The bottom line is to eat the five to nine servings of fruits and vegetables daily that are recommended by the U.S. Department of Agriculture (USDA), including plenty of vitamin C–rich foods like oranges, orange juice, broccoli, cauliflower, sweet red peppers, and cantaloupe.

2. Oil your joints. You can also cool the burn of rheumatoid arthritis with diet. Studies show that the right diet helps relieve pain and stiffness. One key seems to be stepping up your intake of the omega-3 fatty acids found in fish oil. Omega-3 fish oil supplements are the easiest way to get the 3 to 5 grams daily of omega-3 fatty acids used in one very promising study, says Joel Kremer, M.D., head of the division of rheumatology at Albany Medical College in New York. Depending on the potency of the capsules, you would need to take between 6 and 15 capsules a day. "It may be difficult to keep taking capsules for the rest of your life," he adds. "I also tell my patients that they should eat more fish." Adding more Atlantic salmon or Atlantic herring to your diet helps—those two fish are among the highest in omega-3's. "You probably need a serving of such fish every day, which would be hard to do," Dr. Kremer notes. When researchers analyzed 10 of the best-conducted studies, they concluded that at least three months of daily intake of the fish oil supplements provided modest but measurable improvements (less morning stiffness and sore joints) for rheumatoid arthritis sufferers. As always, check with your doctor before making any changes in your medication or diet. Also remember, says Dr. Kremer, that fish and fish oil should be used in addition to your regular medication, not as a substitution for it. Using flaxseed and canola oils also adds the plant form of omega-3's to your diet, though not in as high a concentration as in fish oil supplements.

A different diet strategy that seems to work to ease rheumatoid arthritis symptoms is to cut out all animal proteins except for fish or small amounts of chicken. It's also important to eat fruits, vegetables, grains, legumes (beans, peas, lentils), and soy foods. And keep fat intake down—to no more than 10 percent of total calories, says Edwin H. Krick, M.D., associate professor of medicine at Loma Linda University School of Medicine in Loma Linda, California, who put 45 rheumatoid arthritis sufferers on this regimen. The results? Within three months, symptoms were substantially relieved.

3. **Zap colds with zinc.** They don't taste great, reported most of the 50 people in a study at the Cleveland Clinic Foundation, but those who sucked on zinc lozenges every few hours during a cold had fewer days of congestion, coughing, runny noses, and sore throats than those sucking on fake lozenges. A supposedly tastier version of the lozenge used in the study is available at drugstores and some health food stores. It's marketed under the name Cold-Eeze.

4. **Stop or slow macular degeneration.** This leading cause of noncorrectable vision loss in people over age 50 seems to respond well to spinach and other dark green, leafy vegetables as well as a diet including lots of fruits and vitamin E and protection from ultraviolet and blue light, says Stuart Richer, O.D., Ph.D., principal investigator of the macular degeneration study group at the Veterans Affairs Medical Center in North Chicago. To prove it, Dr. Richer and other researchers studied 71 men in their seventies who had macular degeneration in the early stages. Thirty-nine of them were given a daily capsule containing antioxidant vitamins, minerals, and other compounds from fruits and veggies; the other 32 weren't. After 18 months, the vitamin/mineral group's macular degeneration pretty much had crawled to a halt, while the other group's eyes kept failing. The recommendation? Try to get five to nine servings a day of fruits and vegetables, as recommended by the USDA. Be sure to include 5 ounces of dark green vegetables such as spinach, collard greens, or kale four to seven times a week, suggests Dr. Richer (that's a large spinach salad or about a cup of cooked vegetables per day).

5. **Be a "regular" guy.** If you find yourself struggling on the throne, here's a helpful hint. Toss one, two, or three snack pack–size boxes of raisins (1½ ounces each) in your briefcase each day. You'll need to eat them, of course. Researcher Gene A. Spiller, D.Sc., Ph.D., director of the Health Research and Studies Center in Los Altos, California, fed the equivalent of three packs of raisins daily to 13 men and women who were eating an otherwise low-fiber diet. He found that adding raisins to their diets caused waste to move through their gastrointestinal tracts in half the usual time. Three packs of raisins pack 6 grams of constipation-fighting fiber as well as tartaric acid, another ingredient that may help flush things through the gut, says Dr. Spiller. Just one box daily might be enough for some people, he said.

6. **Ask for the coffee IV.** If you've ever been scheduled for a morning surgery, you know the setup: No food or drink after midnight. This, though, is agonizing for coffee fiends, who are likely to suffer an excruciating postsurgery headache due to caffeine withdrawal, reports a study overseen by anesthesiologist Joseph G. Weber, M.D., of the Mayo Clinic in Rochester, Minnesota. Patients who got intravenous caffeine or a cup of coffee after surgery had fewer headaches. It just took the equivalent of two cups of coffee or two cans of cola to deaden the pain.

7. **Lighten up if you're feeling SAD.** As the days get colder, shorter, and darker, so do some people's tempers. Scientists are calling this wintertime depression seasonal affective disorder, or SAD for short, and it's thought to be brought on by light deprivation. Studies have been inconclusive about whether exposing sufferers to more light or bright light really alleviates symptoms. However, some people swear by light therapy. Physicians working with SAD patients often try it, and it generally is harmless (unless you expose yourself to ultraviolet rays or stare directly into a superbright light source). So try lighting up your life if you think you suffer from winter depression. Here are some commonsense suggestions for easy ways to do it.

- Trim the shrubbery away from your windows to maximize the amount of light that can enter—and keep the curtains open during daylight hours.
- Sit near a window, if you can, if you work in an office.
- Vacation in a sunny area in the winter.
- Incorporate winter sports into your routine. Get outdoors and exercise during daylight hours.

8. **Beat the runs...with yogurt.** Next time your doctor prescribes antibiotics, prescribe yogurt for yourself. Just make sure that it contains live active cultures (the label should tell you). When they enter your body, antibiotics massacre bacteria—including the beneficial bacteria that your stomach needs for normal, healthy digestion. Consequently, sometimes we suffer loose bowels when we take antibiotics. Just a cup of yogurt can replenish the beneficial bacteria, according to a recent study.

9. **Enjoy the daily grind.** Go ahead. Have a cup of joe. Drink filtered coffee—it's good for you. Not what you'd expect to hear doctors say, is it?

Medical scientists now say that coffee is not the bad guy they once suspected it was. In fact, coffee wears many white hats. Filtered coffee does not raise cholesterol levels, as previously thought, and does not contribute to heart disease. On the plus side, coffee is, of course, a temporary cure for fatigue; helps overcome constipation by stimulating the bowels; forestalls forgetfulness; actually improves long-term memory; and, yes, makes us pee a lot. That, researchers at the Harvard School of Public Health say, is a good thing because it washes out the kidneys and reduces kidney stone formation by 10 percent.

In addition, a cup of java can relieve a mild asthma attack because the caffeine acts as a gentle bronchodilator, opening blocked airways, says Marshall Plaut, M.D., chief of the allergic mechanisms section at the National Institute of Allergy and Infectious Disease in Bethesda, Maryland.

10. **Banish bad dreams.** You're on the school bus halfway to River City High. You glance down and suddenly realize you're naked. Just you. Not all the other kids. What's with the bus driver anyway? He saw you get on. Couldn't he have said, "You're naked again, kid. Are you sure you want to go through with this?" But he doesn't say that. Ever. And you have the nightmare over and over.

You don't have to anymore. In one study of dream control, 39 people were told to change the content of a recurrent nightmare. All they had to do was write down a new scenario and rehearse it. Voilà! The bad dreams dried up. It's certainly worth a try. But as a backup, we suggest that you stuff a T-shirt and pair of running shorts in your book bag. And sneer at the bus driver.

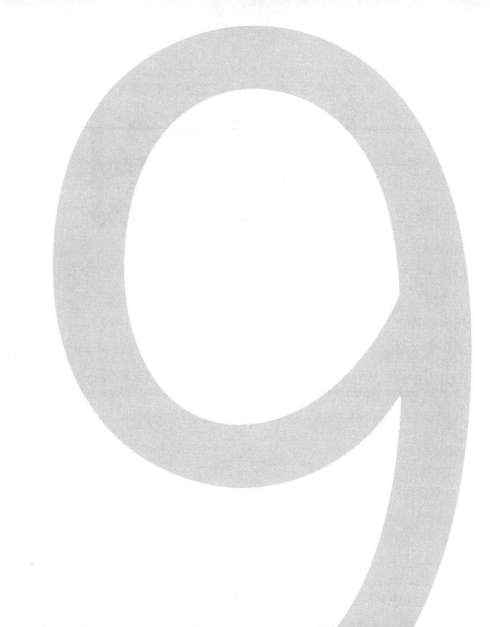

9

SLEEP

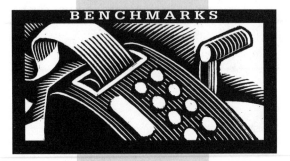

BENCHMARKS

AVERAGES

■ Percentage of sleep spent in dream sleep (REM) each night: 25

■ Duration of average night's sleep in 1910: 9 hours

■ Duration of average night's sleep today: 7 hours

■ Percentage of men who think getting a good night's sleep is most important to feeling good each day: 57

■ Percentage of men who view sleep as one of the things they enjoy most: 15

■ Percentage of men who view sleep as a waste of time they would love to avoid if they could: 27

■ Number of Americans who complain of chronic insomnia: 35 million

■ Percentage of Americans who cite stress or worries as the reason for sleeping difficulty: 46

■ Number of sleeping pill prescriptions filled each year: 14 million

■ Percentage of adults who snore occasionally: 45

■ Percentage of adults who are habitual snorers: 25

■ Number of Americans afflicted with the illness narcolepsy: 1 in 2,000

■ Percentage of fatal police-reported highway crashes that cited driver drowsiness/fatigue: 3.6

■ Number of railroad accidents each year attributed to the employee being asleep: 2

■ Percentage of adults who believe that you can't be successful in a career *and* get enough sleep: 26

■ Percentage of men who admit that they have fallen asleep at work: 18

EXTREMES

■ Longest dream on record: 3 hours, 8 minutes

■ Farthest bed pushing: 3,233 miles by a team of nine from Edinburgh

A New Bedtime Ritual

Flexibility exercises for a sound night of sleep.

Stretching, for the most part, has been designated a daylight activity. It's part of man's morning ritual—coming right after a good burp, a scratch, and a whiz. And in a kinetic sense, it's the prescribed precursor to playing three-on-three basketball or running a 10-K or wrestling a stump out of the backyard.

But stretching at night, just before bed, might be the best idea of all. You should make it a ritual like setting the alarm clock, kicking the dog off the covers, and kissing your better half. Good things can come from a little nighttime flexing.

"Slow, gentle stretching helps move the mind away from worrisome thoughts and onto calming, natural body processes," says one genuinely calm researcher, James Spira, Ph.D., assistant professor of medicine at Duke University School of Medicine in Durham, North Carolina.

What Dr. Spira means, without getting too metaphysical, is that yoga-type stretching is a good way to release pent-up stress so that you can get the kind of deep, restful sleep your body needs. Stress has a way of catching up with a man at day's end, the doctor says.

The following four stretches target the muscles of the back and chest. They encourage you to breathe more fully and release tension. Do them in order, ending with the upside-down stretch, in which you raise your hips and legs above your head and chest. There's a science to this relaxation sequence after all: "The primitive stress response causes blood to be diverted from the organs and into arm and leg muscles, which prepares us to move and act quickly," explains Dr. Spira. "Moving blood out of the legs and back into the torso and organs—as this simple upside-down position does—counteracts that response and calms the nervous system. It signals to your mind and body that it's time to relax."

And if for some reason all this stretching doesn't help you unwind, well, consider this benefit: At least your muscles will be warmed for an athletic roll in the hay, after which sleeping deeply should be no problem.

FORWARD AND BACKWARD STRETCH

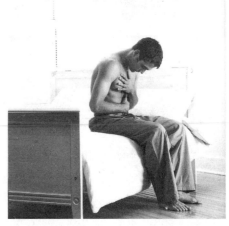

1. Sit on the edge of the bed; place one hand on your chest and the other on your abdomen. As you inhale, gently arch your spine, lifting your chest and collarbone as high as you can. Look up, stopping when you see the ceiling.

2. As you exhale, draw your tailbone under you, and let your back curl forward. Look down. On your next inhale, go to the beginning and slowly repeat the stretch six times. You'll naturally breathe more deeply while doing this.

SIDE-TO-SIDE AND ROTATION STRETCH

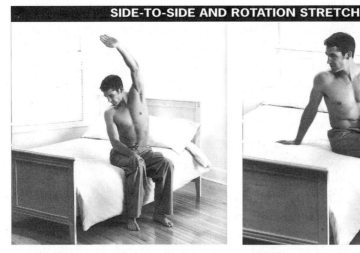
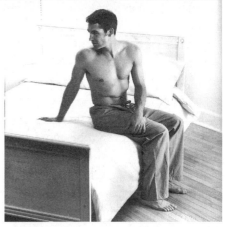

1. Sit on the edge of the bed. Exhale and lift your left arm; shift your rib cage left so your torso forms an inverted C. Shift weight onto your left buttock. Turn your head and look right. Inhale and return to the starting position. Repeat to the right.

2. Remain seated. As you exhale, rotate your torso to the right. Inhale as you lift your chest and rotate it to the right. Turn your chin and look over your right shoulder. Exhale and rotate back to the center. Repeat to the left.

n also be a source of much laughing and pointing.

Stress on your eyes. Solution: Reach out and touch someone. The eyes are ...dows to the soul, said some dead poet. They are also triggers to fatigue when ...t of focus, says Stephen Miller, O.D., director of the clinical care center for the ...merican Optometric Association. "If you're having a hard time focusing, you'll ...vist your body into awkward positions, leaning forward toward the computer ...creen or hunching over your desk," says Dr. Miller. All that hunching can leave ...ou bone-tired. Vision problems also hamper concentration, which can cause ...fatigue.

Take a 5- to 10-minute break from your computer or paperwork every hour. Use the time to do other less stressful visual tasks, such as phone calls.

A boring environment. Solution: Buy a toy fire engine. When London offi-cials decided to paint their black bridges blue, bridge-related suicides reportedly decreased by nearly half. There is no question that colors affect our moods, and surrounding yourself with nothing but somber colors can make you both fa-tigued and depressed, says Leatrice Eiseman, color consultant and director of the Pantone Color Institute in Seabeck, Washington. "Add warm colors of the spectrum to your environment, such as yellow, orange, and especially red."

Sure, it sounds like interior decorator babble, but hard science backs it up. "Red is the color of bloodshed and fire," explains Eiseman. "After eons of associ-ation, we are programmed to respond to it. If you want a quick cure for fa-tigue, focus on something red." A few items placed nearby should do the trick. But don't overdo it. "If you are surrounded by too many items of too many col-ors," says Eiseman, "your environment can become too stimulating. And that, too, can be exhausting."

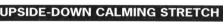

UPSIDE-DOWN CALMING STRETCH

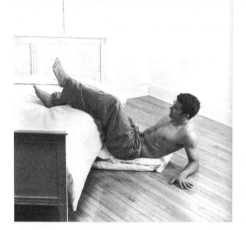
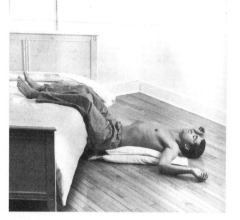

1. Stack several pillows or folded blankets on the floor next to your bed for padding. Sit sideways on one edge of the stack, knees bent, one hip touching the bed. Using your hands to support you, roll back and swing your feet above the bed. You should be sitting on the cushions with your legs hooked over the edge of the bed.

2. Lie back so your upper back and shoulders rest firmly on the floor. Rest your hands beside your head, palms up. Close your eyes, relax, and breathe deeply. You should feel comfortable and strain-free. Relax this way for up to 5 minutes.

Secret Sources of Fatigue

Rid yourself of these energy sappers for good.

When you find yourself nodding off during the boss's slide show, it could be for any number of reasons. Maybe you didn't get your full 8 hours the night be-fore. Maybe it was those three frozen margaritas you washed down last night's dinner with. Or maybe you just don't find "The History of Corporate Tax Shel-ters" terribly stimulating.

But there are days when you feel exhausted for no reason. You had plenty of rest the night before, no one interrupted your REM (rapid eye movement) cycle, and you even Just Said No. Still, it's 11:00 A.M., and you're curling up under the meeting table.

What you don't know is that unseen forces may actually be working against you—at home, at the office, or right inside your body—to drain you of energy and fill you with fatigue. If you can spot them, though, you can beat them.

Here are some of the most common.

Sleep-in-real-late weekends. Solution: Catch up at a better time. Some clever work drone may have said, "I'll catch up on all of my sleep the first year I'm dead," but most of us opt for Saturday mornings. Bad move. "We each have a biological clock that determines when we are sleepy and when we are alert. When you wake up every morning at 7:00 A.M., then sleep until noon on the weekends, you upset your clock and end up feeling more fatigued," says Timothy Roehrs, Ph.D., director of research at the Sleep Disorders Research Center at Detroit's Henry Ford Hospital.

It all has to do with the body's release of cortisol (a hormone that wakes you up), which normally begins between 3:00 and 4:00 A.M. and peaks at about 11:00 A.M. When you lie in bed past this time, you suppress the release of cortisol, dumping your brain into that weekend twilight zone.

Either try to go to bed earlier during the week or play catch-up on the weekend by going to bed early, not sleeping late, suggests Dr. Roehrs. "To keep your biological clock happy, it is critical to wake up every morning at the same time," he says.

Bright lights before bedtime. Solution: Get out of the spotlight before bed. Research from Harvard Medical School and elsewhere suggests that exposure to normal indoor lighting can disrupt your brain's notion of light and dark, putting you in a state of constant jet lag. "As a species, we are designed to be alert by day and to feel tired at night. Normal indoor lights can confuse this natural process, much like when you cross time zones," says Quentin Regestein, M.D., director of the Sleep Clinic at Boston's Brigham and Women's Hospital.

Avoid bright lights, such as those over the bathroom mirror, several hours before bedtime, and install a dimmer switch in your living room.

Not enough water. Solution: Hit the bottle. Once you feel thirsty, you've already lost 1 to 2 percent of the fluid in your body, according to Kristine Clark, R.D., Ph.D., director of sports nutrition at the Pennsylvania State University Center for Sports Medicine in University Park. When you hit the 3 percent mark, you'll start to notice a decline in physical performance. It makes sense. Water is made largely of energizing oxygen, and it also helps carry oxygen in your blood through your body. So keep a container of water at your desk. Drink eight glasses (8 ounces each) a day, or more if you exercise heavily.

Overloading on carbohydrates. Solution: Introduce some culture to every meal. Despite the old Geritol commercials, "iron-poor blood" is not running rampant among American men. But other deficiencies in the diet can lead to fatigue, says Dr. Clark. "Men who eat only high-carbohydrate meals and restrict their protein—so that they're eating only, say, spaghetti, bread, fruits, or salads—will be subject to energy slumps," explains Dr. Clark. "Carbohydrates cause the body to release serotonin, a calming chemical. Protein causes the body

to produce dopamine, which has the opposite effect."

You don't need to reduce your overall carbohydrates or consumption (carbs should make up the bulk of a healthy consume plenty of protein). Just be sure to mix and match. " of a high-protein food such as yogurt, lean meat, low-fat milk sitting," says Dr. Clark. "This will go a long way toward keeping

Unforeseen side effects of medications. Solution: Go altern. know that certain antihistamines, cold medications, and cou make you drowsy. But you may not have known that the list of o energy sappers features many familiar drugs that can cause fatigue in higher-than-recommended doses. These include painkillers, such fen (Advil, Nuprin); some hemorrhoid drugs, such as benzocaine (A. hemorrhoid ointment) and pramoxine (Fleet Relief, ProctoFo: steroidal); and even a few asthma and blood pressure medications. Talk doctor about nonsedating alternatives.

Fear. Solution: Take your brain on a trip. Nothing like a looming, do-o work deadline to leave you wiped for the afternoon. "Fear makes you tense y muscles, which leads to fatigue just as if you were out chopping wood," s. Timothy Smith, Ph.D., psychologist and professor of oral health science at th University of Kentucky Chandler Medical Center College of Dentistry in Lex: ington. "Fear also makes you hold your breath, depriving you of oxygen. This, too, can lead to fatigue."

Next time you're in the hot seat, think about your breathing and try to breathe normally. If possible, close your eyes and envision yourself in a tranquil setting, such as the beach, a sailboat, or a trek through the woods. (Unless, of course, you're deathly afraid of water, boats, or ticks.) Schedule that dental appointment and other discomforting events in the morning so that you don't spend the whole day worrying about them.

Noisy workplace. Solution: Tune it out. If you work amid loud noises, chances are that you end your days feeling bushed. Israeli researchers studied 35 workers in a clamorous textile mill. Some workers wore earmuffs to dull the noise, while others did not. The workers were asked to submit urine samples and fill out questionnaires at regular intervals. By the end of the day, the urine of workers with no sound protection tended to be significantly higher in cortisol, a chemical that indicates stress. Workers with no earmuffs also reported considerably higher levels of afternoon fatigue and crankiness.

If you're surrounded by loud noises exacerbated by loud-mouthed colleagues, suggest that they chill out. If you have a door, shut it. If earmuffs or earplugs are doable, use them. *Caution:* The authors of the Israeli study point out that for many, wearing earmuffs in itself can be a source of fatiguing stress.

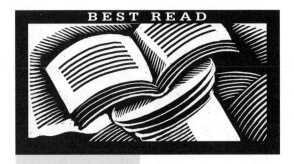

Putting Stress to Sleep

Ever have a truly restless night when you counted so many sheep that you felt like an auditor general for the wool industry? We all have, and we all know that it can drain you and cause more stress for you all the next day. In this excerpt from Stress Blasters *(Rodale Press, 1997), Brian Chichester and Perry Garfinkel examine the relationship between the amount of stress we have and the amount of sleep we get.*

Excluding teenagers, do you know anyone who gets too much sleep? Neither do we. The problem is that whenever we need to cram something into our burgeoning schedules, we lop the minutes or hours off bedtime. Because of this, there's a good chunk of our nation stumbling through life like sleep-deprived zombies.

Health officials say that sleep deprivation may be the most pernicious, undiagnosed medical malady facing Americans today. Chronic deprivation strikes an estimated 40 million of us, with another 20 million to 30 million suffering intermittent problems.

"I don't think that many of us are getting enough sleep, because our lives are so full. People have so many things to do these days," says Martha Davis, Ph.D., psychology professor in the department of psychiatry at Kaiser Permanente Medical Center in Santa Clara, California.

Dr. Davis deals with many stressed-out clients who routinely stay awake until 1:00 or 2:00 A.M., despite having to get up as early as 5:00 A.M. "When they get home from work, they want to exercise. Then they want to eat. Since they have kids, they want to spend time with the kids. Then they want time to themselves," she says. "They feel like there aren't enough hours in the day because there aren't. So they scrimp on sleep."

As a result, Dr. Davis adds, this lack of sleep compounds the stress in our lives. It saps our bodies of the vital recovery time we need, which means our energy can range from low to virtually nonexistent. And being low on sleep makes our tempers flare, our memories falter, and our moods become dour. It's hard to be chipper, optimistic, and energetic—and thus stress-free—when our bodies and minds are crying for a siesta.

Moreover, the problem doesn't seem likely to resolve itself, based on our collective attitude toward sleep. According to one survey from the Better Sleep Council, 88 percent of all adults interviewed ranked nutrition, exercise, and sleep as equally important. Yet, while half exercised regularly, most failed to actually get a good night's sleep. In a previous Better Sleep Council study, more than half the people interviewed got their full 40 winks on a regular basis.

Snooze to Lose Stress

Here's how to hit the hay and send stress packing at the same time.

Sleep for strength. Weight lifters know the importance of what's called the recovery phase. The concept for growing muscle is simple: You work your beefy biceps one day, then let them rest the next. Sleep is life's recovery phase. Because we spend roughly one-third of our lives sleeping, people think that they can prolong productivity by scrimping on their time between the sheets. It just ain't so.

"When does your body get stronger? Not when you're working out; it gets stronger when you're resting," says Pat Etcheberry, a former Olympic javelin thrower, Pan-American Games champion, professional fitness consultant, and motivational speaker for LGE Sport Science in Orlando, Florida.

Find your time. Find out how much sleep you really need by experimenting for the next few weeks. If you're currently getting 5 hours a night, try getting 8 hours for the next week and pay close attention to how it makes you feel. The next week, try 6 hours. Then 9. Tinker around for about a month until you discover just what it takes for you to wake up refreshed, relaxed, and energized. "Most people need 6 to 8 hours of sleep a night—some more, some less—but it's important to recognize what works for you," says Ann McGee-Cooper, Ed.D., international creativity consultant, lecturer, and author of several books, including *You Don't Have to Go Home from Work Exhausted!* and *Building Brain Power.*

Be a regular guy. Once you find your optimal sleep period, stick to it regularly. By going to bed and waking up at roughly the same time every day—including weekends—your body's internal clock stays in sync. So will your stress levels.

Exercise. People who exercise regularly sleep more soundly, says Etcheberry. "Plus, if you're fit, you're going to be able to work longer and handle life's mental and physical stress better," he says. Just don't exercise 2 hours before bed or you'll run the risk of revving your system up so much that it won't be able to unwind when your head hits the pillow.

Be a good manager. Make sure that you're handling your daily schedule as efficiently as possible. Poor time-management skills can lead you to constantly feel rushed and deprive you of the sleep that you need. If you're biting off more than you can chew and it's making you choke sleepwise, put your priorities where they should be: on your health.

Relax before reclining. Take a hot bath, meditate, or ask your spouse for a massage before going to bed. If you're uptight and anxious before bed, your quality of sleep will be at rock bottom, Dr. McGee-Cooper says.

Avoid additives. Avoid alcohol and caffeine 3 hours before bed or they'll interfere with your sleep patterns. While a drink might make you feel drowsy, it'll compromise the soundness of your sleep once you drift off. Caffeine, on the other hand, simply revs up your system, making you toss and turn interminably.

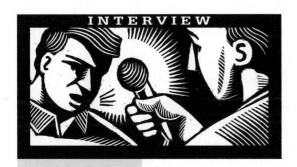

Gary Zammit on
Ending the Sleep Deficit

Men are finally getting the message about taking care of themselves. They're watching what they eat, exercising more, even spending money on grooming aids. But a lot of guys are still neglecting a crucial part of their health regimen: sleep.

We hear you snickering. Sleep is no big deal, you're thinking. Think again. In 1975, there were five sleep centers in the entire country. Today, there are more than 300 accredited sleep disorders clinics. Consider, too, a Louis Harris poll of American workers, commissioned by the National Sleep Foundation, in which 47 percent of those questioned said they have at least occasional sleeplessness. The foundation estimates the cost to employers in lost productivity at more than $18 billion a year.

To find out why Americans are so pooped, we spoke to Gary Zammit, Ph.D., director of the Sleep Disorders Institute at St. Luke's–Roosevelt Hospital Center in New York City and author of Good Nights.

What do you make of that Louis Harris poll?

What's fascinating about those data is that 47 percent of the American workforce said they experienced sleep difficulties in the past three months and two-thirds of them said that the problem interfered with their job performance. And they estimate that their performance falls by 20 percent on those days following a bad night of sleep. The average worker is having eight nights per month of bad sleep. They're functioning (the next day) at 80 percent of capacity. It's a terrible frustration for the worker, and it takes a toll on the employer's bottom line in increased health care costs, increased insurance costs, diminished productivity, absenteeism, tardiness, accidents, and injuries due to fatigue.

What other ramifications does a bad night's sleep have for guys?

People report difficulty with attention, memory, concentration, and even completing simple tasks. They report more mood disturbances—depression, anxiety, and irritability. More difficulty in family and social relationships. They have more problems in all these spheres.

Are men more apt to try and ignore sleep problems than women?

Being men, we tend to be kind of macho and we think that we can just slog through anything. It's not unusual for me to see guys—mostly sleep apnea patients—whose wives are insisting they come in because they see them looking ragged and snoring and not breathing. When you bring these guys face-to-face with the serious health consequences of the disorder, it's very hard for them to accept it sometimes.

Aren't young men better able to cope with too little sleep than those who are older?

I don't think young men are any more capable. Think about the age group in which motor vehicle accident rates are highest. It's in the early twenties, and that's when these kids are sleepy and they're pushing themselves in school and at home and they're experimenting with alcohol. The risk goes way up.

Who more often has sleep difficulties, men or women?

Insomnia tends to be reported more often by women and also tends to be reported in older age groups. That's really the flip side of sleep apnea and snoring, which we know is much more common in men than in women.

Why are so many people having trouble sleeping?

When you ask people what the source of their sleep disturbance is, they will clump it under the category of stress.

What about pain at night?

We know that people commonly report concurrent pain. That could be headache, muscle ache, joint pain, backache, and so on. This is one reason why pain relievers combined with a mild sleep aid, such as Tylenol PM, are used as a source of relief.

What else?

Mood disturbances like depression and anxiety disorders can lead to disturbed nighttime sleep. Some medical disorders, neurologic disorders, some sleep disorders, and some medications can provoke insomnia. Use of stimulants, even what we would consider socially acceptable—such as caffeine and nicotine, and the inappropriate use of alcohol—also causes insomnia.

Why don't sleep problems receive more attention?

It's possible that we have tended to dismiss them because we think that we can control sleep, or many of us intentionally take advantage of our sleep. We work harder, we play harder, we socialize more, and we end up cheating on sleep to do it. It's like we feel we can override this basic bodily need.

Think of the attitude toward sleep. If there's a guy driving down the street and he experiences chest pain, chances are that he's going to pull over his car. But the same guy driving down the street who experiences drowsiness and his head starts to nod, he turns on the radio or rolls down the window and keeps on going. We know that people who have sleep problems, such as people with chronic insomnia, are 2½ times more likely to have fatigue-related automobile accidents. Somebody with sleep apnea, 5 times more likely. Somehow it seems like we're dismissing it.

Does sleep research get short-changed in government funding?

Three or four years ago there was a national commission on sleep disorders research that was set up by Congress. There were professionals as well as patients and people from a variety of sectors who gave testimony to Congress, saying how much we needed more sleep research and that funding was so critical. There is money coming out now in support of sleep research. But when you tally up all the sleep dollars that have been spent versus dollars on other kinds of problems, I would say the expenditures have still been relatively low.

Is sleep loss greater than in the past, or are we just becoming more aware of it now?

There were some statistics cited in the national commission report that indicated that the total nightly average sleep time for Americans has been reduced by about 20 percent since the turn of the century. That's almost 2 hours. This doesn't reflect a change in our basic biological need for sleep but a change in lifestyle and attitude.

Why? Are there more diversions in life keeping us awake?

I think so. We have common electric lighting. We now have 24-hour access to everything—shopping, recreation, socialization, Internet, phones...

How long does the typical person now sleep?

The average reported is somewhere between 7 and 9 hours, but the range is huge. It goes down to 4½ or 5 hours, all the way over to 12-plus hours. I think the key thing is that you don't know what your real sleep need is unless you've tried to assess it. If you're feeling any fatigue or sleepiness during the day, if your performance is impaired, then it may be that you're not allowing yourself enough of an opportunity to sleep and you need more.

What advice would you give men who are chronically tired or who have trouble sleeping?

The first thing they should do is consider their sleep habits, and if they haven't developed good sleep habits, work on doing so.

What are some good sleep habits?

Getting up at the same time every day. Keeping a regular bedtime. Avoiding naps, caffeine, nicotine, and alcohol. Not going to bed too hungry or too full. Making sure that their sleep environment is a good one for them. Exercise regularly in the afternoon or early evening. If they're not improving or getting better, they shouldn't hesitate to call their primary-care doctor. And either through their primary-care doctor or through a referral to a sleep specialist, they'll be able to come to a solution. Only 5 percent of people with insomnia actually go visit their doctor specifically for that problem.

What does the future hold for America's sleep-deprived?

I think we can anticipate some newer and better medications to come out to help people who are suffering from insomnia. But that's not the panacea, the silver bullet. The silver bullet is in having people become more aware that sleep is a basic biological function. They must attend to it just like they attend to their meals and their calorie intake and their weight and what they drink.

They can have good sleep habits, just like they have good eating, exercise, and other kinds of habits. I think with that awareness, people will start to integrate this into their lifestyles.

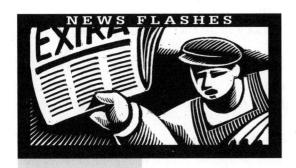

NEWS FLASHES

Sleep Quality Improves with Exercise

STANFORD, Calif.—A Stanford University study has found a way for older adults to get to sleep faster and stay asleep longer—a regular exercise program.

This 16-week study included older adults (ages 50 to 76) who didn't exercise regularly, had no cardiovascular disease, and reported moderate sleep complaints. Volunteers were randomly placed into either an exercise training group or a control group that did no exercise. Those in the exercise group either walked or did low-impact aerobics for 30 to 40 minutes four times each week.

Members of the exercise group reported an increase in the amount of time they slept by almost 1 hour; the nonexercising group reported minimal improvement. Those who exercised also reported falling asleep in half the normal time.

Change in Natural Sleep Pattern Alters Mood

BOSTON—Changing your normal sleep pattern can significantly affect your mood, a Brigham and Women's Hospital study shows.

Researchers interrupted the sleep-wake cycles of 24 healthy people. They asked one group to stay awake for 20 hours and then sleep for 10 and another to stay awake for about 19 hours and sleep for about 9. The study participants stayed on this haywire sleep schedule for about a month.

In both sleep schedules, the researchers found that participants' moods hit rock bottom at 6:00 A.M. when they had already been awake for 8 hours, and soared between the hours of 2:00 P.M. and 10:00 P.M. when they had been awake for the same amount of time.

So, for those of you who work shifts, be wary. Even slight changes to your normal sleep pattern can cause your mood to have extreme highs and lows—especially near 6:00 A.M.

Peppermint Fends Off Sleepiness

CAMBRIDGE, Mass.—Thirty-one percent of adults admit they have at some point dozed off behind the wheel. New research suggests that sleepy drivers should grab a stick of peppermint gum or suck on a peppermint candy to fend off the yawns.

According to a preliminary study from the Institute for Circadian Physiology, peppermint aroma may increase driver alertness. Six healthy men between the ages of 27 and 35 were monitored for two nights while at the controls of a driving simulator.

In one of the two nights, the men were exposed to a peppermint aroma while they were driving. Late at night, when the men were most sleepy, the inhalation of the peppermint aroma increased alertness and improved driving performance.

Further studies are needed to determine administration and dosage of such aromas to increase driver alertness. In the meantime, if you're taking a road trip, don't forget the peppermint candies.

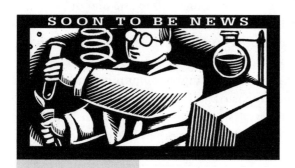

SOON TO BE NEWS

Sleep Better on the Road?

There's no place like home when it comes to getting a good night's sleep. Or is there?

Hilton Hotels, in cooperation with the National Sleep Foundation and an array of sleep-product manufacturers, recently launched a test run of their new Sleep-Tight Rooms: accommodations designed to provide business travelers with the best night's sleep possible on the road.

Rooms are equipped with blackout curtains that have a magnetic strip down the seam to block unwanted light and noise. Guests also get a sleep kit containing earplugs and eyeshades to ease sleep. What's more, travelers can drift off to dreamland while listening to white-noise machines that generate neutral sounds (such as soft radio static) or soothing environmental sounds (such as ocean waves or rain falling). Since our natural sleep cycle (circadian cycle) is based on a 24-hour day and can get thrown off with travel to other time zones, the rooms even include a biorhythm light box designed to realign your body's sleep cycle.

Right now, there are seven rooms in each of the participating test hotels: The Beverly Hills Hilton, Beverly Hills, California; Chicago O'Hare Hilton; New Orleans Hilton Riverside; New York Hilton and Towers, New York City; The Waldorf-Astoria, New York City; Hilton Hawaiian Village at Waikiki Beach; and The Capital Hilton in Washington, D.C.

In the future, Hilton is hoping to expand the Sleep-Tight project to its other hotels, both domestically and internationally, says Bob Dirks, senior vice president of marketing at Hilton Hotels Corporation. Business travelers interested in trying a Sleep-Tight Room should inquire when they check in to one of the participating hotels (the price is the same as another comparable room in the hotel), or call (800) HILTONS.

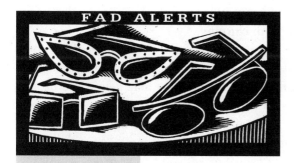

FAD ALERTS

Cat Naps

 You have an important meeting with your boss later in the day, but you had such a bad night's sleep that your brain feels like mush. What to do? Take a short nap.

A team of Swedish researchers studied eight men under three sleep conditions: after a full night's sleep, after 4 hours of sleep, and after 4 hours of sleep followed by a late morning nap that on average lasted 20 minutes.

When tested for alertness, the men quite naturally did best after a good night's sleep, and worst when they had only 4 hours of sleep. But when the men who got 4 hours of sleep took that short nap, they were almost as mentally sharp as when they slept all night.

The positive effects of the nap were observed starting 30 minutes after the nap. How long the benefits of the nap last will vary. "It depends on how sleep-deprived you are in the first place, and how long your nap is," says James Maas, Ph.D., professor of psychology at Cornell University in Ithaca, New York, and author of *The Sleep Advantage: How to Prepare Your Mind for Peak Performance.*

Think of these as power cat naps. Dr. Maas cautions that naps should be brief. "Long naps are going to make you foggy, which will give you sleep inertia when you wake up." In other words, your mind will be more muddled before that big meeting than if you hadn't napped.

"Long naps also are going to interfere with your ability to get to bed on time at night," Dr. Maas says. "You don't want to shift your biological clock by sleeping a lot during the day. We advocate for the tired, exhausted, harried, and hurried person a 20-minute nap. That's enough to get you through the midday trough."

While the men in the Swedish study took their naps in late morning, Dr. Maas says that early afternoon is when most people find a nap beneficial. "You want to catch the trough, which for most people is between 1:00 P.M. and 3:00 P.M."

White Noise Generators

 Perhaps you've seen them advertised: gizmos you place on your night-stand that emit soothing sounds to lull you to sleep. The rain falling. Surf crashing. A heart beating. Birds chirping.

These devices aren't cheap. You can easily spend in the three digits for a gizmo that purports to generate "white noise," the soothing sonic wallpaper that's supposed to make you drowsy. And while they may help some people, they also may be unnecessary, says Dr. Maas. He points out that white noise made by such familiar things as a fan, air conditioning, or the static of a radio can block out unwelcome sounds and help induce sleep, too.

"If spending $300 or $400 on a gadget makes you happy, makes you sleepy, then fine," says Dr. Maas. "But why not take a broken FM radio and put it between two stations?"

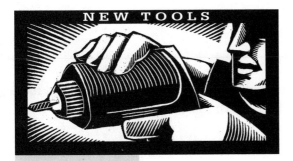

Snoring Snuffer

The Silencer

Its name conjures up images of a hitman and a gun, but makers of The Silencer say that their device is aimed only at snuffing out snoring and sleep apnea. It's an oral appliance that resembles an athletic mouthguard. It fits over the teeth and holds the lower jaw and tongue forward, opening the throat airway.

Its inventor, Canadian dentist L. Wayne Halstrom, D.D.S., says that his plastic appliance is the only one with a titanium hinge, a precision attachment that allows the jaw to move laterally and vertically—making it more comfortable to use during sleep. The Silencer's hinge comes with a lifetime warranty and can only be prescribed and ordered by a specially trained dentist.

Typically, a dentist, after consulting with the patient's physician about the sleep disorder, takes impressions of the patient's mouth, then sends those impressions off to a laboratory, which custom-makes The Silencer to fit a wearer's exact specifications. It can be cleaned by the patient and easily adjusted periodically, if necessary, by the dentist, says Dr. Halstrom's colleague, Michael Gelb, D.D.S., clinical associate professor in the department of oral medicine and pathology at New York University College of Dentistry. Cost starts at $300 but may vary depending on a patient's needs. To find the location of the nearest qualified dentist to prescribe the device, call Integrated Health Technologies at (888) 575-1333, or check out their Web site at http://www.the-silencer.com.

Anti-Snoring Shirt

Sleep-ezzz Nightshirt

John Galgon, M.D., estimates that 10 percent of snorers make their night music only when lying on their backs. So Dr. Galgon, medical director of the Sleep Disorder Center at Lehigh Valley Hospital in Allentown, Pennsylvania, came up with a company and a product called Sleep-ezzz designed to ease snoring—and the sleep of long-suffering partners.

Sleep-ezzz is simply a T-shirt with three pockets sewn down the middle of the back in which the snorer places tennis balls. They, in turn, deter him from rolling on to his back during the night. "This product does nothing more than take the place of the wife's poking," says Dr. Galgon. "If they snore a lot while on their sides, of course, it doesn't work." Sleep-ezzz can be ordered by calling (610) 435-3266. Cost is $24.95, plus shipping. You supply the balls.

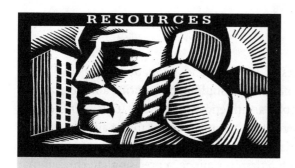

Sleep Disorders

The School of Sleep Medicine's SleepNet Web Site
http://www.sleepnet.com

For "everything you wanted to know about sleep disorders but were too tired to ask," point your browser to Palo Alto's The School of Sleep Medicine Web site, the SleepNet. This site is crammed full of information about the disorders that affect roughly 40 million Americans. Sleep apnea, restless legs syndrome, insomnia, and narcolepsy are just some of the sleep problems you can learn more about. The site's News Links offers current magazine and newspaper articles. You can also find links to other sites offering sleep remedies and treatment ideas.

Dream Analysis

Community Dreamsharing Network
P.O. Box 8032
Hicksville, NY 11802
Harold R. Ellis, Ph.D.
(516) 735-1969

Every man has a dream—several every night, actually. If you want to interpret yours and share them with others, this is the organization for you. The Community Dreamsharing Network, run by Harold R. Ellis, Ph.D., is a collection of hundreds of local and regional groups that meet weekly to discuss and understand their dreams. The Network also sponsors training sessions in methods used to interpret dreams. They even publish a quarterly newsletter, *Dream Switchboard*. Contact them to find a dream group near you.

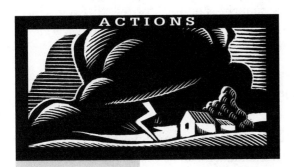

ACTIONS

Whether it's business travel or a vacation, nothing has the potential to ruin a trip like sleep. When you're flying across time zones, lack of sleep—in the form of jet lag—can make you feel like a zombie. If you're driving, the problem is too much sleep—the endless highway and the soothing drone of tires on tarmac can lure you into a dangerous nap behind the wheel.

To combat these travails of travel, James Maas, Ph.D., professor of psychology at Cornell University in Ithaca, New York, and author of *The Sleep Advantage: How to Prepare Your Mind for Peak Performance*, suggests these eight strategies to help you keep your sleep schedule on track in either situation.

1. **Plan your flight.** To avoid jet lag, choose a flight that lets your arrive in the early evening, and stay up until 10:00 P.M. local time. If you simply must sleep during the day, take a nap in the early afternoon, but for no more than two hours. Set an alarm so that you don't oversleep in the morning.

2. **Schedule your sack time.** You can gradually acclimate yourself to a time change—and thus prevent jet lag—before leaving home by going to bed earlier several days prior to an eastward trip and later for a westward sojourn. Try to get on a sleep schedule as close to the ones that people would be on in your destination time zone, Dr. Maas says. And start resetting your biological clock the same number of days you estimate it would take a ship to reach your destination. For instance, cruises to Europe take about one week, so you should start going to bed earlier and earlier about a week before your trip if you were going to, say, London.

3. **Eat light.** During your trip as well as when you reach your destination, avoid heavy meals and alcohol. The digestive track takes longer to absorb food during travel, Dr. Maas says. And also, it takes longer for your biological clock to readjust when your body is occupied with digestion.

4. **Catch some rays.** Try to get outside in the sunlight whenever possible. Generally, 30 minutes of morning sunlight is optimal for resetting your clock, Dr. Maas says. Daylight acts as a stimulant for regulating your biological clock. Staying indoors makes jet lag worse.

5. **Check your room.** Examine your room for possible distractions: light coming in through a crack in the drapes, for example, or unwanted sounds like a dripping faucet.

6. **Avoid driving during downtime.** On the road, take a mid-afternoon break and find a place to sleep between midnight and 6:00 A.M., your body's usual downtime. Remember that the peak hour for fatigue-related collisions is 2:00 A.M.

7. **Talk with your passenger.** A passenger can also tell you when you are showing signs of sleepiness and perhaps take the wheel if you are drowsy.

8. **Set break times.** Schedule a break every 2 hours or 100 miles. During your break, take a nap, stretch, take a walk, and get some exercise before resuming driving.

10

HEALTH MANAGEMENT

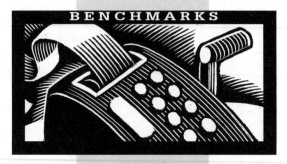

BENCHMARKS

AVERAGES

■ Percentage of a man's happiness that stems from his genetic makeup: 80

■ Percentage of male patients who have bad breath, according to dentists: 81

■ How long a 1-year-old boy can expect to live today: 72.4 years

■ How long a 1-year-old girl can expect to live today: 78.8 years

■ Average number of U.S. workers who die on the job each day as a result of workplace injuries: 18

■ Average number of emergency room visits nationwide each day for toilet seat–related injuries: 120

■ Percentage by which regular self-examinations can reduce deaths from skin cancer: 63

■ Average increase in the number of annual work hours from 1969 to 1987: 163

■ Average age at which a man first notices that his hair is turning gray: 39

■ Average length of time Americans ages 18 to 24 spend in the shower: 16.4 minutes

■ Estimated number of Americans who have high cholesterol: 96 million

EXTREMES

■ Times per year a physician is asked to stretch sick leaves unnecessarily: 100

■ How much more likely you are to die from a volcanic eruption than from a snakebite: more than three times

■ Average number of times a man passes gas daily: 13.63

■ Daily average for a woman: 3.28

■ America's least healthy state, according to statistics for infant mortality, child immunizations, and smoking: Arkansas

VITAL READING

The True Measure of a Man

Discover which body-fat measurement tests are accurate.

It's not what you weigh that's important; it's what percentage of that weight is composed of pure lard. You can be 6 feet tall and weigh 250 and look like Mr. America, but you can have those same statistics and look like a Bartlett pear. To really know (and be able to brag about) your fitness level, you need to measure what at first would seem immeasurable. And there's no end of manufacturers and marketers lining up to help you. But which of the ever-expanding arsenal of body-fat tests and gizmos are most accurate? We went and found out.

Skinfold Testing

We started where most men start: at the gym. Kevin Heidel, strength-training coordinator at Manhattan's West Side YMCA, explained that healthy, though not necessarily aesthetically pleasing, body-fat levels for men range from about 15 to 20 percent; for women, 20 to 25 percent. (The numbers differ slightly depending on whom you ask.) Elite male runners and bodybuilders can drop as low as 5 percent.

Then Heidel unboxed a pair of calipers. The caliper test is the most widely used method of body-fat testing; it's also, say experts, the least accurate. "There's a lot of variety in testers," Heidel explained, nabbing a chunk of our guinea pig staff writer's thigh between the calipers' pincers. "What I'm doing is gathering all the tissue that's above muscle—skin and fat. If a tester grabs too much, or grabs too little, it can throw off the test."

Heidel put the calipers to seven sites on the body, repeating each pinch three times for accuracy. Then he punched the data into the computer, which yielded 21 percent. "Reduction advised!" the printout cautioned.

We wanted a second opinion.

Bioelectrical Impedance Analysis

Many upscale health clubs are using bioelectrical impedance analysis (BIA) machines. BIAs estimate your overall percentage of body fat by shooting electrical current through your flesh and measuring the resistance it meets. If your club doesn't have a machine, the test might cost you $50 at an exercise physiology laboratory. We went to the Nicholas Institute of Sports Medicine and Athletic Trauma at Lenox Hill Hospital in New York City.

There, sports nutritionist Beth Glace said BIA results are remarkably consistent both from test to test and from one tester to another but can be inaccurate if the subject is dehydrated. And both BIA and skinfold tests are less reliable than underwater weighing, which Glace and others still call the gold standard. The advantage of BIAs is that you don't have to get wet.

To do the BIA test, Glace taped electrodes to the left wrist and ankle and threw the switch. Our subject didn't feel anything as the machine flashed "13 percent."

There was a pair of calipers nearby—one with a built-in computer—and we asked Glace to use it on our tester. Compared with Heidel's, her grip was more assertive and probing. It read 16.9 percent, virtually equidistant from each of the two prior results. "Always pick the lowest number," Glace helpfully suggested. "We only use the numbers we like."

X-ray Absorptiometry

We were beginning to suspect that body-fat testing was more of an art than a science when we heeded Glace's suggestion and checked out the Body Composition Lab at New York City's St. Luke's–Roosevelt Hospital. At the lab, five different body-fat testing procedures are performed—a state-of-the-art analysis that usually costs $225.

Research associate Chris Nunez seemed most eager to show off the lab's $100,000 Lunar Dual-Energy X-Ray Absorptiometry (DXA) machine. It's similar to a computerized tomography scan and takes three-dimensional pictures of your body's adipose tissue. Call it a fat scan. For the DXA exam, you lie motionless on an open-air table for about 20 minutes while x-rays emitted from below pass through your body to a detector on tracks overhead. Then the machine prints out a picture of you as a skeleton, which is weird, with the body-fat percentages of your different "compartments" and an overall figure—in our subject's case, 19.7 percent.

Next, Nunez used two different BIAs. The first, called a Tanita Body Fat Analyzer, has two metal footpads with built-in electrodes that you stand on. This prevents mistakes in electrode placement, which Nunez says is common. This test yielded a reading of 17 percent.

The second BIA machine was similar to the one at Lenox Hill Hospital, except its electrodes always go on the right side of the body. Result: 15.3 percent.

Hydrostatic Weighing

Weighing yourself underwater is the truest gauge of blubber.

"It's based on the principles of Archimedes," Nunez explained. "We figure out your volume by taking the difference between your weight on land and your weight underwater." But then this difference is factored into an equation to derive your body density, which is plugged into a formula based on the measurements of melted corpses. "It's a little complex," he admitted.

It's not such a good measurement if you have gas. "If you're really gassy, that's going to add to your weight in water and lead to an error in your estimate of body fat," Nunez said.

The tank was metal and rectangular, but it looked like your average suburban above-ground pool—an impression heightened by the blue inflatable dolphin propped against one corner. Wearing a weight belt, a person being tested positions himself on the gridlike scale on the tank's bottom. You have to completely submerge yourself and expel all the air in your lungs through your mouth.

Since this 10- to 15- second process feels like drowning, some people can't handle it—and some really big people have trouble staying down. Our wet guinea pig stayed under long enough to get a reading of 18.9 percent.

"Do different machines ever give wildly different results for one person?" we asked. "Say, 10 and 25 percent?"

"That does occur," he said. If certain tests are done wrong, some people get negative numbers.

"Is anything 100 percent accurate?"

"Yes," said Nunez earnestly. "But we'd have to dissect you."

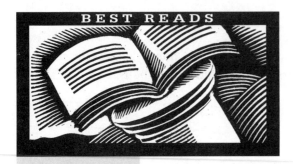

How to Choose the Break You Need

Six months off. Those three words are as ripe with fabulous possibilities as they are cruelly taunting. After all, who can take that much time off? After reading Six Months Off *(Henry Holt and Company, 1996) by Hope Dlugozima, James Scott, and David Sharp, you'll be amazed at how attainable this fantasy is. In this excerpt, the authors explain how to figure out what to do during your sabbatical.*

If you were given six months off—all expenses paid—to do whatever you like, what would you choose?

Maybe you'd like to walk across England. Or perhaps jerry-rig an old Nissan Pathfinder and drive it from Paris to Dakar. Or rent a house in Ireland and play traditional music. Or head off to Zagreb to aid in the war-refugee effort. Or maybe just crawl into bed with the complete collection of Jane Austen. The problem, you quickly find, is not a lack of possibilities. It is, instead, a veritable ocean of choices.

The solution is an elegant and intriguing one: Get to know yourself as you never have before.

Begin by approaching your time off the way you might approach any big decision: Hatch a big idea, research the subject, get advice from knowledgeable people, ask what your friends and family think, determine what you can afford (in both dollars and days), and then make some inevitable, though not necessarily hard, compromises. Do all this carefully and the right time off will gradually float to the top.

So grab a pencil and several sheets of paper, and prepare yourself for some intensive—and intensely enjoyable—brainstorming. Once the metaphorical skies are clear again, your sabbatical choice should be, too.

What Will You Do?

First, pick a quiet time, a Sunday afternoon or an early evening out on the balcony, to sit and think about what you might do with your time off. Bring along any adventure brochures you may have stuffed away, prospectuses on fellowships you've dreamed of applying for, notes you've written to yourself about big ideas or getaways, coffee-table books about your favorite places or pastimes, maybe even your high school and college yearbooks. Take a deep breath and lean back. You'll soon begin writing down anything and everything you can possibly imagine doing on an extended break. If you're planning a sabbatical with your family or a friend, you might try this as a group experience.

Don't censor any ideas or do any nay-saying at this point. The aim is to generate volume, not to distill. If it helps, think of this step as driving a car at night with the headlights on. Since it's dark outside, you can't see your final destination at first. But the simple act of driving through the darkness illuminates areas you wouldn't have seen otherwise. Likewise, the simple act of writing down random thoughts will lead you to ideas you hadn't imagined.

Your list might contain some generic sabbatical goals, such as "Learn an exotic language," "Help the poor," "Win the such-and-such fellowship," or "Get into shape." But before you start scribbling more of your imaginings, read on for a bit. We've assembled a batch of idea-generating techniques that you may not have considered.

Create an extensive self-profile. What likes, dislikes, and attitudes define you? For example, do you prefer the outdoors? Do you blossom at the notion of devoting yourself to the arts? Are you a stoic loner who thrives in wide-open spaces, or do you crave more time with your buddies? Is there a certain challenge that would test your skills to the maximum—but that you've not yet found the time to try?

Write down all the traits that describe you. Add to that list any special skills or talents you possess. Then combine your entries into some logical groupings and see what experiences or activities they translate into. Let's say your descriptive list features "like to be in charge," "a generous person," and "gutsy" and your skills list includes "good with tools" and "a whiz at math." Maybe the group Habitat for Humanity could use you for five or six months.

Or take an expandable folder and, over a period of a month, write notes to yourself about anything that captures your imagination—a movie, a newspaper article, a TV documentary, a memorable experience, a long talk with someone—and put those notes in the folder. At the end of the month, empty the folder, spread the notes out over a big table, and group together the ones that are part of overall themes and patterns. What might have seemed to you a collection of random thoughts could actually turn out to have sublime order and symmetry.

Take the case of Sean Plottner, a magazine editor. More than a year before Plottner embarked on his five-month African odyssey, he assessed the pluses and minuses of his current situation, his finances, and his job, and asked himself the question, "How can I make myself happy?" "I wrote down things that I wanted to do, mostly deep-rooted things," he says. "I wanted to learn to fly. Climb a mountain. Do some serious white-water rafting. A lot of my thoughts had to do with the outdoors—crazy adventures. I even put down something like 'more exercise.' I realized that a lot of these things could be done, and if you added them all up, they equaled a major trip."

Take a look at what other people have tried as a way to jog your own ideas. Sabbatical counselor Cornelius Bull sends a list of opportunities to new clients. "When I sit down with people," Bull says, "I don't think most of them have any idea what's out there. But if you give them a lot of options and ask them to talk about them, more often than not they'll see something that they hadn't even thought about that turns out to be exactly what they're going to do." By having clients go through a list of 32 varied options, Bull says he gets an idea of what sorts of experiences he should hunt up for them. And those same clients are able to recognize opportunities that may not have been clear before.

Revisit your childhood dreams. Turn the clock back to when you were 10 or 12 years old. If someone had asked you to name your future occupation, what would you have said? Okay, take "astronaut" and "president" off the list. Do any of the other jobs still appeal to you? Can you update them for the nineties? If so, write them down. You might try tracking down people you knew as a kid. Not only parents and family members but friends from your yearbooks, store owners you used to visit, people who knew you well. By telling them of your future plans you fulfill two purposes: First, those people, when found, are absolutely enchanted to hear from you; and second, they usually have fairly vivid memories of what you used to talk about as a child—things that you may have submerged later in life because there were other expectations. Maybe you spent your youth putting on plays in the backyard—and perhaps it's not too late to enroll in drama school. Or perhaps you thought you'd ford the world's greatest rivers when you grew up—and could now plan an expedition down the Nile.

Ask yourself what you'd do if you had only six months to live. Few imagined scenarios will better focus your thinking about your real priorities in life than the one in which your life is about to end. On your deathbed, what are your regrets going to be? You're probably not going to regret the things you did but rather the things you *didn't* do. You're not going to say, "Gee, I wish I had advanced my career in 1996," or "Gee, I wish I had visited fewer foreign countries or learned fewer new skills."

You might divide the "things I must do before I no longer exist" list into several categories: (1) goals that you absolutely, positively must accomplish before the end—these are your likely sabbatical plans; (2) things you would have liked to have done before departing—these might be folded in; and (3) parts of your lifestyle you'd stop doing right away if you had only six months left—this may help solidify your decision to leave behind your regular life for a while. They don't have to be grandiose achievements, like sailing the Pacific solo or climbing to the highest point of elevation in each of the 50 states. Your goal could be simply to write the history of your hometown or drive a camper to all of California's state parks or spend the summer with your oldest daughter before she goes away to college.

Consider making your pastime into your time off. What are your hobbies? Maybe you can ratchet them up a few notches. If you're really good at something, you might find it gratifying to seek out tougher competition in a place where the surroundings are less familiar and the stakes are higher. For example, if you like tennis, hook up with a high-powered pro for a few months of lessons and start entering city tourneys. If you paint, take five months and do nothing but that, and then start offering your efforts at art and crafts shows. If you're not a smashing success, so what? You had fun trying and have honed a lifelong skill. And after all, nobody says you have to junk your present career and rely on your hobby to cover the mortgage—though wouldn't it be poetic if things turned out that way?

Take the case of Kite Giedraitis of Portland, Oregon. He was a computer programmer, but deep inside he saw himself as a full-time marimba player. Finally, he quit his computer job, went on a year-long sabbatical to southern Africa to hone his musical skills in the instrument's homeland, and embraced marimba playing as a life's occupation. "I passionately love it, and I can't imagine life without it at this point," says Giedraitis. Today, he teaches marimba back in Portland and is a founding member of the Village Spirit Marimba Band.

Staying Healthy on the Swing Shift

Anyone who has worked the swing shift knows what a grind it can be. Merely maintaining your health becomes a daunting task. Don't let the clock punch you. In this chapter from Stronger Faster *(Rodale Press, 1997), Brian Paul Kaufman and Sid Kirchheimer tell you how to stay strong and healthy even while working the graveyard shift.*

It's a dilemma facing some 20 million American shift workers—from emergency services personnel and overnight delivery workers to clerical staff and computer programmers. How do you stay healthy, eat right, get a good workout, plenty of sleep, and still have some semblance of a life?

Shift work–related mishaps alone cost an estimated $70 billion annually in lost productivity, lost wages, medical expenses, property damage, and insurance costs, says Lynne Lamberg, author of *Bodyrhythms: Chronobiology and Peak Performance* and *The American Medical Association Guide to Better Sleep*.

The toll on workers' health is also high. Two-thirds of shift workers complain of disrupted sleep; twice as many shift workers as regular folks develop gastrointestinal problems such as ulcers, diarrhea, or constipation—symptoms derisively called graveyard gut. Half of all shift workers smoke—twice that of the national average. And after five years on the job, shift workers are twice as likely to suffer heart attacks and heart disease as day workers of the same age and sex, Lamberg says.

"There's really no other conclusion here that you can draw. The human body is not designed to work through the night. Most of us are what's called diurnal—programmed to be awake and alert during the day," says Jack Connolly, Ph.D., president of ShiftWork Consultants, a consulting firm based in Springfield, Missouri, that provides support services to 24-hour operations.

Avoiding Occupational Hazards

All economic trends point to an increase in the use of shift workers—with some guys actually volunteering for duty, albeit reluctantly. "Rather than bringing on extra workers, employers are just making the people they have work longer," says Timothy H. Monk, Ph.D., professor of psychiatry and director of the Human Chronobiology Program at the University of Pittsburgh. "And in an environment where real wages are falling, people are taking on second and third jobs to maintain their standard of living. By definition, the second job is usually a shift-working job."

But whether you're new to shift work or an old pro, experts say that there are several practical things you can do to maintain a healthy lifestyle while working odd hours. Here's what they suggest.

Ease in a regular workout. For people who sleep at night, Lamberg says, physical performance is best around 5:00 P.M. Reflexes are faster, and coordination is smoother then. For people who sleep in the daytime, particularly those who frequently change schedules, the optimal performance time is harder to predict. The best time to work out, Lamberg says, is whenever it's most convenient. Having a special time is not as important as making time to do it. But if you can fit exercise into a regular time slot in your daily schedule, she says—right before or after work, for example—that's a plus. It will help keep your body clock in line and should improve your sleep, mood, and overall fitness.

Take your treadmill with you. During a visit to the control room of an electrical power company, Dr. Connolly observed that the shift workers had installed a rowing machine. "It looked like they would be able to exercise without ever being too far away from where they needed to be," Dr. Connolly says.

Go into morning. Those who punch out at around 7:00 A.M. should try to eat breakfast with the family, then read the paper and relax—literally puttering around the house for an hour or two before going to bed, says Lamberg. "The main thing is to try to get on a schedule and keep it so that your body can adapt as much as possible."

Go gentle into that good night. Guys who get off at 11:00 P.M. should probably forsake lengthy after-hours socializing—not to mention booze—and opt to hit the sack instead.

Other shift workers simply use alcohol as a sleep aid. In one small study, 32 percent of the shift workers reported using alcohol to fall asleep after their 12-hour day shifts, while 20 percent used it to sleep after their night shifts. It's far better, says Joanne Curran-Celentano, R.D., Ph.D., associate professor of nutrition and food science at the University of New Hampshire in Durham, to eat a healthful meal containing complex carbohydrates—a bowl of cereal, for example—than to depend on alcohol to encourage sleep.

Cut the caffeine. And you thought the cast of *Friends* sucked down a lot of coffee? The typical shift worker drinks between seven and eight cups of joe a day—twice the national average.

"Obviously, they're trying to keep themselves awake, but too much caffeine has well-known negative effects on the cardiovascular system. It increases resting heart rate and blood pressure, and it can create arrhythmias in people with tendencies toward irregular heartbeats," says Dr. Connolly.

Not only that, but caffeine stays in your bloodstream for 5 hours, disrupting sleep patterns, Dr. Monk warns. His recommendation: If you're on the night shift, don't take any caffeine after about 4:00 A.M. If you're on the evening shift, avoid it.

Put some light on the subject. Instead of having the boss pay for another industrial-size bag of coffee, ask him to spring for brighter lights, which studies show may help keep shift workers more alert, Lamberg says.

Lay down the law. Social taboos prevent us from calling anyone at 2:00 A.M. unless it's an emergency. So why aren't shift workers spared afternoon calls—for some, their prime sleeping time? Often it's because family and friends haven't taken their sleeping schedule seriously. Make sure that people understand that calls and other interruptions aren't appreciated. Point out that you'd probably be more fun to talk to after some rest anyway, Dr. Monk says.

Nap if you need it. Since evening shift workers actually report better sleep than those who work 9:00 A.M. to 5:00 P.M., they probably won't need a nap. But studies show that those who work the night shift may benefit from a 2-hour afternoon nap, says Dr. Monk. "We're not talking about 10 to 20 minutes here. The research shows that you'd need a much longer nap to see any benefit," he says.

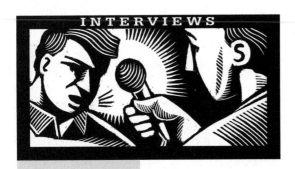

Ralph Keyes on
Making Time Your Friend

No matter how you try to stretch it, there is only so much time. Each week you have 168 hours, 10,080 minutes, or 604,800 seconds to work, play, and sleep. But more than likely you spend a good chunk of your day feeling rushed. Being constantly time-crunched is more than stressful—it's a never-ending fight against an enemy that can't be beaten—the clock. Eventually, this one-sided battle can wear you down and cause or aggravate many serious medical conditions, including heart disease and digestive disorders. In this interview, Ralph Keyes, author of Timelock: How Life Got So Hectic and What You Can Do about It, *discusses how you can learn to feel less harried.*

Your basic argument is that men have been taught to conquer time, manage time, cope with time, and these things really don't address the problem in a way that is constructive. Does that about sum it up?

Yes. We seem to think that controlling time is a very manly thing to do. I think when men are confronted with time pressure—feeling like they don't have enough time, feeling that things are moving too fast—their intuitive reaction is to say, "Time is my enemy. I'll beat it to a pulp." The only problem is that that doesn't work. The harder we try to beat up time, the more time beats us up.

Why?

I think that it is an illusion that we can control time in the first place. I think that illusion grows out of the fact that about four centuries ago we learned how to measure time mechanically. Before we had mechanical clocks that were dependable, we really had little idea of exactly what time it was. And when we didn't know exactly what time it was, we couldn't make appointments, we couldn't all show up to work at the same time, we couldn't say at exactly what time a condemned prisoner was to be executed. Which is why the traditional time to execute someone is at dawn because that is one of the few times you can put your finger on without a clock. So before we could measure time, we had a much more relaxed, much more circumspect, much more realistic attitude toward time. We knew we couldn't control it and didn't try. And as a result, I think we led healthier lives time-wise. But once we learned to measure time—first to the hour, then to the minute, second, and now the nanosecond—we developed this notion that if we can measure it, we can control it, which is not true at all.

And that's what leads to what you call speed inflation?

Yes, that's exactly it. Once we could measure time, that led inevitably to the notion that we could get better use of our time. One way to do this obviously is to create labor-saving devices, which can free up more time, at least in theory. In fact, it seems like the more labor-saving and supposedly time-saving devices we have, the less time we have in our day. And there's a reason for that.

Which is?

I call it the convenience catch. It's the paradox that once we can do a job more easily with mechanical or electronic help, we tend to do that job more often. We also set our standards higher. How many times have you stood in front of a microwave watching the timer count down thinking, "Come on, come on"? And just a few years ago, we would think, "Wow, only 30 seconds to reheat a muffin." Now, we're standing there going "25...24...23...come on, what's taking so long?" That's speed inflation. Our tempo just accelerates to match the new conveniences, and expectations go up. That's true of many things we use—washing machines, computers, fax machines.

What the convenience catch also has done is eliminate downtime. You used to have to wind your watch every day, for instance, rather than having a battery to keep it going constantly. Winding your watch isn't a big deal. It just takes a few seconds. But it was one among many points in the day when you would stop and take a moment or two to catch your breath. Filling your fountain pen was another breath-catching moment, along with stropping your razor. Giving up any one of these little mini-moments in the day doesn't mean a lot. But when you give them all up, when do you catch your breath? The result is that we've basically become a breathless society. We're always rushing to do something because our so-called time-saving devices don't give us a moment to stop so that we can catch our breath.

What does speed inflation do to a man's mental and physical health?

I don't think it is healthy either mentally or physically to feel like you don't have a second to spare in your calendar. The doctors I interviewed for my book came up with a surprisingly long list of ailments including headaches, digestive problems, clogged arteries, heart disease, poor nutrition, and insomnia that can result from too much time pressure.

You say that one of the toughest things for men to do is listen to their bodies. What does that have to do with time pressure?

As I get older, I find that if I'm pushing myself too hard, working too many hours, rushing too fast, I get indigestion. One response to that is to reach for the Mylanta. But in the process of doing that, I try to ask myself: Why am I getting indigestion? How can I alter the way that I'm living so that I don't get indigestion? I think we all get little signals like that that are telling us we're trying to do too much. A few years ago, I got irregular heart beats—what they call premature ventricular contractions. This was probably from working too many hours, drinking too much caffeine, taking too many decongestants, and consuming too much alcohol. So I cut back on my hours. I don't work until 1:00 or 2:00 in the morning anymore. I don't drink nearly as much coffee as I once did. I don't drink soda at all. I don't ever take decongestants. I generally allow time for my body to relax, and it hasn't been a problem since. So I think all of these things that go wrong in our bodies are very good in one sense because they are warnings that we need to alter the way that we are living.

You say we have fewer sanctuaries away from the busy world. Why?

Just look at the up-to-date man today. He has a fax machine. He has a computer. He has an answering machine. He has a pager and a cellular phone. He has a laptop. Now it used to be that you got on a plane, you could relax. You could say, nobody can reach me here, and I really don't have the tools I need to work, so I'll just read this novel I have. Now, you get on a plane and there might be a phone in the seatback in front of you. You might have your laptop computer with you; you might have your tape recorder with you. Now, there is no place in the world that you can go today without being reachable by some of these so-called conveniences.

What are some things men can do to lessen their sense of time pressure?

One of the things I say in *Timelock* is that you should never add something to your calendar without first subtracting something else. Better yet, subtract two. But how often do we add a new activity to our lives without thinking that you have to give something up in order to take on this new task? Where are those hours going to come from? Am I going to get less sleep? Am I going to spend less time playing with my kids? Am I going to spend less time talking with my wife? Am I going to spend less time reading in the evening? That time has to come from somewhere—time, after all, is finite. So to stay in a healthy relationship with time, I think it is important to avoid taking on new time-consuming activities without first eliminating other ones.

What are some other ways that men can help themselves stay sane in a time-crunched world?

First, it is important to acknowledge that time can't be controlled. I think this is a particularly hard one for men. We see ourselves to be men who can control the environment, including time, but we're just fooling ourselves.

You have to learn to create periods in the day when you are not driven to do anything. I think it really helps men to take 15-minute breaks twice a day when they aren't allowed to do anything except listen to relaxing music. One of the best things that I've learned from a doctor I spoke to for my book is when you are unavoidably delayed—when there is a long line at the bank, when your flight is postponed—don't get into an uproar. Treat it as downtime. It's a nice time to sit, relax, meditate, jot down some ideas. I was one of these people who would go crazy whenever I was trapped in a long line or delayed at the airport. And ever since I learned this technique, I've calmed down in those situations. I finally have learned to realize that even if I can't control the situation, I certainly can control my reaction.

Why is it important to reduce background noise like radios and television?

Even at its best, TV tends to be a fast-paced medium. It's quick scene after quick scene. My heart gets racing, my skin gets tense. So I think that when we have the TV on, even just in the background, it is going to a fast beat, and I think that our nervous systems unconsciously try to keep up with that beat. We pay a price for that. I don't think it is a healthy beat.

It's interesting that you suggest using more prehistoric timekeeping methods like sunrise, dusk, and watching shadows. What does that accomplish?

I think we're way too time-conscious in this society. Look around. Count up how many clocks you have in your household, including clocks in appliances. For most people, it is an amazing number. I did that and it turned out I had something like 23 in my house. Ever since then, I've tried to do three things.

First, I've tried to reduce the number of clocks in my house altogether. I try studiously to avoid buying any appliance that has a clock in it. They're just a nuisance. If nothing else, you have to reset all of those clocks twice a year for daylight savings time. But the worst thing is whenever you turn around you are faced with the time. Why? What good does it do us to constantly know what time it is?

Second, when we do get a clock now, we get a small one. We put it off to one side so that the time is there when we need it, but it isn't staring us in the face. We don't have any big wall clocks because that makes time more prominent than I want it to be in my life.

The third thing is that I almost never wear a watch these days. It's amazing what you discover once you stop wearing a watch. At first, it is very hard because most of us are addicted to checking the time on our wrists. But once you stop doing that, once you don't have the time on your wrist, it's really amazing how seldom you actually need to know the time. You're almost never in a setting where you can't find out the time if you really need it.

Another part of that process is to use other means of telling time. It's funny, but I eat a banana every morning around 11:30. There are two ways of approaching this. I can look at the clock and when it is 11:30 I can go into the kitchen and have a banana. Or, when I get hungry for a banana, I know that it is 11:30. Well, I'd much rather do the latter. So I don't even look at the clock when I get hungry. I know that it is 11:30 and it is time for a banana. It's more fun to tell time that way. I use an egg timer to cook soft-boiled eggs. I try to guess by the shadows or dusk approximately what time it is. It is just one more way of keeping time in its place. Keeping it from becoming the precise, ominous thing that it can be when we are always looking at clocks and watches.

Do you think men can feel more youthful or energized if we don't rely on precise time?

I know I certainly do. It allows me to work in a much more modulated way. Sometimes I work fast; other times I go slow. My body tells me every day around midafternoon that it is time for a nap. And if I'm lucky and don't have too many things to do, I take a nap. Now, granted, I'm blessed by working at home. And most people still don't have that option. If I can't take a nap, my energy level goes way down later in the day. But if I can nap, even if it is just for 15 minutes, my energy level soars. It's like drinking 10 cups of coffee, but it's much more natural. I feel much more youthful and productive. For some reason, we view naps as a very lazy, unmanly thing to do. But a lot of very productive guys learned to do it. Just look at the presidents—Harry Truman, Lyndon Johnson, Ronald Reagan—they were great nap takers. Winston Churchill took naps every day even at the peak of World War II. This is just not some lazy guy's approach to life. This is a way to be a refreshed, energetic, and productive leader.

So your basic bottom line is that the world is going at a certain pace, but you don't necessarily have to live at that pace?

No, you don't. But you can't just say, I can organize time better and I'll have it licked. You have to make fundamental choices. I think the single best thing you can do to get the pace of life at a healthy momentum and reduce time stress in your life is to grab your calendar and start crossing things off. It's amazing how many of the things you cross off will be things that you really didn't want to do that much anyway.

Matt James on
Talking to Your Kids about Tough Issues

The talk. Few of us escaped it—the mandatory moment when your father sat you down and explained the facts of life. It was awkward for him. It was awkward for you.

It hasn't gotten any easier. In fact, talking about the birds and bees is just the beginning these days. In an era when children as young as 11 are sexually active, drinking, smoking, and exposed to drugs and violence every day, talking about these tough issues is one of the most important and influential health-management roles a father can fulfill, says Matt James, senior vice president for communications and media programs at the Kaiser Family Foundation, an independent health care philanthropy. In 1997, the foundation published a pamphlet, Talking with Kids about Tough Issues *(for ordering information, see Resources on page 317). Here James, a father of two, discusses how dads can make the most of conversations with their preteen and teenage children.*

From reading your pamphlet, we understand that the earlier you start communicating with your children about these issues, the better. But suppose you've missed that opportunity. Say you're now dealing with a teenager

who already may be sexual active and exposed to drugs. What is the message that you should try to get out to kids who are between 13 and 17?

My first message to fathers in this situation would be: Never think it's too late. You can and should have these kinds of discussions with your kids, particularly during the teen years. The decisions that kids make in their teen years have a dramatic impact on the rest of their lives. So even if you missed the boat when your kids were young, you should try to open those lines of communication now. It's tougher as they get older, but you can do it.

How do you prepare yourself to be comfortable during these conversations?

That's the difficult part. I think the best way to prepare yourself is to be familiar with the information that you want to convey. Let's just take an example: Say your child is sexually active and you're concerned about her protecting herself from unintended pregnancy, sexually transmitted diseases, and AIDS. You as a parent need to read up and be familiar with the information that you want to teach her. Kids are smart. If they sense that you don't understand what you are talking about, then you're going to have much less influence on them.

Some fathers will say, "My kids are learning this stuff at school. Why should I bother with it at home?"

School provides your kids with the basics on the birds and the bees. Where a dad has a big opportunity, particularly when it comes to relationships, is in imparting his own values to his sons and daughters. He can teach his sons respect for women and that sexual activity should not be the be-all and end-all in a relationship. Hearing those things from Dad can really make a difference in how your son views sex. As for daughters, the kind of dad you are can have a dramatic influence on the kind of man that your daughter is eventually attracted to. And that's something that every father is concerned about.

How important is it for you to live the lifestyle that you preach?

If you are a nonsmoker, keep yourself in shape, don't abuse alcohol, and don't do drugs, that will send a strong message to your kids about how you think they should live their lives. The behavior that your kids observe is going to have more of an impact than what you did 20 years ago. They are naturally going to be interested in what you did, why you now think it was a positive or negative experience—but it's how you live your everyday life that really has an impact on kids.

Suppose, despite your best efforts, they start drinking alcohol, smoking pot, or having sex at a young age. How do you get across to them that you don't approve of it?

The best thing you can do is to try to not be overly judgmental and harsh, because at that point communication shuts down. You can still forcefully state to your kids, "I don't approve of what you are doing. I think it's wrong; here are the reasons." But you always have to end it with "but I love you and I'm going to be there for you, and if you want to talk about this or you feel that you want help with this situation, I'm here to help you."

All of us made mistakes when we were growing up. One of the questions that probably worries a lot of fathers is what to tell your kids about your own choices about using drugs. Suppose you choose to tell your child, "I smoked marijuana or snorted cocaine." What should the rest of that message be?

Well, the message can be "I smoked marijuana and I thought it was a mistake later in life because it slowed me down," or "I realize now that there were health dangers of cocaine that I didn't know about at the time. I made mistakes just like you're going to make mistakes, and the one thing I would like to see you do is not make the same mistakes that I did." Whatever the response, it has to be honest. So fathers must think this through carefully before kids talk to them about these subjects. Otherwise, you'll have that deer-in-the-headlights look and end up being less than truthful. And your kids see right through it.

So the bottom line message is?

As a dad, if you want your kids to be sexually responsible and stay away from sex, drugs, and violence, you really need to be a part of their lives. That's something that men have traditionally had difficulty doing. I think a lot of times we've held up the notion that we're the hunter/gatherers as an excuse. I have a job that demands that I travel, and I work long hours. There are many dads out there in similar situations, but that's still no excuse. You have to find time to be involved with your kids.

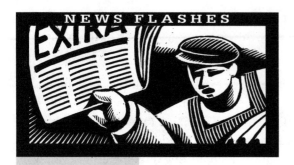

Driving while Phoning Takes Its Toll

TORONTO—Talking on your cell phone while driving is about as risky as drinking and driving.

In a recent study, Canadian researchers analyzed nearly 27,000 phone calls placed by hundreds of cellular phone users over a 14-month period. They found that using a cellular phone while driving quadruples your chances of getting into an accident. They also found that phones which allow your hands to be free were no safer than handheld phones. That could be because even though handheld phones don't limit the use of your hands, they do limit your attention, say the researchers.

Most of the phone calls made during the study period were brief and infrequent, which explains why even though millions of people have bought cell phones in the past few years, there has not been a tremendous increase in the number of car accidents.

But some countries feel that the safety hazard is great enough to warrant banning the use of cellular phones while driving. Brazil, Israel, and Australia have all passed laws against phoning and driving. It's not illegal yet in the United States, but you still may want to pull over before making your next call.

Law Protects HMO Doctors, Patients from Gag Clauses

WASHINGTON, D.C.—Health maintenance organizations (HMOs) may have cut the costs of medical care services and slowed medical inflation, but some doctors say that they're also cutting off vital information from patients. A number of doctors claim that the contracts they must sign to become HMO members include "gag clauses," which prohibit them from telling patients about treatment options that aren't covered by the HMO.

The Department of Health and Human Services recently placed a ban on gag clauses within Medicare HMOs, and Congress is considering 6 bills that would regulate HMOs, a number of which would prohibit gag clauses. In 1997, President Clinton named a commission to develop guidelines to protect all health care consumers, not just those in HMOs. The guidelines, to be submitted by March 1998, are to ensure that doctors can discuss all medical options with their patients—and that caregivers will not be rewarded for withholding care.

Airline Gets Heart-Smart

FORT WORTH, Tex.—Oxygen masks and seat belts aren't the only safety devices on airplanes anymore. American Airlines has recently equipped 249 of its planes with automatic external defibrillators (AEDs). Currently, only three other airlines in the world have portable defibrillators on board their planes. AEDs work like this: The defibrillator delivers an electric current that can jump-start a heart and jolt a heart attack sufferer back to life. Cardiopulmonary resuscitation can only keep the brain alive for a short time—too short on international flights.

Recently approved for use on aircraft, the portable AED is a "smart" device: You attach it to the heart attack victim and flip the switch. It knows whether a shock is needed and how powerful that shock needs to be.

For now, the airline has trained more than 2,000 of its flight attendants to administer the treatment and to contact the airline's doctor on call for further advice on how to handle the patient. Someday, American Airlines may install technology so that the defibrillators can automatically transmit the patient's vital signs to a doctor on the ground via the Internet or an air phone.

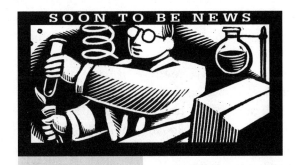

SOON TO BE NEWS

A Toothpaste That Reverses Cavities?

Cavities aren't just for kids anymore. In fact, because people are keeping their own teeth longer, tooth decay is becoming a bigger problem for adults than for children. In an effort to stop this dental scourge, researchers with the American Dental Association Health Foundation have developed a treatment that actually rebuilds tooth structure in the early stages of decay by remineralizing (rehardening) and strengthening the tooth.

This tooth treatment uses a compound of calcium phosphate—a compound found naturally in saliva—to rebuild tooth enamel after plaque acids have begun to destroy it. The extra calcium phosphate in the treatment accelerates the process of remineralization and supposedly creates a tooth surface harder than the original structure, according to Brooks Cole, president of Enamelon, the company that holds marketing rights for this method. The tooth-building compound may also reduce pain in teeth that are sensitive to hot, cold, air pressure, and touch.

Plans to create an entire product line including toothpaste, mouthwash, gum, and even candies are currently in the works. A toothpaste could be nationally available this year, while a chewing gum may be available by 1999.

Will Insurance Cover a Massage?

As massage therapists, acupuncturists, homeopathic doctors, and other practitioners of alternative medicine gain more popularity and credibility, more consumers are asking their insurers to pay for visits to these unconventional healers.

A 1993 study in the *New England Journal of Medicine* showed that Americans spent $13.7 billion on alternative care in 1990, most of which was not covered by insurance. But now, more insurance companies are cautiously looking into the possibility of covering alternative health therapies. They believe that members who choose alternative care may go to medical doctors less often, and could reduce costs by up to 20 percent. A few major insurers now reimburse for alternative medical practices, and the American Medical Association is encouraging its doctors to educate themselves about these practices.

Some states are also beginning to mandate coverage of some alternative health practices. Washington state has led the charge with a 1996 state law mandating insurers to pay for visits to all categories of health care providers licensed or certified by the state. More states are currently looking into creating similar laws.

Currently, there's little more than personal testimonies to vouch for the effectiveness of some therapies. That's why the National Institutes of Health's Office of Alternative Medicine is funding evaluation of roughly 42 alternative medical treatments. In the future, it may well become standard practice for your doctor to refer you to an acupuncturist, naturopath—or even write you a prescription for a massage.

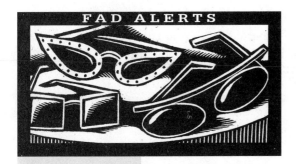

"Fast" Emergency Care

 "Thirty minutes or it's free" has long been a mantra in the pizza delivery business. Now, this concept is cropping up in an unlikely place: emergency rooms.

A few hospitals in Phoenix; San Jose, California; and other parts of the United States are promising to begin care for minor emergencies within 30 minutes. If they don't, the service is free. In comparison, typical emergency room waits are about 90 minutes, experts say.

At Columbia Medical Center Phoenix, for instance, emergency doctors treat about 15,000 cases a year. But after an advertising campaign promoting the 30-minute guarantee began, weekday emergency room visits increased 5 to 10 percent, says hospital spokeswoman Caroline Berger. On weekends, the number of emergency rooms visits jumped 20 percent. So far, the hospital has not had to pick up the tab for a single patient.

"We still do triage. The people with the most severe injuries are still seen first," Berger says. "So this program doesn't affect quality of care at all."

But while some emergency physicians laud the trend toward more efficient care, they worry that doctors and nurses trying to beat the clock will be more apt to make questionable medical decisions.

"Trying to put a guarantee on anything when it comes to medicine is misleading. It's just not the nature of this profession because emergency medicine is absolutely unpredictable. I'm concerned that physicians or nurses might ignore things that they should be doing in order to meet some artificial deadline," says Todd B. Taylor, M.D., an emergency physician in Phoenix and former president of the Arizona chapter of the American College of Emergency Physicians.

Other physicians fret that some ill people are reportedly driving more than 20 miles—past other emergency rooms—to take advantage of Columbia's guarantee.

"If what you think is minor indigestion turns out to be a heart attack, you could be compounding the problem by not seeking immediate care at the nearest emergency room," says Larry Bedard, M.D., president of the American College of Emergency Physicians, based in Dallas. "This fast-food approach to medicine is disconcerting for many reasons. It may be quick, but is it quality?"

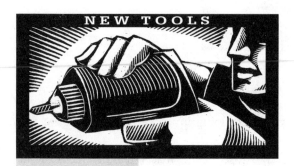

Instant Medical Data

The LIFE-FAX Card

If you're not a fan of those clunky silver medical-alert chains, we understand. Not only do they feel a bit like wearing a toe tag when you're still alive, they also advertise your weaknesses to an all-too-curious world. Now you can be more discreet yet still be assured that your medical information will be available to rescuers worldwide in an instant. The solution, developed by a company called LIFE-FAX, is a handy credit card–size version of your vital statistics. If you take a tumble and get knocked cold while on a biking tour of the Alps, the medical personnel who find this card in your pocket can dial a toll-free number to access your medical history, blood type, emergency contact numbers, and allergies. They can even get a copy of a living will if the crash was worse than you thought. The cost of membership is $75 a year, with an option to renew at a reduced annual rate. The system has a fax-on-demand service that prompts callers in English, Spanish, French, and Japanese. A multilingual operator also is available 24 hours a day. Call LIFE-FAX at (800) 487-0329.

Less Typing Strain

Ergonomic Keyboards

Every computer store has odd little gadgets that only a true cybergeek could love. From monitors shaped like modern art to a mouse shaped like Pamela Lee's...well, let's just say that most of them aren't that practical. But ergonomic keyboards—the ones allegedly easier on your wrists because the keys are split and slanted to match the "natural" angle of your arms—are a notable exception. Experts don't know if the new keyboards prevent carpal tunnel syndrome, but they say that many users find them more comfortable. And that's benefit enough.

"This keyboard design can reduce awkward wrist and arm postures, which may be indirectly related to musculoskeletal pain," says David Rempel, M.D., director at the Berkeley ergonomics research laboratory of the University of California, San Francisco. When one of our more skeptical *Men's Health* editors tried it for a week, he found that he easily adapted to the cockeyed design within hours. Better yet, his stiff pecking gave way to a sit-back, let-your-fingers-fly word stream. Try one of these next-generation boards (they're available in computer stores for $75 to $160), and even if you're using a 12-year-old personal computer that pulls its software off cassette tapes, everyone will think you're high-tech.

But even this modern marvel can only do so much. To ensure that your hands and wrists stay in tip-top shape, you also must maintain proper posture at the keyboard and take frequent breaks, cautions Sidney Blair, M.D., professor emeritus of orthopedics at Loyola University Medical Center in Chicago.

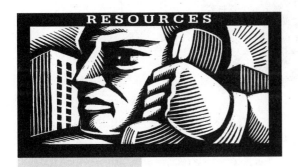

Online Doctor Finder

American Medical Association Physician Select Web Search
http://www.ama-assn.org

Now you can check out the doctor before he checks you out, thanks to this service on the official American Medical Association (AMA) Web site. Search a database of more than 650,000 physicians by name, specialty, and location. Find the office address and phone number. Discover where he studied, when he graduated, where he has practiced before, and whether he's board-certified. In addition, this site offers access to other medical sites and any of 12 AMA journals and association press releases. You can even look into the new Asthma Information Center and browse AMA catalogs.

Tackling Tough Issues

Kaiser Family Foundation
2400 Sand Hill Road
Menlo Park, CA 94025

In an era when children as young as 11 are sexually active, drinking, smoking, and exposed to drugs and violence every day, talking about tough issues with your kids is one of the most influential health-management roles a father can fulfill, says the Kaiser Family Foundation, an independent health care philanthropy. In 1997, the foundation published "Talking with Kids about Tough Issues" to help you play that role perfectly. To make the most of conversations with your preteen or teenage kids, write to the address above for a free copy or call (800) 244-5344.

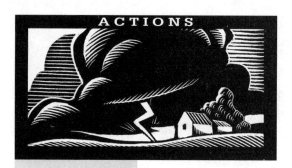

On his 100th birthday, songwriter Eubie Blake quipped, "If I'd known I was gonna live this long, I'd have taken better care of myself." Well, it's never too late to start. Here are 11 ideas that will help you manage your health wisely.

1. Be a master of disaster. Whether your kid swallows a quarter or you get nailed in the family jewels by a line drive during a softball tournament, have a battle plan drawn up before you head for the emergency room. It will save you plenty of time and anguish, says Todd B. Taylor, M.D., an emergency physician in Phoenix and former president of the Arizona chapter of the American College of Emergency Physicians. Here's how.

- First, get a family physician that you trust. Then find out in advance which hospital he wants you to go to so that he can help make medical decisions when an emergency does occur.
- If possible, call your doctor before going to the emergency room, since many minor emergencies can be handled at home, Dr. Taylor says.

- Keep a list of your medical conditions, allergies, and medications; or bring the medications with you to the emergency room.
- Finally, if you are ever away from your children overnight, make sure to give another responsible adult medical power of attorney in writing so that your child can be treated in an emergency, suggests Dr. Taylor.

2. **Never let your drugs sweat.** Store your drugs away from your bathroom, the Food and Drug Administration recommends. Since heat and moisture can lessen a drug's effectiveness, most medicines should be stored in a cool, dry place. That's not exactly the bathroom, especially during long, hot showers. For more free advice on medications, write to About Medicines, Consumer Information Center, Pueblo, CO 81009.

3. **Brown-bag it.** When you go in for a complete physical exam, don't forget to perform the "the brown-bag test," says Isaac Kleinman, M.D., associate professor of family medicine at Baylor College of Medicine in Houston. Sweep all of your prescription and over-the-counter medications into a paper bag and take them to your physician. If your doctor detects a medical problem, having all of your medications with you will help him determine if drug interactions are complicating the situation.

4. **Watch your altitude.** If you plan to go skiing or hiking in altitudes much higher than you are accustomed to—say, 8,000 to 12,000 feet above sea level—ask your doctor about flu vaccination, suggests Steven R. Mostow, M.D., chairman of the department of medicine at Rose Medical Center at the University of Colorado in Denver. "Higher altitudes stress the body and make you extremely susceptible to influenza," Dr. Mostow explains.

5. **Get traveler's insurance.** Before traveling overseas, ask your doctor about getting a hepatitis A vaccination, urges Eric G. Anderson, M.D., a family-practice physician in San Diego. Hepatitis A is a highly contagious virus of the liver that can result in serious flu symptoms, permanent liver damage, and, in severe cases, even death. It is known as a traveler's disease because Americans get it most often when they visit foreign countries like Mexico, parts of the Caribbean, and other developing countries where the disease is common. You can become infected with hepatitis A even at some of the best resorts and hotels from contaminated water, ice, fruits, salads, shellfish, or any food item touched by unwashed human hands. Given in a series of two shots, the hepatitis A vaccine may provide immunity for as long as 20 years.

Who should take it? "Anyone who will be taking three or more trips within 10 years to a place of moderate or high risk, but of late I've been liberalizing that view and giving in more to patient's requests," says David N. Spees, M.D., a medical author and travel-clinic doctor in San Diego, specializing in international medicine.

6. **Lessen the ouch factor.** When you do get a vaccination or other needle work, ask the nurse to apply firm pressure to the injection site for about 10 seconds before sticking you. A study in the *Journal of Pain and Symptom Management* found that people who were injected this way reported about one-third less pain than another group who were poked in the usual manner. Pressing the skin prior to the jab seems to impair transmission of pain signals to the brain, which lessens the ouch.

7. **Play a game of chants.** The next time you're stuck in traffic and begin to feel your blood boil, try meditation. Meditation may be as effective as drug therapy at lowering your blood pressure, according to research at the West Oakland Health Center in Oakland, California. During a three-month study, African-American men and women who practiced meditation for 20 minutes two times a day lowered their blood pressure by 11 systolic points (the top number) and 6 diastolic points (the bottom number). It was twice the decrease that others attained through simple relaxation. And with a compliance rate of 97 percent, the men and women who meditated stuck with the program longer than most people stay with other blood-lowering techniques like drug therapy or aerobic exercise.

To get some meditation practice, lift your tongue to the roof of your mouth and gently press it up against your front teeth, suggests Jackie Valdez, a meditation instructor and intuitive counselor in Encinitas, California. Then begin breathing more deeply. Each time you inhale, repeat a phrase like "cool, calm mind." When you exhale, think, "peaceful, relaxed body." Whenever your mind starts to wander and you start to worry about deadlines, schedules, or urgent errands, refocus your attention on your breathing. Repeat this simple meditation exercise a couple of minutes several times a day. It can be done anywhere, Valdez says. You can meditate while you're stuck in traffic, eating a meal, or getting ready for bed.

8. **Live the sweat life.** Exercising can not only extend your life; it can prevent you from becoming the loneliest guy in town. The 28-year Alameda County Study, which followed the lives of 6,131 people in northern California, found that four to five times as many sedentary men died over the course of the study (usually of cardiovascular disease) as men who exercised the most. But they also found that the least active people were more socially isolated than those who exercised most.

9. **Lengthen your fuse.** To make it to 100, you'd better learn to count to 10. Harvard School of Public Health researchers who studied 1,305 men ages 40 to 90 found that men with the highest anger scores on a personality test were three times as likely to develop heart disease. The researchers believe that anger may trigger the release of toxic stress hormones into the blood. If you're in a situation that normally triggers irritation, like standing in a long line at the grocery store, take a time-out. Practice observing other people or read a magazine, rather than focusing on your aggravation. You can also recollect a very pleasant event that made you feel calm or peaceful, says Barton Sparagon, M.D., director of the Meyer Friedman Institute in San Francisco, a world-renowned center for research in the treatment of type A behavior.

10. **Check the equipment.** Before getting out of the shower, do a testicular exam, Dr. Anderson suggests. You're naked anyway, and the warm water helps make the scrotum more supple and relaxed. Although testicular cancer is rare, it still ranks as the number one solid cancer in males up to the age of 35.

Roll each testicle between your thumb and the first two fingers of your hand, feeling for any lumps, hardness, or irregularities. Except for the epididymis (the cords that your testicles are attached to), you should feel only the smooth surface of the testicles, says Dr. Anderson. Also be sure to note any pain, tenderness, or sensation of heaviness.

11. **Have a tall, cold...water.** Dehydration may trigger fatigue because it handicaps cells, says E. Wayne Askew, Ph.D., director of the division of foods and nutrition at the University of Utah in Salt Lake City. So stay ahead of dehydration by drinking 8 to 16 ounces of cold water as soon as you wake up, since your body is already facing a water deficit from the night. Then, keep a bottle of ice water on your desk to sip from throughout the day.

Credits

"The Blended Workout" on page 13 was adapted and reprinted from *Body Engineering: How to Reinvent the Way You Look and Feel*. Copyright © 1997 by John Abdo and Kenneth A. Dachman. Permission granted by the Berkley Publishing Group. All rights reserved. Permission for United Kingdom granted by John Abdo and Kenneth A. Dachman.

"Waist Not, Want Not" on page 82 was adapted from *Sex Appeal: The Art and Science of Sexual Attraction* by Kate and Douglas Botting. Copyright © 1995 by Kate and Douglas Botting. Reprinted by permission of St. Martin's Press Incorporated. Permission for United Kingdom granted by Boxtree Ltd.

"Three Age Erasers" on page 144 was adapted from "Natural Age-Erasers" by Stephen Rae, which appeared in *Men's Health* magazine (July/August 1996). Copyright © 1996 by Stephen Rae.

"Don't Be an Old Fogey" on page 157 was adapted from "How to Stave Off Fogeydom" from *A Man's Life: The Complete Instructions* by Denis Boyles. Copyright © 1996 by Denis Boyles. Reprinted by permission of HarperCollins Publishers, Inc.

"Maximizing Mind and Memory" on page 158 was reprinted, with slight changes, by permission of Macmillan General Reference, a Simon & Schuster Macmillan Company, from *12 Steps to a Better Memory* by Carol A. Turkington.

An Arco book. Copyright © 1996 by Carol Turkington.

"For Those at Risk for Cardiovascular Disease" on page 185 was adapted from *Eight Weeks to Optimum Health* by Andrew Weil, M.D. Copyright © 1997 by Andrew Weil, M.D. Reprinted by permission of Alfred A. Knopf, Inc.

"Cultivating Confidence" on page 221 was adapted and reprinted with the permission of Simon & Schuster from *Golf Is Not a Game of Perfect* by Robert Rotella. Copyright © 1995 by Robert Rotella.

"Self-Care Massage of the Head and Face" on page 254 was adapted from *Massage for Pain Relief: A Step-by-Step Guide* by Peijian Shen. Text Copyright © 1996 by Peijian Shen. Reprinted by permission of Random House, Inc. and Gaia Books Limited, UK.

"How to Choose the Break You Need" on page 298 was adapted from *Six Months Off: How to Plan, Negotiate, and Take the Break You Need without Burning Bridges or Going Broke* by Hope Dlugozima, James Scott, and David Sharp. Copyright © 1996 by Hope Dlugozima, James Scott, and David Sharp. Reprinted by permission of Henry Holt & Co., Inc.

Index

Boldface page references indicate main discussions of topics. Underscored references indicate photographs.

Cures, **248–70**. *See also* Disease prevention; Health management
alternatives to open-heart surgery, 261
anti-arthritis supplements, 262
banishing boredom, 256–59
for cancer, 261–62
dietary cures to symptoms, 249–52
echinacea, for colds and flu, 263–64
ground flaxseed, for high cholesterol, 264
for headaches, 252–53
for heart attacks, 260–61
for hemorrhoids, 259–60
for periodontal disease, 259
for neck pain, 264–65
resources for, 265–66
self-massage of head and face, 254–55
statistics on, 294
strategies for, 267–69
Curiosity and long life, 163
Curvature of penis, 74–75
Cytomegalovirus (CMV), 180–81

D

Defibrillators, portable, 200–201, 313
Definitive Penis Size Survey Web site, 100
Dehydration, 211
avoiding, 143
fatigue and, 276, 321
Dehydropiandrosterone (DHEA), 170–71

Depression
colors and, 278
countering with houseplants, 246
omega-3 fatty acids and, 67
Saint-John's-Wort for, 205–6
subsyndromal symptomatic depression (SSD), 236–37
Dermatologists, 195–96
Dessert(s)
low-calorie substitutes for, 66
low-fat chocolate bars, 130
yogurts, 60
Desyrel, 81
DHEA, 170–71
Diabetes
erections and, 94–95
National Institute of Diabetes and Digestive and Kidney Disorders, 266
resources for, 266
Diagnostic Center for Men, 99
Diarrhea, 249–50
Dihydrotestosterone, 80
Dining out
for breakfast, 119
foods for avoiding overeating, 46
weight loss and, 65
Dinner, for 8-hour revitalization plan, 154–55
Disease prevention, **178–212**. *See also* Cures; *specific diseases*
boredom and health, 257
for cardiovascular disease, 185–89, 197–201

combating surgical infections, 203
with exercise prescription, **190–94**
for heart disease
for skin cancer, 194–97
products for
blue-green algae, 205
flu vaccinations, 204–5
Saint-John's-Wort, 205–6
for rectal bleeding, 202–3
resources for, 99, 100–101, 206–7
for headaches, 207
for lung problems, 207
Safe Drinking Water Hotline, 206–7
for sexually transmitted diseases, 207
for salmonella, 202
statistics on, 178
strategies for maintaining health, 208–12
strengthening your immune system, 182–84, 203–4
Dogs, relaxation and, 209
Door Gym, 33
Dopamine, 276–77
Dreaming
Community Dreamsharing Network, 290–91
controlling nightmares, 270
Driving
cellular phones and, 312
eating breakfast while, 119
meditation in traffic jams, 320
relieving stress of, 217–18, 245
Drugs. *See* Prescription drugs

blending anaerobic and aerobic, 13–16
for breathing, 242
burning body fat with, 111–13
cardiovascular disease and, 188
for 8-hour revitalization plan, 151–52
for face, 171–72
fitting in, 35–38, 132
free weight, 3, 3–9, 7
as fun, 18
goals of, 16–20
high-altitude training, 28–29
for improving
metabolism, 116–17
posture, 143
sleep, 280–81, 285
interval training, 111–13
with Macarena workout videos, 129
mental, 158, 164
motivation and, 244
with partners of opposite sex, 13
personal workout plans, 34
as preventive medicine, 190–94
social benefits of, 320
spiritual, 29–30
strengthening immune system with, 184
strength training, 20–24
stress release and, 193
stretching, 273–76
for swing shift workers, 302–3
time of day and, 27–28
Exercise prescription, **190–94**
for decreasing risk of heart attack, 194
for duration of exercise, 190–91

for improving cholesterol levels, 192–93
stress and, 193
Eyebrows, clipping, 142
Eye(s)
effect of dietary fat on contact lenses, 55
macular degeneration, 268–69
strain, fatigue and, 278
vision training, 172

F

Face
creams for, 167–69
exercises for, 171–72
self-massage for, 254–55
Fat, body
burning, 111–13
combining exercises for, 36
measurement tests for, 295–97
Fat, dietary
breakfasts high in, 119
in EatRight program, 124
effect of, on contact lenses, 55
low-fat foods, 110
migraine headaches and, 64–65
Fat-free diets, 59
Fatigue
dehydration and, 276, 321
sleep disorders and, 281–85
sources of, 251, 275–78
Fear
sexual arousal and, 102–3
as source of fatigue, 277
Fiber
curbing hunger with, 121
disease prevention and, 56, 57

preventing cardiovascular disease with, 187
sources of
ground flaxseed, 264
high-fiber cereals, 45
Fish
omega-3 fatty acids in, 67
relieving rheumatoid arthritis with, 267–68
Fitness, **2–38**. *See also* Exercise(s); Strength training; Weight lifting
Door Gym, 33
heart monitors, 33
high-altitude training, 28–29
increased sex drive and, 81
inline skating, 27
maximizing workout time, 35–38
muscle-building supplements and, 24–26
Otomix Bodybuilding Shoes, 33
resources for, 34
Rowbikes, 32
sports drinks and, 65
statistics on, 2
strategies for, 35–38
Fitness Connection, The, 34
Fitness Zone Web site, 35
Flossing teeth, 210
Flu
echinacea and, 263–64
vaccinations for, 204–5, 319
Fluorescent light, headache and, 252–53
Fluoxetine, 81, 205–6, 248
Folic acid, 107, 199
Food colors, nutrition and, 41–44
Food diaries, 109

W